Respiratory Diseases and Infections: A Clinical Guide to Diagnosis and Treatment

Respiratory Diseases and Infections: A Clinical Guide to Diagnosis and Treatment

Editor: Ramonita Samson

AMERICAN
MEDICAL PUBLISHERS
www.americanmedicalpublishers.com

AMERICAN
MEDICAL PUBLISHERS
www.americanmedicalpublishers.com

Cataloging-in-Publication Data

Respiratory diseases and infections : a clinical guide to diagnosis and treatment / edited by Ramonita Samson.
p. cm.
Includes bibliographical references and index.
ISBN 979-8-88740-435-6
1. Respiratory organs--Diseases. 2. Respiratory infections. 3. Respiratory organs--Diseases--Diagnosis.
4. Respiratory organs--Diseases--Treatment. 5. Respiratory infections--Diagnosis. 6. Respiratory infections--Treatment.
I. Samson, Ramonita.
RC731 .R47 2023
616.2--dc23

American Medical Publishers,
41 Flatbush Avenue,
1st Floor, New York,
NY 11217, USA

ISBN 979-8-88740-435-6 (Hardback)

Contents

Preface

Respiratory diseases and infections refer to those diseases that inhibit the lungs and respiratory system from functioning normally. These conditions negatively impact the tissues and organs which are responsible for exchanging gas in lungs. Respiratory diseases include conditions like influenza, bacterial pneumonia, tuberculosis, lung cancer and acute asthma. Respiratory infections are conditions such as pharyngitis, common cold, laryngotracheitis, and epiglottitis. These diseases and infections can be diagnosed by the performance of various tests, such as blood test, chest X-ray, pleura or lung biopsy, pulmonary function test, CT scan, ventilation-perfusion scan and ultrasound scanning. Treatment generally includes antipyretics, decongestants, bed rest, and consumption of sufficient fluids. Severe respiratory diseases can be treated with lung transplantation. Preventive measures like quitting smoking, eating well and getting vaccinated can help to reduce the progression of respiratory diseases and infections. This book provides comprehensive insights on respiratory diseases and infections. Also included herein is a detailed explanation of diagnosis and treatment of these medical conditions. This book will serve as a valuable source of reference for graduate and post graduate students.

This book is the end result of constructive efforts and intensive research done by experts in this field. The aim of this book is to enlighten the readers with recent information in this area of research. The information provided in this profound book would serve as a valuable reference to students and researchers in this field.

At the end, I would like to thank all the authors for devoting their precious time and providing their valuable contribution to this book. I would also like to express my gratitude to my fellow colleagues who encouraged me throughout the process.

Editor

1

Targeting Aging Pathways in Chronic Obstructive Pulmonary Disease

Molly Easter [1], Seth Bollenbecker [1], Jarrod W. Barnes [1,2] and Stefanie Krick [1,2,*]

1 Division of Pulmonary, Allergy and Critical Care Medicine, Department of Medicine, The University of Alabama at Birmingham, Birmingham, AL 35294, USA; measter@uab.edu (M.E.); setheb@uab.edu (S.B.); jbarnes@uabmc.edu (J.W.B.)

2 Gregory Fleming James Cystic Fibrosis Center, The University of Alabama at Birmingham, Birmingham, AL 35294, USA

* Correspondence: skrick@uabmc.edu

Abstract: Chronic obstructive pulmonary disease (COPD) has become a global epidemic and is the third leading cause of death worldwide. COPD is characterized by chronic airway inflammation, loss of alveolar-capillary units, and progressive decline in lung function. Major risk factors for COPD are cigarette smoking and aging. COPD-associated pathomechanisms include multiple aging pathways such as telomere attrition, epigenetic alterations, altered nutrient sensing, mitochondrial dysfunction, cell senescence, stem cell exhaustion and chronic inflammation. In this review, we will highlight the current literature that focuses on the role of age and aging-associated signaling pathways as well as their impact on current treatment strategies in the pathogenesis of COPD. Furthermore, we will discuss established and experimental COPD treatments including senolytic and anti-aging therapies and their potential use as novel treatment strategies in COPD.

Keywords: COPD; aging; senescence; inflammation; senolytics; cigarette smoke

---

1. Introduction

COPD is a progressive and debilitating respiratory condition that affects millions of people worldwide and represents a large medical and financial burden [1]. The worldwide population is living longer by 2050, 21% of the world population will be 60 years or older [2] and the prevalence of age-related chronic diseases like COPD is also increasing along with morbidity, mortality, and a greater degree of disability [3–6]. There is a five-fold increased risk for those aged over 65 years compared with patients aged less than 40 years of developing COPD [7]. In a recent report analyzing a cohort of 126,283 COPD patients (≥45 years), the prevalence of COPD was 3.6% and it increased greatly with age (1.9% in 45–64 years, 4.8% in 65–74 years, 6.8% in 75–84 years and 5.6% in ≥ 85 years) [8]. In addition, the elderly showing age-associated changes of the lung [9], which are per se not a pathological but it is unclear, whether those alterations might predispose to COPD development.

The Global Initiative of Obstructive Lung Disease (GOLD) has proposed guidelines for management and treatment of COPD; however, therapeutic interventions targeting the elderly population still need to be evaluated and translated into clinical practice [10,11]. COPD is considered a disease of accelerated aging with several aging pathways involved in its pathogenesis [12–14]. Current therapies mainly focus on symptomatic treatment. Thus, the understanding of age-related pathomechanisms associated with COPD is critical to uncover novel disease specific treatment strategies.

Impact and Pathophysiology of COPD in the Elderly

COPD has become the third leading cause of death worldwide with the incidence increasing with age [15]. It has been reported that COPD is 2–3 times more prevalent in the elderly, and given that the world population is aging, age will become an even more significant risk factor for COPD [16].

COPD is a chronic inflammatory disease, and it is known that increased inflammation results in a progressive decline in lung function over time [17,18]. Its pathophysiology includes irreversible airway limitation caused by long term inhalation of noxious gases and/or cigarette smoke [17,19]. Classically, COPD has been defined by two main pathologies: (1) emphysema with parenchymal destruction and loss of alveolar septa; and (2) chronic bronchitis that consists of chronic bronchial inflammation of the bronchi, which is clinically defined as a chronic cough and sputum production for 3 months for two continuous years [20]. The diagnosis is usually based on symptoms and obstructive lung function test (spirometry) values with patients often having various degrees of severity of chronic bronchitis, emphysema, or an overlap of both [11].

Particularly elderly patients with COPD suffer from additional chronic diseases such as coronary artery disease, thyroid dysfunction, hypertension, congestive heart failure, atrial fibrillation, and other cardiovascular diseases [21]. Individuals with COPD have a four-fold increase risk for cardiovascular disease, and a significantly increased risk of psychiatric, renal, neurological, gastrointestinal, and metabolic comorbidities [22,23]. These aforementioned COPD-associated comorbidities have been linked to aging-associated pathomechanisms including chronic inflammation, cell senescence and telomere shortening [23–29]. In addition to these mechanisms, dysregulation of the extracellular matrix including protease/anti-protease balance and dysregulated matrix metalloproteinases [30,31] also play a role in the pathogenesis of COPD in the elderly [13]. Those comorbidities and their associated pharmacological treatments make COPD therapies in the elderly even more complex and challenging.

2. Aging-Associated Molecular Mechanisms in the Pathogenesis of COPD

Aging is a progressive degeneration of tissues that has negative effects on structure and function of vital organs [32]. Age-related diseases develop when physiological anti-inflammatory and antioxidant mechanisms fail to protect the body from damage due to a persistent low-grade inflammation and increased reactive oxygen species (ROS). This imbalance leads to cell and/or tissue injury, which contributes to COPD in the elderly in combination with the general risk factors for COPD such as cigarette smoking.

Additionally, there is an age-associated decline in lung function and structural dysfunction starting in the third decade of life [33]. For example, the lung function of normal aging individuals resembles an accelerated aging profile of lung function decline (e.g., mild airflow limitation severity) in COPD consistent with early stages of the disease [12]. This loss of function in the elderly can be contributed to an underlying phenomenon that has been called the "senile lung", which is characterized by alveolar enlargement in the absence of wall destruction [12,34,35]. In addition to lung function decline and these structural changes with age, the pulmonary defense mechanisms are less effective, leading to an increased risk of lung infections and a decreased protective response against oxidative stress and inflammation [36]. The senile lung, however, is pathophysiologically different from emphysema in COPD [9]. Several mouse models have been generated in an attempt to recapitulate the senile lung, including knockout mice deficient in klotho, the senescence marker protein-30 (SMP30), or the "Senescence-Accelerated Mouse" protein (SAM) [12,37–39]. In addition, Schulte and colleagues found age-related structural and functional changes in an aged mouse lung [39]. COPD animal models are a valuable tool for understanding the underlying molecular mechanisms due to the potential of genetic as well as pharmacological pathway modulation [40]. In conclusion, these mouse models demonstrate the age-associated molecular mechanisms involved in lung aging and their potential contribution to COPD independently of known mechanisms such as cigarette smoking.

2.1. *Inflammaging*

Aging-associated chronic low-grade inflammation (inflammaging) plays a major role in the pathogenesis of COPD and stems from an imbalance of inflammatory and anti-inflammatory networks [41]. This discrepancy increases with age, leading to increased disease susceptibility [41]. COPD-associated inflammaging is characterized by an increase in immune cells (e.g., alveolar macrophages, neutrophils, and T lymphocytes) that secrete cytokines, chemokines, growth factors and lipid mediators, which perpetuate the inflammatory process and destruction of the lung parenchyma [42]. In particular, interleukin-6 (IL-6) has been characterized as an age-related pro-inflammatory cytokine and is associated with negative health outcomes and mortality, and linked to persistent, low grade activation of chronic inflammation [43,44]. IL-6 also plays a major role in sepsis with IL-6 levels in serum correlating with onset and progression of the disease [45,46]. In addition, IL-6 was found to be increased in COPD patients with acute exacerbations [47] and was associated with the development of emphysema in COPD [48]. COPD lung cells exhibit a "senescence-associated secretory phenotype" (SASP), which is characterized by senescent lung cells secreting pro-inflammatory molecules such as IL-6, IL-8, monocyte chemoattractant protein-1, and plasminogen-activated inhibitor-1 [49,50], which further contribute to the pathogenesis of COPD.

2.2. *Cell Senescence*

Cell senescence is defined as an irreversible growth arrest in response to stressors such as telomere shortening, oxidative stress, stem cell depletion and persistent DNA damage [12]. Cell senescence was originally discovered in the 1960s by Hayflick when he observed that primary culture cells lost replicative capacity after several passages [51]. More recently, cellular senescence has shown to contribute to the loss of tissue homeostasis leading to the accumulation of senescent cells and contributing to the aging process [52–54]. Cell senescence has also been shown to contribute to the accelerated aging process in COPD [55,56]. Cigarette smoke can induce expression of the cell senescence marker p21 in epithelial cells and fibroblasts. Emphysematous lungs show increased expression of p16, p19 and p21, all of which are cyclin kinase inhibitors and markers of cell senescence [56]. Furthermore, senescent cells lose regenerative capacity and prevent cell repair in the COPD lung contributing to the progression of emphysema and worsening lung function over time.

2.3. *Stem Cell Exhaustion*

Stem cells play an important role in replacing cells lost to homeostatic turnover, injury, and disease [57]. With age, stem cell function and regenerative capacity decrease. Age-related decline in stem cell capacity in tissues that have regenerative potential can contribute to the development of age-associated diseases [57,58]. The lung is considered a slow renewing organ with a stable cell pool of differentiated cells and infrequent proliferation of stem cells [59]. Therefore, extensive lung injury results in limited proliferative capacity of stem cells and its consecutive depletion [60]. For example, airway basal progenitor cells play an important role in the lung's response to injury, as they are multipotent cells that can differentiate into basal, secretory, and ciliated cells [61]. In COPD, the differentiation ability of airway basal cells is decreased, which is accompanied by an early exhaustion of airway basal progenitor cells [61,62]. Therefore, stem cell regenerative therapy could potentially benefit COPD patients, especially the elderly subpopulation.

2.4. *Oxidative Stress*

The free radical theory states that oxidative stress is a key driver of accelerated aging [63]. Oxidative stress arises from endogenous antioxidant defense mechanisms being overwhelmed by the presence of ROS [64]. This imbalance between pro-oxidants and anti-oxidants increases with age and leads to an accumulation of oxidative damage contributing to senescence-associated tissue injury [63]. Several studies have demonstrated that a reduction in oxidative stress leads to a longer lifespan in

C. elegans, drosophila, and mice [63,65–70]. Furthermore, cigarette smoke exposure and mitochondrial dysfunction have been shown to lead to oxidative stress in COPD [71]. Oxidative stress causes DNA damage to lung cells thereby inducing additional aging hallmarks such as cellular senescence and inflammaging [72]. In summary, oxidative stress plays a role in age-associated pathomechanisms of COPD such as cellular senescence and inflammaging. Therefore, antioxidant treatments might be effective in targeting the accelerated aging process in COPD.

3. Current Treatment Options for Individuals with COPD

There is no cure for COPD; however, there are a variety of therapies that alleviate symptoms, mitigate the risk of complications, and enhance the quality and quantity of life. Current standard therapies include smoking cessation, bronchodilator therapy, oxygen supplementation, pulmonary rehabilitation, and lung transplantion [73–77].

Smoking cessation, when done effectively, can result in long term quit rates of up to 25% [78]. Smoking cessation is achieved through pharmacotherapies combined with counseling [77]. Pharmacotherapies consist of nicotine replacement products, including nicotine gum, nasal spray, transdermal patches, tablets, and lozenges; however, use of these products alone has a low success rate [79,80]. Counseling in combination with pharmacological products like varenicline, bupropion, and nortriptyline have been shown to be effective therapies for smoking cessation [81].

Both short- and long-acting inhaled bronchodilators, including beta adrenergic receptor agonists, and muscarinic antagonists are mainstay therapies in the pharmacological treatment regimen of COPD patients [43]. They achieve bronchodilation through the following different mechanisms: (1) muscarinic antagonists bind to M3 receptors in airway smooth muscle cells to block acetylcholine-mediated bronchoconstriction [82]; and (2) B2 agonists stimulate B2-adrenergic receptors inducing smooth muscle relaxation [83,84]. There is growing evidence that combination treatment of these long-acting bronchodilators is more beneficial than monotherapies for improving health-related quality of life, lung function, and decreasing COPD exacerbation frequency [85]. Inhaled corticosteroids (ICSs) are commonly used to treat asthma, but are also used for COPD in combination with bronchodilators, leading to a decrease in COPD exacerbations but an increased risk of pneumonia in some cases [86]. Furthermore, triple combinations are now available to treat therapy-refractory COPD patients or those with frequent exacerbations [85,87].

COPD patients with hypoxemia show an increased survival rate with supplemental oxygen therapy [88]. A more comprehensive therapy for COPD is pulmonary rehabilitation, which is a patient-tailored therapy that consists of exercise training, education and behavioral interventions. It is designed to improve the overall physical and psychological condition of COPD patients [89]. In addition, lung transplantation can be a treatment option for patients with end-stage COPD or rapidly progressing disease. Lung transplantation does not prolong survival; however, it can improve functional capacity and overall health, but advanced age is normally an exclusion criteria [90]. Double lung versus single lung transplant has been shown to provide longer survival, especially in patients older than 60 years [91]. COPD patients with severe emphysema can be treated with lung reduction surgery or endobronchial valve or coil placement to remove or reduce the emphysematous tissue, thereby decreasing hyper-inflation and providing the space of more functional lung tissue. These procedures have been shown to be beneficial for certain subgroups of COPD patients [92–97].

Together these therapies are effective in treating the symptoms of COPD, but they have not been shown to attenuate disease progression, and it is not clear whether they are as effective in the elderly population.

4. Anti-Aging Treatment Strategies in COPD

4.1. Repurposed Drugs as Potential Anti-Aging Therapies

4.1.1. Resveratrol

Resveratrol (3,4,5-trihydroxystilbene) is a plant polyphenol that is part of a family of antibiotic compounds called phytolaxins that are produced by plants in response to infections [98]. Resveratrol can be found in many common foods such as grapes, red wine, and peanuts [98]. Previous studies have shown that resveratrol can extend the life span of certain organism including yeast, drosophila, *C. elegans*, and fish [99–101]. Resveratrol has anti-inflammatory and antioxidant properties, which make it a potentially useful treatment for age-associated COPD [102,103]. Specifically, in COPD patients, resveratrol has been shown to inhibit the release of IL-8 in alveolar macrophages by 94% and 88% in smokers and patients with COPD respectively [18]. Another study showed that treatment with resveratrol reduced C-reactive protein levels and increased total antioxidant status values in smokers [102]. In a COPD rat model, resveratrol demonstrated anti-inflammatory and anti-oxidant properties by decreasing IL-6 and IL-8 production, upregulating Sirtuin1 and proliferator-activated receptor-γ coactivator-1α (PGC-1α), lowering levels of malondialdehyde and increasing superoxide dismutase activity [104]. Sirtuins are well known for their anti-aging properties [105–107]. Additionally, resveratrol has shown to have therapeutic effects in a COPD mouse model by decreasing the levels of the pro-inflammatory cytokines IL-17, IL-6, TNF-α, and TGF-β, attenuating fibrosis and mucus hypersecretion [108]. Together, these studies suggest that resveratrol has anti-inflammatory and anti-aging properties and could be a potential future treatment for COPD patients.

4.1.2. Metformin

Metformin is a drug widely used for the treatment of type 2 diabetes and polycystic ovary syndrome [109]. Metformin belongs to the drug class of biguanides. It suppresses endogenous glucose production mainly in the liver and increases glucose uptake in the muscle [110]. Metformin has been characterized as a 'geroprotector', a class of molecules that are known to have anti-aging properties [105]. Anisimov and colleagues showed that treatment with metformin increased life span by 14% and delayed tumor progression in female SHR mice [109]. Metformin activates the 5′ AMP-activated protein kinase (AMPK), which has downstream effects on the Sirtuin-forkhead box (FOXO) axis and Sirtuin-mTOR signaling. These are two important pathways for cellular response to oxidative stress which leads to attenuation of airway inflammation and lung function improvement as well as extends life span [111]. COPD is often associated with type 2 diabetes [112]. Two studies examined the effects of metformin on COPD outcomes. Hitchings and colleagues conducted a randomized control trial to examine the effects of short-term treatment with metformin on the frequency of severe COPD exacerbations in COPD patients without type 2 diabetes [113]. There was no difference in CRP and blood glucose levels after hospitalization from a severe exacerbation. This study suggests that short-term treatment with metformin is not sufficient to improve COPD symptoms. The long-term effects of metformin were not examined, which would be interesting to study since COPD is a chronic illness. A study by Bishwakarma et al. observed that patients with COPD and diabetes treated with metformin were less sick, less likely requiring oxygen, and had fewer hospitalizations when compared to patients that did not receive metformin [114].

4.1.3. Melatonin

Melatonin, *N*-acetyl-5-methoxytryptamine, is a hormone produced in the pineal gland that plays a key role in circadian rhythm control [115]. In addition, melatonin is a free radical scavenger for OH, O_2^-, and NO [116,117]. Melatonin supplementation has been shown to increase the lifespan of mice, rats, and fruit flies [117–119]. In patients with COPD, melatonin levels were shown to be decreased during exacerbations in combination with an increase in oxidative stress and decreases in antioxidant enzymes [120]. A randomized, double-blinded controlled trial focusing on the treatment of COPD patients with melatonin showed a decrease in oxidative stress and dyspnea after melatonin treatment and an increase in IL-8 levels in non-treated control COPD patients [121]. Additionally, melatonin treatment has been shown to reduce MUC5AC, a mucin involved in COPD-associated mucus hypersecretion [122] and IL-6 production [123]. Another report demonstrated that mice exposed to cigarette smoke and treated intraperitoneally with melatonin showed decreased total cell counts in bronchoalveolar lavage fluid (BALF), as well as decreased transforming growth factor (TGF)-β1 [124]. Together, these studies suggest that melatonin has anti-oxidative and anti-inflammatory properties and therefore might be useful in the treatment of COPD after validation in appropriate clinical trials.

4.2. The FGF23/Klotho Signaling Pathway

In 1997, Kuro-o et al. fortuitously discovered that deletion of the protein α-klotho (klotho) in a mouse model led to a premature aging phenotype including features such as skin atrophy, osteoporosis, soft tissue calcification, gonadal dysplasia, infertility, hypoglycemia, arteriosclerosis, and pulmonary emphysema [125]. Furthermore, these mice died within 8–12 weeks of age. On the other hand, overexpression of klotho in mice extended their lifespan by approximately 30% [126–128]. In humans, serum levels of klotho decrease with age [128] and klotho seems to play a protective role in age-related neurodegenerative disorders such as Alzheimer's Disease [129]. Klotho is a co-receptor for fibroblast growth factor (FGF) 23, a pro-inflammatory and phosphaturic hormone, which signals through two main receptors: FGF receptor 1 (klotho dependent signaling) and FGF receptor 4 (klotho independent signaling) [130–132]. FGF23 is secreted by osteocytes and is important for regulating phosphate [131]. The FGF23/klotho signaling pathway has been studied in several inflammatory diseases such as heart disease, chronic kidney disease (CKD), and inflammatory airway diseases including COPD [132–136]. FGF23 levels have also been shown to be higher in COPD patients with more frequent exacerbations [137]. In COPD, where FGF23 levels have been shown to be elevated, klotho levels were found to be reduced. These results align with the finding that airway inflammation is modulated via the FGFR4/NFAT signaling pathway [133].

Klotho has been shown to exert anti-oxidative, anti-inflammatory, and anti-proliferative functions in the heart, lung, and kidney [135,138,139]. In the lung, klotho was shown to inhibit bronchial IL-8 secretion via attenuation of TGF-β signaling. Furthermore, klotho deficiency in the lung led to impaired mucociliary clearance [135,138]. Thus, klotho supplementation could be a useful treatment for chronic airway inflammation associated with COPD. In addition, FGFR blocking antibodies could become a novel treatment strategy to target airway inflammation. There are several FGFR inhibitors in phase 2 clinical trials for hepatocellular carcinoma [140]. Taken together, FGF23/klotho signaling may have the potential to be an amenable target pathway in the development of anti-aging and anti-inflammatory treatments in COPD.

4.3. IL-6 as an Anti-Inflammatory Therapy in COPD

Since IL-6 plays a key role in the pathogenesis of COPD, novel therapies targeting the inhibition of IL-6 would be reasonable. Previous clinical trials have used IL-6 receptor blockers in diseases such as rheumatoid arthritis and Crohn's disease [43,141]. Furthermore, current clinical trials are investigating the use of IL-6 receptor blockers for the treatment of diseases associated with chronic inflammation such as chronic kidney disease, rheumatoid arthritis, polycystic ovarian syndrome, and Crohn's disease. In particular, clinical trials using the IL-6 receptor blocker tocilizumab for rheumatoid arthritis were effective in decreasing circulating IL-6 levels and improving symptoms and disease activity scores [43]. To date, IL-6 receptor blockers have not been explored in COPD, but they represent a potential novel direction, requiring detailed studies to define correct timing, for an anti-aging/anti-inflammatory COPD phenotype.

A subset of COPD patients present with a predominantly IL-5 mediated eosinophilic inflammation, which has shown to contribute to exacerbation frequency and lung function decline [142–144]. IL-5 mediated eosinophilic inflammation plays a critical role in asthma [142,145,146] and treatments with mepolizumab [147] and reslizumab [148], which both target IL-5, are approved for asthma therapy. Age-associated differences in eosinophil activity is unclear [149,150], but for the subset of COPD patients with eosinophilic inflammation, IL-5 therapy represents a promising anti-inflammatory treatment and needs to be further explored as a potential COPD treatment strategy.

5. Potential Novel Anti-Aging Treatments for COPD

5.1. Senolytics

In recent years, senolytics have been explored as a possible treatment to "therapeutically remove" senescent cells. The ability to reduce senescent cells may result in decreased inflammation and increase the efficacy of stem and progenitor cells for tissue repair [49]. It has been shown that elimination of senescent cells might prevent or delay age-related functional impairments and extend life span [151]. Baker et al. demonstrated the ability to specifically target senescent cells in a mouse model of inducible elimination of p16-positive cells (p16Ink4a- apoptosis through targeted activation of caspase) using AP20187, which was shown to augment apoptosis [152]. Elimination of p16-positive cells has been shown to delay age-related pathologies such as sarcopenia, cataracts, and loss of adipose tissue [49,152]. Moreover, Zhu et al. discovered that senescent cells had an increased expression of pro-survival networks that confer apoptotic resistance in senescent cells [153]. Using siRNA to silence expression of key players in this pathway including ephrins (EFNB1 or 3), PI3Kd, p21, BCL-xL, and plasminogen-activated inhibitor-2, eradication of senescent cells was successfully achieved. In addition, drugs like Dasatinib and Quercetin were characterized as senolytic agents. Treatment with Dasatinib and Quercetin reduced senescent cells in aged mice and improved cardiac function and carotid vascular reactivity after single treatment [154] Recently, clinical trials examined Dasatinib and Quercetin as senolytic treatment strategies for idiopathic pulmonary fibrosis (IPF) and diabetic kidney disease [155]. Results for the IPF clinical trial showed that treatment was feasible and senolytics alleviated physical dysfunction in IPF [156]. In these studies, Dasatinib and Quercetin reduced senescent cells in the skin and SASP proteins in the blood (IL-1, IL-6, and MMP-9) [155,157]. Other senolytics such as Navitoclax, which targets BCL-2, BCL-X(l) and BCL-w, was also demonstrated to be effective in removing senescent cells, but was associated with high toxicity causing blood cell dyscrasias [155]. Moreover, cardiac glycosides such as Ouabain and Digoxin exhibit senolytic effects by inhibiting BCL-2 family proteins via inhibition of Na+/K+ ATPase [155,158]. They also exhibit selective senolytic effects on p16-expressing human airway epithelial cells [155,158]. However, to date, there are no current clinical trials assessing senolytic therapies for COPD, which may be a valid future option to investigate. Collectively, these findings demonstrate that senescent cells can be targeted and eliminated in preclinical models and patients with age-related diseases (see Table 1). Targeting senescent cells may be a potential therapy for aging-associated diseases such as COPD.

Table 1. A table of senolytic drugs. This table includes the molecular targets of each of the drugs and the progress to becoming a therapy for senescence.

Senolytics	Target	Model
Dasatinib	Tyrosine Kinases	Phase 2 Clincal Trial
Quercetin	Tyrosine Kinases	Phase 2 Clincal Trial
Navitovlax	BCL–2 Family	Animal Models
Cardiag Glycosides	BCL–2 Family	Animal Models

5.2. Stem Cell Therapies

In recent years, mesenchymal stem cells (MSCs) have been studied as a potential treatment for COPD [159]. MSCs are multi-potent stem cells that have fibroblast-like morphology and the capacity to differentiate into chondrocytes, osteoblasts, adipocytes, and muscle cells under different environmental conditions [160]. In addition to their regenerative properties, MSCs have distinctive anti-inflammatory properties that make them a potential treatment option for a variety of inflammatory disorders including COPD [160]. MSCs secrete anti-inflammatory molecules such as IL-10 and modulate the release of the pro-inflammatory cytokines IL-1β, TNF-α, IL-6, and prostaglandin (PG)E2 [160–162]. MSCs release growth factors important for tissue repair like VEGF, HGF, EGF, and TGF-β1 [160,163–165]. Another approach to employ stem cell therapy in COPD is through "ex vivo bioengineering" of functional lung tissue for implantation [166], which uses 3D matrices or scaffolds seeded with lung stem cells cultured to form functional lung tissue capable of gas-exchange [167]. This method has been shown to be feasible in rodents, pigs, and human lungs; however, it has yet to produce lung tissue with robust gas-exchange capacity [166–168]. Bioengineering of the lung has great potential as a therapy for progressive COPD due to its ability to restore damaged lung tissue and improve lung function.

5.3. Antioxidant Therapy

Antioxidant agents such as thiol molecules, especially glutathione and polyphenols, can reduce inflammatory gene expression and inhibit cigarette smoke-induced inflammatory responses [99]. Moreover, sputum from patients with stable moderate-to-severe COPD and control subjects showed increased glutathione disulfides and nitrosothiols [169]. Several clinical trials have been investigating the effects of antioxidants in different diseases (e.g., the potential of oral supplementation of glutathione in pediatric cystic fibrosis patients) and have shown a significant decrease in bowel inflammation scores following glutathione supplementation [170]. Unfortunately, lung function tests were not performed. A different clinical trial investigated inhaled glutathione as a treatment strategy for cystic fibrosis but found no clinically relevant improvements in lung function, exacerbation frequency, and patient-reported outcomes [171]. However, Lamson and colleagues published a case study using nebulized glutathione for treatment of acute respiratory crisis secondary to emphysema and found rapid resolution and improvement in respiratory function [172]. Moreover, the erdosteine thiol compound has muco-active, antioxidant and anti-inflammatory properties in addition to functioning as a modulator for bacterial adhesiveness [173]. The EQUALIFE study found that treatment with erdosteine led to a significant decrease in exacerbations and shortened hospital stay [174]. Erdosteine could prove to be an effective treatment for elderly COPD patients, especially since they are more susceptible to respiratory tract infections. In summary, more studies are needed to determine whether antioxidant therapies are useful to combat the aging process in COPD.

6. Conclusions

The lifespan of the world population is increasing, which will further enhance the prevalence of age-related diseases such as COPD. The increased lifespan and age-related diseases will ultimately put a burden on our healthcare systems and significantly affect the quality of life of these patients. Current treatments for COPD are mainly addressing COPD-associated symptoms, but alternative treatment strategies are needed to evaluate the underlying mechanisms that lead to the development of COPD, especially in the elderly (Figure 1). Therefore, it is of high interest to focus on anti-aging treatment strategies, since the numbers of the elderly with COPD will continue to rise. There are already promising therapeutic targets for aging-associated COPD pathomechanisms; however, more research needs to be conducted to better understand these mechanisms and help to develop safe and effective anti-aging therapies.

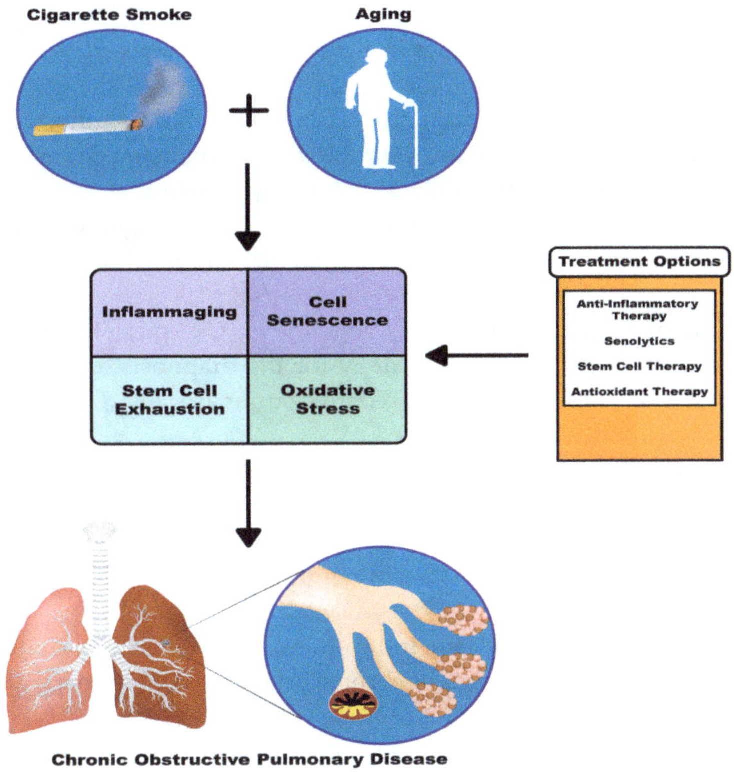

Figure 1. Diagram depicting two major risk factors for COPD cigarette smoke and aging. These risk factors cause downstream pathologies such as inflammaging, cell senescence, stem cell exhaustion and oxidative stress, which can be targeted with the treatment options shown in the orange and white box: anti-inflammatory therapy, senolytics, stem cell therapy and antioxidant therapy.

Author Contributions: M.E. and S.K. wrote the initial draft, S.B. and M.E. designed the figures and all authors edited the draft. All authors have read and agreed to the published version of the manuscript.

References

1. May, S.M.; Li, J.T. Burden of chronic obstructive pulmonary disease: Healthcare costs and beyond. *Allergy Asthma Proc.* **2015**, *36*, 4–10. [CrossRef] [PubMed]
2. Divo, M.J.; Martinez, C.H.; Mannino, D.M. Ageing and the epidemiology of multimorbidity. *Eur. Respir. Soc.* **2014**, *44*, 1055–1068. [CrossRef] [PubMed]
3. Guilleminault, L.; Rolland, Y.; Didier, A. Characteristics of non-pharmacological interventions in the elderly with COPD. Smoking cessation, pulmonary rehabilitation, nutritional management and patient education. *Rev. Mal. Respir.* **2018**, *35*, 626–641. [CrossRef] [PubMed]
4. Kennedy, B.K.; Berger, S.L.; Brunet, A.; Campisi, J.; Cuervo, A.M.; Epel, E.S.; Franceschi, C.; Lithgow, G.J.; Morimoto, R.I.; Pessin, J.E.; et al. Geroscience: Linking aging to chronic disease. *Cell* **2014**, *159*, 709–713. [CrossRef]
5. Fragoso, C.A.V.; Gill, T.M. Defining chronic obstructive pulmonary disease in an aging population. *J. Am. Geriatr. Soc.* **2010**, *58*, 2224. [CrossRef]
6. Dall, T.M.; Gallo, P.D.; Chakrabarti, R.; West, T.; Semilla, A.P.; Storm, M.V. An aging population and growing disease burden will require alarge and specialized health care workforce by 2025. *Health Aff.* **2013**, *32*, 2013–2020. [CrossRef]
7. Raherison, C.; Girodet, P.-O. Epidemiology of COPD. *Eur. Respir. Rev.* **2009**, *18*, 213–221. [CrossRef]

8. Anecchino, C.; Rossi, E.; Fanizza, C.; De Rosa, M.; Tognoni, G.; Romero, M. Prevalence of chronic obstructive pulmonary disease and pattern of comorbidities in a general population. *Int. J. Chronic Obs. Pulm. Dis.* **2007**, *2*, 567–574.
9. Bellia, M.; Benfante, A.; Menozzi, M.; Augugliaro, G.; Scichilone, N.; Cannizzaro, F.; Midiri, M.; Bellia, V. Validation of lung densitometry threshold at CT for the distinction between senile lung and emphysema in elderly subjects. *Monaldi Arch. Chest Dis.* **2011**, *75*, 162–166. [CrossRef]
10. Pistelli, R.; Ferrara, L.; Misuraca, C.; Bustacchini, S. Practical management problems of stable chronic obstructive pulmonary disease in the elderly. *Curr. Opin. Pulm. Med.* **2011**, *17* (Suppl. S1), S43–S48. [CrossRef] [PubMed]
11. Vestbo, J.; Hurd, S.S.; Agustí, A.G.; Jones, P.W.; Vogelmeier, C.; Anzueto, A.; Barnes, P.J.; Fabbri, L.M.; Martinez, F.J.; Nishimura, M.; et al. Global strategy for the diagnosis, management, and prevention of chronic obstructive pulmonary disease: GOLD executive summary. *Am. J. Respir. Crit. Care Med.* **2013**, *187*, 347–365. [CrossRef] [PubMed]
12. Meiners, S.; Eickelberg, O.; Königshoff, M. Hallmarks of the ageing lung. *Eur. Respir. J.* **2015**, *45*, 807–827. [CrossRef] [PubMed]
13. Ito, K.; Barnes, P.J. COPD as a disease of accelerated lung aging. *Chest* **2009**, *135*, 173–180. [CrossRef]
14. Mercado, N.; Ito, K.; Barnes, P.J. Accelerated ageing of the lung in COPD: New concepts. *Thorax* **2015**, *70*, 482–489. [CrossRef] [PubMed]
15. Chapman, K.; Mannino, D.; Soriano, J.; Vermeire, P.; Buist, A.S.; Thun, M.; Connell, C.; Jemal, A.; Lee, T.; Miravitlles, M.; et al. Epidemiology and costs of chronic obstructive pulmonary disease. *Eur. Respir. J.* **2006**, *27*, 188–207. [CrossRef]
16. Ito, K.; Mercado, N. STOP accelerating lung aging for the treatment of COPD. *Exp. Gerontol.* **2014**, *59*, 21–27. [CrossRef]
17. Hikichi, M.; Mizumura, K.; Maruoka, S.; Gon, Y. Pathogenesis of chronic obstructive pulmonary disease (COPD) induced by cigarette smoke. *J. Thorac. Dis.* **2019**, *11*, S2129–S2140. [CrossRef]
18. Culpitt, S.V.; Rogers, D.F.; Fenwick, P.S.; Shah, P.; De Matos, C.; Russell, R.E.K.; Barnes, P.J.; Donnelly, L.E. Inhibition by red wine extract, resveratrol, of cytokine release by alveolar macrophages in COPD. *Thorax* **2003**, *58*, 942–946. [CrossRef]
19. Hogg, J.C. Pathophysiology of airflow limitation in chronic obstructive pulmonary disease. *Lancet* **2004**, *364*, 709–721. [CrossRef]
20. Sethi, S. Infectious etiology of acute exacerbations of chronic bronchitis. *Chest* **2000**, *117*, 380S–385S. [CrossRef]
21. Marengoni, A.; Rizzuto, D.; Wang, H.X.; Winblad, B.; Fratiglioni, L. Patterns of chronic multimorbidity in the elderly population. *J. Am. Geriatr. Soc.* **2009**, *57*, 225–230. [CrossRef] [PubMed]
22. Soriano, J.B.; Visick, G.T.; Muellerova, H.; Payvandi, N.; Hansell, A.L. Patterns of comorbidities in newly diagnosed COPD and asthma in primary care. *Chest* **2005**, *128*, 2099–2107. [CrossRef] [PubMed]
23. Pedone, C. Comorbidities of COPD as a function of age: Evidence and practical recommendations. *J. Gerontol. Geriatr.* **2016**, *64*, 126–130.
24. De Miguel Díez, J.; Morgan, J.C.; García, R.J. The association between COPD and heart failure risk: A review. *Int. J. Chronic Obstr. Pulm. Dis.* **2013**, *8*, 305. [CrossRef] [PubMed]
25. Incalzi, R.A.; Corsonello, A.; Pedone, C.; Battaglia, S.; Paglino, G.; Bellia, V. Extrapulmonary Consequences of COPD in the Elderly Study Investigators. S. Chronic renal failure: A neglected comorbidity of COPD. *Chest* **2010**, *137*, 831–837. [PubMed]
26. Maurer, J.; Rebbapragada, V.; Borson, S.; Goldstein, R.; Kunik, M.E.; Yohannes, A.M.; Hanania, N.A. Anxiety and depression in COPD: Current understanding, unanswered questions, and research needs. *Chest* **2008**, *134*, 43S–56S. [CrossRef] [PubMed]
27. Graat-Verboom, L.; Wouters, E.; Smeenk, F.; Van Den Borne, B.; Lunde, R.; Spruit, M. Current status of research on osteoporosis in COPD: A systematic review. *Eur. Respir. J.* **2009**, *34*, 209–218. [CrossRef]
28. Barnes, P.J. Senescence in COPD and Its Comorbidities. *Annu. Rev. Physiol.* **2017**, *79*, 517–539. [CrossRef]
29. Córdoba-Lanús, E.; Cazorla-Rivero, S.; Espinoza-Jiménez, A.; de-Torres, J.P.; Pajares, M.J.; Aguirre-Jaime, A.; Celli, B.; Casanova, C. Telomere shortening and accelerated aging in COPD: Findings from the BODE cohort. *Respir. Res.* **2017**, *18*, 59. [CrossRef]
30. Churg, A.; Zhou, S.; Wright, J.L. Series "matrix metalloproteinases in lung health and disease": Matrix metalloproteinases in COPD. *Eur. Respir. J.* **2012**, *39*, 197–209. [CrossRef]

31. Shapiro, S.D.; Ingenito, E.P. The pathogenesis of chronic obstructive pulmonary disease: Advances in the past 100 years. *Am. J. Respir. Cell Mol. Biol.* **2005**, *32*, 367–372. [CrossRef] [PubMed]
32. MacNee, W. Is Chronic Obstructive Pulmonary Disease an Accelerated Aging Disease? *Ann. Am. Thorac. Soc.* **2016**, *13* (Suppl. S5), S429–S437. [CrossRef] [PubMed]
33. Fragoso, C.A.V. Epidemiology of Chronic Obstructive Pulmonary Disease (COPD) in Aging Populations. *COPD J. Chronic Obstr. Pulm. Dis.* **2016**, *13*, 125–129. [CrossRef] [PubMed]
34. Teramoto, S.; Ishii, M. Aging, the aging lung, and senile emphysema are different. *Am. J. Respir. Crit. Care Med.* **2007**, *175*, 197–198. [CrossRef] [PubMed]
35. Janssens, J.-P.; Pache, J.-C.; Nicod, L. Physiological changes in respiratory function associated with ageing. *Eur. Respir. J.* **1999**, *13*, 197–205. [CrossRef] [PubMed]
36. Brandsma, C.-A.; de Vries, M.; Costa, R.; Woldhuis, R.R.; Königshoff, M.; Timens, W. Lung ageing and COPD: Is there a role for ageing in abnormal tissue repair? *Eur. Respir. Rev.* **2017**, *26*, 170073. [CrossRef]
37. Sato, A.; Hirai, T.; Imura, A.; Kita, N.; Iwano, A.; Muro, S.; Nabeshima, Y.; Suki, B.; Mishima, M. Morphological mechanism of the development of pulmonary emphysema in klotho mice. *Proc. Natl. Acad. Sci. USA* **2007**, *104*, 2361–2365. [CrossRef]
38. Teramoto, S.; Fukuchi, Y.; Uejima, Y.; Teramoto, K.; Oka, T.; Orimo, H. A novel model of senile lung: Senescence-accelerated mouse (SAM). *Am. J. Respir. Crit. Care Med.* **1994**, *150*, 238–244. [CrossRef]
39. Schulte, H.; Mühlfeld, C.; Brandenberger, C. Age-Related Structural and Functional Changes in the Mouse Lung. *Front. Physiol.* **2019**, *10*, 1466. [CrossRef]
40. Vandivier, R.W.; Ghosh, M. Understanding the Relevance of the Mouse Cigarette Smoke Model of COPD: Peering through the Smoke. *Am. J. Respir. Cell. Mol. Biol.* **2017**, *57*, 3–4. [CrossRef]
41. Franceschi, C.; Garagnani, P.; Vitale, G.; Capri, M.; Salvioli, S. Inflammaging and 'Garb-aging'. *Trends Endocrinol. Metab.* **2017**, *28*, 199–212. [CrossRef] [PubMed]
42. Barnes, P.J. Inflammatory mechanisms in patients with chronic obstructive pulmonary disease. *J. Allergy Clin. Immunol.* **2016**, *138*, 16–27. [CrossRef] [PubMed]
43. Garth, J.; Barnes, J.W.; Krick, S. Targeting cytokines as evolving treatment strategies in chronic inflammatory airway diseases. *Int. J. Mol. Sci.* **2018**, *19*, 3402. [CrossRef] [PubMed]
44. Franceschi, C.; Capri, M.; Monti, D.; Giunta, S.; Olivieri, F.; Sevini, F.; Panourgia, M.P.; Invidia, L.; Celani, L.; Scurti, M.; et al. Inflammaging and anti-inflammaging: A systemic perspective on aging and longevity emerged from studies in humans. *Mech. Ageing Dev.* **2007**, *128*, 92–105. [CrossRef]
45. Remick, D.G.; Bolgos, G.; Copeland, S.; Siddiqui, J. Role of Interleukin-6 in Mortality from and Physiologic Response to Sepsis. *Infect. Immun.* **2005**, *73*, 2751–2757. [CrossRef]
46. Damas, P.; Ledoux, D.; Nys, M.; Vrindts, Y.; De Groote, D.; Franchimont, P.; Lamy, M. Cytokine serum level during severe sepsis in human IL-6 as a marker of severity. *Ann. Surg.* **1992**, *215*, 356. [CrossRef]
47. Wedzicha, J.A.; Seemungal, T.A.; MacCallum, P.K.; Paul, E.A.; Donaldson, G.C.; Bhowmik, A.; Jeffries, D.J.; Meade, T.W. Acute exacerbations of chronic obstructive pulmonary disease are accompanied by elevations of plasma fibrinogen and serum IL-6 levels. *Thromb. Haemost.* **2000**, *84*, 210–215.
48. Song, W.; Zhao, J.; Li, Z. Interleukin-6 in bronchoalveolar lavage fluid from patients with COPD. *Chin. Med. J.* **2001**, *114*, 1140–1142.
49. Kirkland, J.L.; Tchkonia, T.; Zhu, Y.; Niedernhofer, L.J.; Robbins, P.D. The Clinical Potential of Senolytic Drugs. *J. Am. Geriatr. Soc.* **2017**, *65*, 2297–2301. [CrossRef]
50. Freund, A.; Orjalo, A.V.; Desprez, P.Y.; Campisi, J. Inflammatory networks during cellular senescence: Causes and consequences. *Trends Mol. Med.* **2010**, *16*, 238–246. [CrossRef]
51. Hayflick, L.; Moorhead, P.S. The serial cultivation of human diploid cell strains. *Exp. Cell Res.* **1961**, *25*, 585–621. [CrossRef]
52. Wang, C.; Jurk, D.; Maddick, M.; Nelson, G.; Martin-Ruiz, C.; Von Zglinicki, T. DNA damage response and cellular senescence in tissues of aging mice. *Aging Cell* **2009**, *8*, 311–323. [CrossRef] [PubMed]
53. Herbig, U.; Ferreira, M.; Condel, L.; Carey, D.; Sedivy, J.M. Cellular senescence in aging primates. *Science* **2006**, *311*, 1257. [CrossRef] [PubMed]
54. Passos, J.F.; Nelson, G.; Wang, C.; Richter, T.; Simillion, C.; Proctor, C.J.; Miwa, S.; Olijslagers, S.; Hallinan, J.; Wipat, A. Feedback between p21 and reactive oxygen production is necessary for cell senescence. *Mol. Syst. Biol.* **2010**, *6*, 347. [CrossRef] [PubMed]

55. Chilosi, M.; Carloni, A.; Rossi, A.; Poletti, V. Premature lung aging and cellular senescence in the pathogenesis of idiopathic pulmonary fibrosis and COPD/emphysema. *Transl. Res.* **2013**, *162*, 156–173. [CrossRef]
56. Tuder, R.M.; Kern, J.A.; Miller, Y.E. Senescence in Chronic Obstructive Pulmonary Disease. *Proc. Am. Thorac. Soc.* **2012**, *9*, 62–63. [CrossRef]
57. Signer, R.A.; Morrison, S.J. Mechanisms that regulate stem cell aging and life span. *Cell Stem Cell* **2013**, *12*, 152–165. [CrossRef]
58. Ruzankina, Y.; Asare, A.; Brown, E.J. Replicative stress, stem cells and aging. *Mech. Ageing Dev.* **2008**, *129*, 460–466. [CrossRef]
59. Stripp, B.R.; Reynolds, S.D. Maintenance and repair of the bronchiolar epithelium. *Proc. Am. Thorac. Soc.* **2008**, *5*, 328–333. [CrossRef]
60. Ghosh, M.; Miller, Y.E.; Nakachi, I.; Kwon, J.B.; Barón, A.E.; Brantley, A.E.; Merrick, D.T.; Franklin, W.A.; Keith, R.L.; Vandivier, R.W. Exhaustion of airway basal progenitor cells in early and established chronic obstructive pulmonary disease. *Am. J. Respir. Crit. Care Med.* **2018**, *197*, 885–896. [CrossRef]
61. Staudt, M.R.; Buro-Auriemma, L.J.; Walters, M.S.; Salit, J.; Vincent, T.; Shaykhiev, R.; Mezey, J.G.; Tilley, A.E.; Kaner, R.J.; Ho, M.W.; et al. Airway Basal stem/progenitor cells have diminished capacity to regenerate airway epithelium in chronic obstructive pulmonary disease. *Am. J. Respir. Crit. Care Med.* **2014**, *190*, 955–958. [CrossRef] [PubMed]
62. Zhang, Y.; Unnikrishnan, A.; Deepa, S.S.; Liu, Y.; Li, Y.; Ikeno, Y.; Sosnowska, D.; Van Remmen, H.; Richardson, A. A new role for oxidative stress in aging: The accelerated aging phenotype in Sod1−/− mice is correlated to increased cellular senescence. *Redox Biol.* **2017**, *11*, 30–37. [CrossRef] [PubMed]
63. Kirkham, P.A.; Barnes, P.J. Oxidative stress in COPD. *Chest* **2013**, *144*, 266–273. [CrossRef]
64. Pérez, V.I.; Bokov, A.; Van Remmen, H.; Mele, J.; Ran, Q.; Ikeno, Y.; Richardson, A. Is the oxidative stress theory of aging dead? *Biochim. Biophys. Acta* **2009**, *1790*, 1005–1014. [CrossRef] [PubMed]
65. Lithgow, G.J.; White, T.M.; Melov, S.; Johnson, T.E. Thermotolerance and extended life-span conferred by single-gene mutations and induced by thermal stress. *Proc. Natl. Acad. Sci. USA* **1995**, *92*, 7540–7544. [CrossRef]
66. Johnson, T.E.; Lithgow, G.J.; Murakami, S. Hypothesis: Interventions that increase the response to stress offer the potential for effective life prolongation and increased health. *J. Gerontol. Ser. A Biol. Sci. Med Sci.* **1996**, *51*, B392–B395. [CrossRef]
67. Murakami, S.; Salmon, A.; Miller, R.A. Multiplex stress resistance in cells from long-lived dwarf mice. *FASEB J.* **2003**, *17*, 1565–1576. [CrossRef]
68. Migliaccio, E.; Giorgio, M.; Mele, S.; Pelicci, G.; Reboldi, P.; Pandolfi, P.P.; Lanfrancone, L.; Pelicci, P.G. The p66 shc adaptor protein controls oxidative stress response and life span in mammals. *Nature* **1999**, *402*, 309–313. [CrossRef]
69. Holzenberger, M.; Dupont, J.; Ducos, B.; Leneuve, P.; Géloën, A.; Even, P.C.; Cervera, P.; Le Bouc, Y. IGF-1 receptor regulates lifespan and resistance to oxidative stress in mice. *Nature* **2003**, *421*, 182–187. [CrossRef]
70. Boukhenouna, S.; Wilson, M.A.; Bahmed, K.; Kosmider, B. Reactive Oxygen Species in Chronic Obstructive Pulmonary Disease. *Oxid. Med. Cell Longev.* **2018**, *2018*, 5730395. [CrossRef]
71. Aoshiba, K.; Tsuji, T.; Yamaguchi, K.; Itoh, M.; Nakamura, H. The danger signal plus DNA damage two-hit hypothesis for chronic inflammation in COPD. *Eur. Respir. J.* **2013**, *42*, 1689–1695. [CrossRef] [PubMed]
72. Hanania, N.A.; Ambrosino, N.; Calverley, P.; Cazzola, M.; Donner, C.F.; Make, B. Treatments for COPD. *Respir. Med.* **2005**, *99*, S28–S40. [CrossRef] [PubMed]
73. Mulhall, P.; Criner, G. Non-pharmacological treatments for COPD. *Respirology* **2016**, *21*, 791–809. [CrossRef] [PubMed]
74. Thabut, G.; Dauriat, G.; Stern, J.B.; Logeart, D.; Levy, A.; Marrash-Chahla, R.; Mal, H. Pulmonary hemodynamics in advanced COPD candidates for lung volume reduction surgery or lung transplantation. *Chest* **2005**, *127*, 1531–1536. [CrossRef] [PubMed]
75. Stoller, J.K.; Panos, R.J.; Krachman, S.; Doherty, D.E.; Make, B.; Group, Long-term Oxygen Treatment Trial Research Group. Oxygen therapy for patients with COPD: Current evidence and the long-term oxygen treatment trial. *Chest* **2010**, *138*, 179–187. [CrossRef]
76. Willemse, B.W.; ten Hacken, N.H.; Rutgers, B.; Lesman-Leegte, I.G.; Postma, D.S.; Timens, W. Effect of 1-year smoking cessation on airway inflammation in COPD and asymptomatic smokers. *Eur. Respir. J.* **2005**, *26*, 835–845. [CrossRef]

77. van Eerd, E.A.; van der Meer, R.M.; van Schayck, O.C.; Kotz, D. Smoking cessation for people with chronic obstructive pulmonary disease. *Cochrane Database Syst. Rev.* **2016**, *2016*, Cd010744. [CrossRef]
78. Frishman, W.H.; Mitta, W.; Kupersmith, A.; Ky, T. Nicotine and non-nicotine smoking cessation pharmacotherapies. *Cardiol. Rev.* **2006**, *14*, 57–73. [CrossRef]
79. CADTH. CADTH Rapid Response Reports. In *Nicotine Replacement Therapy for Smoking Cessation or Reduction: A Review of the Clinical Evidence*; Canadian Agency for Drugs and Technologies in Health: Ottawa, ON, Canada, 2014.
80. Aubin, H.J.; Luquiens, A.; Berlin, I. Pharmacotherapy for smoking cessation: Pharmacological principles and clinical practice. *Br. J. Clin. Pharmacol.* **2014**, *77*, 324–336. [CrossRef]
81. Buels, K.S.; Fryer, A.D. Muscarinic receptor antagonists: Effects on pulmonary function. In *Handbook of Experimental Pharmacology*; Spinger: Berlin/Heidelberg, Germany, 2012; pp. 317–341.
82. Lipson, D.A.; Barnacle, H.; Birk, R.; Brealey, N.; Locantore, N.; Lomas, D.A.; Ludwig-Sengpiel, A.; Mohindra, R.; Tabberer, M.; Zhu, C.-Q.; et al. FULFIL Trial: Once-Daily Triple Therapy for Patients with Chronic Obstructive Pulmonary Disease. *Am. J. Respir. Crit. Care Med.* **2017**, *196*, 438–446. [CrossRef]
83. Rossi, A.; Khirani, S.; Cazzola, M. Long-acting β2-agonists (LABA) in chronic obstructive pulmonary disease: Efficacy and safety. *Int. J. Chronic Obstr. Pulm. Dis.* **2008**, *3*, 521. [CrossRef] [PubMed]
84. Singh, D. New combination bronchodilators for chronic obstructive pulmonary disease: Current evidence and future perspectives. *Br. J. Clin. Pharmacol.* **2015**, *79*, 695–708. [CrossRef]
85. Agusti, A.; Fabbri, L.M.; Singh, D.; Vestbo, J.; Celli, B.; Franssen, F.M.; Rabe, K.F.; Papi, A. Inhaled corticosteroids in COPD: Friend or foe? *Eur. Respir. J.* **2018**, *52*, 1801219. [CrossRef] [PubMed]
86. Lipson, D.A.; Barnhart, F.; Brealey, N.; Brooks, J.; Criner, G.J.; Day, N.C.; Dransfield, M.T.; Halpin, D.M.G.; Han, M.K.; Jones, C.E.; et al. Once-Daily Single-Inhaler Triple versus Dual Therapy in Patients with COPD. *N. Engl. J. Med.* **2018**, *378*, 1671–1680. [CrossRef]
87. McDonald, C.F. Oxygen therapy for COPD. *J. Thorac. Dis.* **2014**, *6*, 1632–1639. [PubMed]
88. Reardon, J.; Casaburi, R.; Morgan, M.; Nici, L.; Rochester, C. Pulmonary rehabilitation for COPD. *Respir. Med.* **2005**, *99*, S19–S27. [CrossRef]
89. Patel, N.; DeCamp, M.; Criner, G.J. Lung transplantation and lung volume reduction surgery versus transplantation in chronic obstructive pulmonary disease. *Proc. Am. Thorac. Soc.* **2008**, *5*, 447–453. [CrossRef]
90. Subramanian, M.P.; Meyers, B.F. Bilateral versus single lung transplantation: Are two lungs better than one? *J. Thorac. Dis.* **2018**, *10*, 4588–4601. [CrossRef]
91. National Emphysema Treatment Trial Research Group. A Randomized Trial Comparing Lung-Volume–Reduction Surgery with Medical Therapy for Severe Emphysema. *N. Engl. J. Med.* **2003**, *348*, 2059–2073. [CrossRef]
92. Refaely, Y.; Dransfield, M.; Kramer, M.; Gotfried, M.; Leeds, W.; McLennan, G.; Tewari, S.; Krasna, M.; Criner, G. Biologic lung volume reduction therapy for advanced homogeneous emphysema. *Eur. Respir. J.* **2010**, *36*, 20–27. [CrossRef]
93. Fishman, A.; Fessler, H.; Martinez, F.; McKenna, R.J., Jr.; Naunheim, K.; Piantadosi, S.; Weinmann, G.; Wise, R. Patients at high risk of death after lung-volume-reduction surgery. *N. Engl. J. Med.* **2001**, *345*, 1075–1083.
94. Criner, G.J.; Delage, A.; Voelker, K.; Hogarth, D.K.; Majid, A.; Zgoda, M.; Lazarus, D.R.; Casal, R.; Benzaquen, S.B.; Holladay, R.C.; et al. Improving Lung Function in Severe Heterogenous Emphysema with the Spiration Valve System (EMPROVE). A Multicenter, Open-Label Randomized Controlled Clinical Trial. *Am. J. Respir. Crit. Care Med.* **2019**, *200*, 1354–1362. [CrossRef] [PubMed]
95. Sciurba, F.C.; Criner, G.J.; Strange, C.; Shah, P.L.; Michaud, G.; Connolly, T.A.; Deslée, G.; Tillis, W.P.; Delage, A.; Marquette, C.H.; et al. Effect of Endobronchial Coils vs Usual Care on Exercise Tolerance in Patients With Severe Emphysema: The RENEW Randomized Clinical Trial. *JAMA* **2016**, *315*, 2178–2189. [CrossRef] [PubMed]
96. Dransfield, M.T.; Garner, J.L.; Bhatt, S.P.; Slebos, D.J.; Klooster, K.; Sciurba, F.C.; Shah, P.L.; Marchetti, N.T.; Sue, R.D.; Wright, S.; et al. Effect of Zephyr Endobronchial Valves on Dyspnea, Activity Levels, and Quality of Life at One Year. Results from a Randomized Clinical Trial. *Ann. Am. Thorac. Soc.* **2020**, *17*, 829–838. [CrossRef] [PubMed]
97. Knutson, M.D.; Leeuwenburgh, C. Resveratrol and novel potent activators of Sirt1: Effects on aging and age-related diseases. *Nutr. Rev.* **2008**, *66*, 591–596. [CrossRef] [PubMed]
98. Rahman, I. Antioxidant therapies in COPD. *Int. J. Chronic Obs. Pulm. Dis.* **2006**, *1*, 15–29. [CrossRef]

99. Zou, S.; Carey, J.R.; Liedo, P.; Ingram, D.K.; Müller, H.G.; Wang, J.L.; Yao, F.; Yu, B.; Zhou, A. The prolongevity effect of resveratrol depends on dietary composition and calorie intake in a tephritid fruit fly. *Exp. Gerontol.* **2009**, *44*, 472–476. [CrossRef]
100. Tatar, M. Diet restriction in Drosophila melanogaster. Design and analysis. *Interdiscip. Top. Gerontol.* **2007**, *35*, 115–136.
101. Bo, S.; Ciccone, G.; Castiglione, A.; Gambino, R.; De Michieli, F.; Villois, P.; Durazzo, M.; Cavallo-Perin, P.; Cassader, M. Anti-inflammatory and antioxidant effects of resveratrol in healthy smokers a randomized, double-blind, placebo-controlled, cross-over trial. *Curr. Med. Chem.* **2013**, *20*, 1323–1331. [CrossRef]
102. Beijers, R.; Gosker, H.R.; Schols, A. Resveratrol for patients with chronic obstructive pulmonary disease: Hype or hope? *Curr. Opin. Clin. Nutr. Metab. Care* **2018**, *21*, 138–144. [CrossRef]
103. Wang, X.-L.; Li, T.; Li, J.-H.; Miao, S.-Y.; Xiao, X.-Z. The effects of resveratrol on inflammation and oxidative stress in a rat model of chronic obstructive pulmonary disease. *Molecules* **2017**, *22*, 1529. [CrossRef] [PubMed]
104. Ito, K.; Colley, T.; Mercado, N. Geroprotectors as a novel therapeutic strategy for COPD, an accelerating aging disease. *Int. J. Chronic Obstr. Pulm. Dis.* **2012**, *7*, 641. [CrossRef]
105. Ghosh, H.S. The anti-aging, metabolism potential of SIRT1. *Curr. Opin. Investig. Drugs* **2008**, *9*, 1095–1102. [PubMed]
106. Grabowska, W.; Sikora, E.; Bielak-Zmijewska, A. Sirtuins, a promising target in slowing down the ageing process. *Biogerontology* **2017**, *18*, 447–476. [CrossRef] [PubMed]
107. Chen, J.; Yang, X.; Zhang, W.; Peng, D.; Xia, Y.; Lu, Y.; Han, X.; Song, G.; Zhu, J.; Liu, R. Therapeutic effects of resveratrol in a mouse model of LPS and cigarette smoke-induced COPD. *Inflammation* **2016**, *39*, 1949–1959. [CrossRef] [PubMed]
108. Anisimov, V.N.; Berstein, L.M.; Popovich, I.G.; Zabezhinski, M.A.; Egormin, P.A.; Piskunova, T.S.; Semenchenko, A.V.; Tyndyk, M.L.; Yurova, M.N.; Kovalenko, I.G.; et al. If started early in life, metformin treatment increases life span and postpones tumors in female SHR mice. *Aging* **2011**, *3*, 148–157. [CrossRef]
109. Rena, G.; Hardie, D.G.; Pearson, E.R. The mechanisms of action of metformin. *Diabetologia* **2017**, *60*, 1577–1585. [CrossRef]
110. Piskovatska, V.; Stefanyshyn, N.; Storey, K.B.; Vaiserman, A.M.; Lushchak, O. Metformin as a geroprotector: Experimental and clinical evidence. *Biogerontology* **2019**, *20*, 33–48. [CrossRef]
111. Ho, T.W.; Huang, C.T.; Ruan, S.Y.; Tsai, Y.J.; Lai, F.; Yu, C.J. Diabetes mellitus in patients with chronic obstructive pulmonary disease-The impact on mortality. *PLoS ONE* **2017**, *12*, e0175794. [CrossRef]
112. Hitchings, A.W.; Lai, D.; Jones, P.W.; Baker, E.H. Metformin in severe exacerbations of chronic obstructive pulmonary disease: A randomised controlled trial. *Thorax* **2016**, *71*, 587–593. [CrossRef]
113. Bishwakarma, R.; Zhang, W.; Lin, Y.-L.; Kuo, Y.-F.; Cardenas, V.J.; Sharma, G. Metformin use and health care utilization in patients with coexisting chronic obstructive pulmonary disease and diabetes mellitus. *Int. J. Chronic Obstr. Pulm. Dis.* **2018**, *13*, 793. [CrossRef] [PubMed]
114. Reiter, R.J.; Tan, D.-X.; Poeggeler, B.; Menendez-Pelaez, A.; Chen, L.-D.; Saarela, S. Melatonin As a Free Radical Scavenger: Implications for Aging and Age-Related Diseasesa. *Ann. N. Y. Acad. Sci.* **1994**, *719*, 1–12. [CrossRef] [PubMed]
115. Poeggeler, B.; Thuermann, S.; Dose, A.; Schoenke, M.; Burkhardt, S.; Hardeland, R. Melatonin's unique radical scavenging properties—Roles of its functional substituents as revealed by a comparison with its structural analogs. *J. Pineal Res.* **2002**, *33*, 20–30. [CrossRef] [PubMed]
116. Anisimov, V.N.; Popovich, I.G.; Zabezhinski, M.A.; Anisimov, S.V.; Vesnushkin, G.M.; Vinogradova, I.A. Melatonin as antioxidant, geroprotector and anticarcinogen. *Biochim. Biophys. Acta* **2006**, *1757*, 573–589. [CrossRef]
117. Anisimov, V.N.; Alimova, I.N.; Baturin, D.A.; Popovich, I.G.; Zabezhinski, M.A.; Rosenfeld, S.V.; Manton, K.G.; Semenchenko, A.V.; Yashin, A.I. Dose-dependent effect of melatonin on life span and spontaneous tumor incidence in female SHR mice. *Exp. Gerontol.* **2003**, *38*, 449–461. [CrossRef]
118. Bonilla, E.; Medina-Leendertz, S.; Díaz, S. Extension of life span and stress resistance of Drosophila melanogaster by long-term supplementation with melatonin. *Exp. Gerontol.* **2002**, *37*, 629–638. [CrossRef]
119. Gumral, N.; Nazıroglu, M.; Ongel, K.; Beydilli, E.D.; Ozguner, F.; Sutcu, R.; Calıskan, S.; Akkaya, A. Antioxidant enzymes and melatonin levels in patients with bronchial asthma and chronic obstructive pulmonary disease during stable and exacerbation periods. *Cell Biochem. Funct.* **2009**, *27*, 276–283. [CrossRef]

120. de Matos Cavalcante, A.G.; de Bruin, P.F.C.; de Bruin, V.M.S.; Nunes, D.M.; Pereira, E.D.B.; Cavalcante, M.M.; Andrade, G.M. Melatonin reduces lung oxidative stress in patients with chronic obstructive pulmonary disease: A randomized, double-blind, placebo-controlled study. *J. Pineal Res.* **2012**, *53*, 238–244. [CrossRef]
121. Kesimer, M.; Ford, A.A.; Ceppe, A.; Radicioni, G.; Cao, R.; Davis, C.W.; Doerschuk, C.M.; Alexis, N.E.; Anderson, W.H.; Henderson, A.G.; et al. Airway Mucin Concentration as a Marker of Chronic Bronchitis. *N. Engl. J. Med.* **2017**, *377*, 911–922. [CrossRef]
122. Shin, I.-S.; Park, J.-W.; Shin, N.-R.; Jeon, C.-M.; Kwon, O.-K.; Lee, M.-Y.; Kim, H.-S.; Kim, J.-C.; Oh, S.-R.; Ahn, K.-S. Melatonin inhibits MUC5AC production via suppression of MAPK signaling in human airway epithelial cells. *J. Pineal Res.* **2014**, *56*, 398–407. [CrossRef]
123. Shin, N.-R.; Park, J.-W.; Lee, I.-C.; Ko, J.-W.; Park, S.-H.; Kim, J.-S.; Kim, J.-C.; Ahn, K.-S.; Shin, I.-S. Melatonin suppresses fibrotic responses induced by cigarette smoke via downregulation of TGF-β1. *Oncotarget* **2017**, *8*, 95692–95703. [CrossRef] [PubMed]
124. Kuro-o, M.; Matsumura, Y.; Aizawa, H.; Kawaguchi, H.; Suga, T.; Utsugi, T.; Ohyama, Y.; Kurabayashi, M.; Kaname, T.; Kume, E.; et al. Mutation of the mouse klotho gene leads to a syndrome resembling ageing. *Nature* **1997**, *390*, 45–51. [CrossRef] [PubMed]
125. Kurosu, H.; Yamamoto, M.; Clark, J.D.; Pastor, J.V.; Nandi, A.; Gurnani, P.; McGuinness, O.P.; Chikuda, H.; Yamaguchi, M.; Kawaguchi, H.; et al. Suppression of aging in mice by the hormone Klotho. *Science* **2005**, *309*, 1829–1833. [CrossRef] [PubMed]
126. Chen, T.H.; Kuro, O.M.; Chen, C.H.; Sue, Y.M.; Chen, Y.C.; Wu, H.H.; Cheng, C.Y. The secreted Klotho protein restores phosphate retention and suppresses accelerated aging in Klotho mutant mice. *Eur. J. Pharmacol.* **2013**, *698*, 67–73. [CrossRef] [PubMed]
127. Xu, Y.; Sun, Z. Molecular basis of Klotho: From gene to function in aging. *Endocr. Rev.* **2015**, *36*, 174–193. [CrossRef]
128. Torbus-Paluszczak, M.; Bartman, W.; Adamczyk-Sowa, M. Klotho protein in neurodegenerative disorders. *Neurol. Sci.* **2018**, *39*, 1677–1682. [CrossRef]
129. Erben, R.G. Update on FGF23 and Klotho signaling. *Mol. Cell Endocrinol.* **2016**, *432*, 56–65. [CrossRef]
130. Grabner, A.; Amaral, A.P.; Schramm, K.; Singh, S.; Sloan, A.; Yanucil, C.; Li, J.; Shehadeh, L.A.; Hare, J.M.; David, V.; et al. Activation of Cardiac Fibroblast Growth Factor Receptor 4 Causes Left Ventricular Hypertrophy. *Cell Metab.* **2015**, *22*, 1020–1032. [CrossRef]
131. Lu, X.; Hu, M.C. Klotho/FGF23 Axis in Chronic Kidney Disease and Cardiovascular Disease. *Kidney Dis.* **2017**, *3*, 15–23. [CrossRef]
132. Krick, S.; Grabner, A.; Baumlin, N.; Yanucil, C.; Helton, S.; Grosche, A.; Sailland, J.; Geraghty, P.; Viera, L.; Russell, D.W.; et al. Fibroblast growth factor 23 and Klotho contribute to airway inflammation. *Eur. Respir. J.* **2018**, *52*, 1800236. [CrossRef]
133. Singh, S.; Grabner, A.; Yanucil, C.; Schramm, K.; Czaya, B.; Krick, S.; Czaja, M.J.; Bartz, R.; Abraham, R.; Di Marco, G.S.; et al. Fibroblast growth factor 23 directly targets hepatocytes to promote inflammation in chronic kidney disease. *Kidney Int.* **2016**, *90*, 985–996. [CrossRef] [PubMed]
134. Krick, S.; Baumlin, N.; Aller, S.P.; Aguiar, C.; Grabner, A.; Sailland, J.; Mendes, E.; Schmid, A.; Qi, L.; David, N.V.; et al. Klotho Inhibits Interleukin-8 Secretion from Cystic Fibrosis Airway Epithelia. *Sci. Rep.* **2017**, *7*, 14388. [CrossRef] [PubMed]
135. Barnes, J.W.; Duncan, D.; Helton, S.; Hutcheson, S.; Kurundkar, D.; Logsdon, N.J.; Locy, M.; Garth, J.; Denson, R.; Farver, C.; et al. Role of fibroblast growth factor 23 and klotho cross talk in idiopathic pulmonary fibrosis. *Am. J. Physiol. Lung Cell. Mol. Physiol.* **2019**, *317*, L141–L154. [CrossRef] [PubMed]
136. Gulati, S.; Wells, J.M.; Urdaneta, G.P.; Balestrini, K.; Vital, I.; Tovar, K.; Barnes, J.W.; Bhatt, S.P.; Campos, M.; Krick, S. Fibroblast Growth Factor 23 is Associated with a Frequent Exacerbator Phenotype in COPD: A Cross-Sectional Pilot Study. *Int. J. Mol. Sci.* **2019**, *20*, 2292. [CrossRef] [PubMed]
137. Garth, J.; Easter, M.; Skylar Harris, E.; Sailland, J.; Kuenzi, L.; Chung, S.; Dennis, J.S.; Baumlin, N.; Adewale, A.T.; Rowe, S.M.; et al. The Effects of the Anti-aging Protein Klotho on Mucociliary Clearance. *Front. Med. (Lausanne)* **2019**, *6*, 339. [CrossRef] [PubMed]
138. Doi, S.; Zou, Y.; Togao, O.; Pastor, J.V.; John, G.B.; Wang, L.; Shiizaki, K.; Gotschall, R.; Schiavi, S.; Yorioka, N.; et al. Klotho inhibits transforming growth factor-beta1 (TGF-beta1) signaling and suppresses renal fibrosis and cancer metastasis in mice. *J. Biol. Chem.* **2011**, *286*, 8655–8665. [CrossRef]

139. Raja, A.; Park, I.; Haq, F.; Ahn, S.-M. FGF19-FGFR4 Signaling in Hepatocellular Carcinoma. *Cells* **2019**, *8*, 536. [CrossRef]
140. Choy, E.; Isenberg, D.; Garrood, T.; Farrow, S.; Ioannou, Y.; Bird, H.; Cheung, N.; Williams, B.; Hazleman, B.; Price, R.; et al. Therapeutic benefit of blocking interleukin-6 activity with an anti–interleukin-6 receptor monoclonal antibody in rheumatoid arthritis: A randomized, double-blind, placebo-controlled, dose-escalation trial. *Arthritis Rheum.* **2002**, *46*, 3143–3150. [CrossRef]
141. Saha, S.; Brightling, C.E. Eosinophilic airway inflammation in COPD. *Int. J. Chronic Obs. Pulm. Dis.* **2006**, *1*, 39–47. [CrossRef]
142. Narendra, D.K.; Hanania, N.A. Targeting IL-5 in COPD. *Int. J. Chronic Obs. Pulm. Dis.* **2019**, *14*, 1045–1051. [CrossRef]
143. Singh, D.; Kolsum, U.; Brightling, C.E.; Locantore, N.; Agusti, A.; Tal-Singer, R. Eosinophilic inflammation in COPD: Prevalence and clinical characteristics. *Eur. Respir. J.* **2014**, *44*, 1697–1700. [CrossRef] [PubMed]
144. Zeiger, R.S.; Schatz, M.; Li, Q.; Chen, W.; Khatry, D.B.; Gossage, D.; Tran, T.N. High Blood Eosinophil Count Is a Risk Factor for Future Asthma Exacerbations in Adult Persistent Asthma. *J. Allergy Clin. Immunol. Pract.* **2014**, *2*, 741–750. [CrossRef] [PubMed]
145. Tran, T.N.; Khatry, D.B.; Ke, X.; Ward, C.K.; Gossage, D. High blood eosinophil count is associated with more frequent asthma attacks in asthma patients. *Ann. Allergy Asthma Immunol.* **2014**, *113*, 19–24. [CrossRef] [PubMed]
146. Fala, L. Nucala (Mepolizumab): First IL-5 Antagonist Monoclonal Antibody FDA Approved for Maintenance Treatment of Patients with Severe Asthma. *Am. Health Drug Benefits* **2016**, *9*, 106–110.
147. Hom, S.; Pisano, M. Reslizumab (Cinqair): An Interleukin-5 Antagonist for Severe Asthma of the Eosinophilic Phenotype. *Pharm. Ther.* **2017**, *42*, 564–568.
148. Mathur, S.K.; Schwantes, E.A.; Jarjour, N.N.; Busse, W.W. Age-related changes in eosinophil function in human subjects. *Chest* **2008**, *133*, 412–419. [CrossRef]
149. Busse, P.J.; Zhang, T.F.; Srivastava, K.; Schofield, B.; Li, X.M. Effect of ageing on pulmonary inflammation, airway hyperresponsiveness and T and B cell responses in antigen-sensitized and -challenged mice. *Clin. Exp. Allergy* **2007**, *37*, 1392–1403. [CrossRef] [PubMed]
150. Cazzola, M.; Matera, M.G.; Rogliani, P.; Calzetta, L. Senolytic drugs in respiratory medicine: Is it an appropriate therapeutic approach? *Expert Opin. Investig. Drugs* **2018**, *27*, 573–581. [CrossRef]
151. Baker, D.J.; Wijshake, T.; Tchkonia, T.; LeBrasseur, N.K.; Childs, B.G.; van de Sluis, B.; Kirkland, J.L.; van Deursen, J.M. Clearance of p16Ink4a-positive senescent cells delays ageing-associated disorders. *Nature* **2011**, *479*, 232–236. [CrossRef] [PubMed]
152. Zhu, Y.; Tchkonia, T.; Pirtskhalava, T.; Gower, A.C.; Ding, H.; Giorgadze, N.; Palmer, A.K.; Ikeno, Y.; Hubbard, G.B.; Lenburg, M.; et al. The Achilles' heel of senescent cells: From transcriptome to senolytic drugs. *Aging Cell* **2015**, *14*, 644–658. [CrossRef] [PubMed]
153. Baker, J.R.; Donnelly, L.E.; Barnes, P.J. Senotherapy: A New Horizon for COPD Therapy. *Chest* **2020**, *158*, 562–570. [CrossRef]
154. Roos, C.M.; Zhang, B.; Palmer, A.K.; Ogrodnik, M.B.; Pirtskhalava, T.; Thalji, N.M.; Hagler, M.; Jurk, D.; Smith, L.A.; Casaclang-Verzosa, G.; et al. Chronic senolytic treatment alleviates established vasomotor dysfunction in aged or atherosclerotic mice. *Aging Cell* **2016**, *15*, 973–977. [CrossRef] [PubMed]
155. Justice, J.N.; Nambiar, A.M.; Tchkonia, T.; LeBrasseur, N.K.; Pascual, R.; Hashmi, S.K.; Prata, L.; Masternak, M.M.; Kritchevsky, S.B.; Musi, N.; et al. Senolytics in idiopathic pulmonary fibrosis: Results from a first-in-human, open-label, pilot study. *EBioMedicine* **2019**, *40*, 554–563. [CrossRef] [PubMed]
156. Hickson, L.J.; Prata, L.G.L.; Bobart, S.A.; Evans, T.K.; Giorgadze, N.; Hashmi, S.K.; Herrmann, S.M.; Jensen, M.D.; Jia, Q.; Jordan, K.L.; et al. Senolytics decrease senescent cells in humans: Preliminary report from a clinical trial of Dasatinib plus Quercetin in individuals with diabetic kidney disease. *EBioMedicine* **2019**, *47*, 446–456. [CrossRef] [PubMed]
157. Guerrero, A.; Herranz, N.; Sun, B.; Wagner, V.; Gallage, S.; Guiho, R.; Wolter, K.; Pombo, J.; Irvine, E.E.; Innes, A.J.; et al. Cardiac glycosides are broad-spectrum senolytics. *Nat. Metab.* **2019**, *1*, 1074–1088. [CrossRef]
158. Broekman, W.; Khedoe, P.P.; Schepers, K.; Roelofs, H.; Stolk, J.; Hiemstra, P.S. Mesenchymal stromal cells: A novel therapy for the treatment of chronic obstructive pulmonary disease? *Thorax* **2018**, *73*, 565–574. [CrossRef]

159. Liu, X.; Fang, Q.; Kim, H. Preclinical studies of mesenchymal stem cell (MSC) administration in chronic obstructive pulmonary disease (COPD): A systematic review and meta-analysis. *PLoS ONE* **2016**, *11*, e0157099. [CrossRef]
160. Zhang, W.-G.; He, L.; Shi, X.-M.; Wu, S.-S.; Zhang, B.; Mei, L.; Xu, Y.-J.; Zhang, Z.-X.; Zhao, J.-P.; Zhang, H.-L. Regulation of transplanted mesenchymal stem cells by the lung progenitor niche in rats with chronic obstructive pulmonary disease. *Respir. Res.* **2014**, *15*, 33. [CrossRef]
161. Gu, W.; Song, L.; Li, X.-M.; Wang, D.; Guo, X.-J.; Xu, W.-G. Mesenchymal stem cells alleviate airway inflammation and emphysema in COPD through down-regulation of cyclooxygenase-2 via p38 and ERK MAPK pathways. *Sci. Rep.* **2015**, *5*, 8733. [CrossRef]
162. Zhen, G.; Xue, Z.; Zhao, J.; Gu, N.; Tang, Z.; Xu, Y.; Zhang, Z. Mesenchymal stem cell transplantation increases expression of vascular endothelial growth factor in papain-induced emphysematous lungs and inhibits apoptosis of lung cells. *Cytotherapy* **2010**, *12*, 605–614. [CrossRef]
163. Kim, Y.-S.; Kim, J.-Y.; Huh, J.W.; Lee, S.W.; Choi, S.J.; Oh, Y.-M. The therapeutic effects of optimal dose of mesenchymal stem cells in a murine model of an elastase induced-emphysema. *Tuberc. Respir. Dis.* **2015**, *78*, 239–245. [CrossRef] [PubMed]
164. Guan, X.J.; Song, L.; Han, F.F.; Cui, Z.L.; Chen, X.; Guo, X.J.; Xu, W.G. Mesenchymal stem cells protect cigarette smoke-damaged lung and pulmonary function partly via VEGF–VEGF receptors. *J. Cell. Biochem.* **2013**, *114*, 323–335. [CrossRef] [PubMed]
165. Weiss, D.J. Cell-based Therapy for Chronic Obstructive Pulmonary Disease. Rebuilding the Lung. *Ann. Am. Thorac. Soc.* **2018**, *15* (Suppl. S4), S253–S259. [CrossRef] [PubMed]
166. Wagner, D.E.; Bonvillain, R.W.; Jensen, T.; Girard, E.D.; Bunnell, B.A.; Finck, C.M.; Hoffman, A.M.; Weiss, D.J. Can stem cells be used to generate new lungs? Ex vivo lung bioengineering with decellularized whole lung scaffolds. *Respirology* **2013**, *18*, 895–911. [CrossRef] [PubMed]
167. Horváth, L.; Umehara, Y.; Jud, C.; Blank, F.; Petri-Fink, A.; Rothen-Rutishauser, B. Engineering an in vitro air-blood barrier by 3D bioprinting. *Sci. Rep.* **2015**, *5*, 7974. [CrossRef] [PubMed]
168. Beeh, K.M.; Beier, J.; Koppenhoefer, N.; Buhl, R. Increased glutathione disulfide and nitrosothiols in sputum supernatant of patients with stable COPD. *Chest* **2004**, *126*, 1116–1122. [CrossRef]
169. Ciofu, O.; Smith, S.; Lykkesfeldt, J. Antioxidant supplementation for lung disease in cystic fibrosis. *Cochrane Database Syst. Rev.* **2019**, *10*, Cd007020. [CrossRef]
170. Griese, M.; Kappler, M.; Eismann, C.; Ballmann, M.; Junge, S.; Rietschel, E.; van Koningsbruggen-Rietschel, S.; Staab, D.; Rolinck-Werninghaus, C.; Mellies, U.; et al. Inhalation treatment with glutathione in patients with cystic fibrosis. A randomized clinical trial. *Am. J. Respir. Crit. Care Med.* **2013**, *188*, 83–89. [CrossRef]
171. Lamson, D.W.; Brignall, M.S. The use of nebulized glutathione in the treatment of emphysema: A case report. *Altern. Med. Rev.* **2000**, *5*, 429–431.
172. Dal Negro, R.W.; Wedzicha, J.A.; Iversen, M.; Fontana, G.; Page, C.; Cicero, A.F.; Pozzi, E.; Calverley, P.M. Effect of erdosteine on the rate and duration of COPD exacerbations: The RESTORE study. *Eur. Respir. J.* **2017**, *50*, 1700711. [CrossRef]
173. Moretti, M.; Bottrighi, P.; Dallari, R.; Da Porto, R.; Dolcetti, A.; Grandi, P.; Garuti, G.; Guffanti, E.; Roversi, P.; De Gugliemo, M.; et al. The effect of long-term treatment with erdosteine on chronic obstructive pulmonary disease: The EQUALIFE Study. *Drugs Exp. Clin. Res.* **2004**, *30*, 143–152. [PubMed]
174. Meyer, K.C. Lung infections and aging. *Ageing Res. Rev.* **2004**, *3*, 55–67. [CrossRef] [PubMed]

2

Cryptides Identified in Human Apolipoprotein B as New Weapons to Fight Antibiotic Resistance in Cystic Fibrosis Disease

Rosa Gaglione [1,3], Angela Cesaro [1], Eliana Dell'Olmo [1], Rocco Di Girolamo [1], Luca Tartaglione [1], Elio Pizzo [2] and Angela Arciello [1,3,*]

1 Department of Chemical Sciences, University of Naples Federico II, Via Cintia 21, I-80126 Naples, Italy; rosa.gaglione@unina.it (R.G.); angela.cesaro@unina.it (A.C.); eliana.dellolmo@unina.it (E.D.); rocco.digirolamo@unina.it (R.D.G.); luca.tartaglione.lt@gmail.com (L.T.)

2 Department of Biology, University of Naples Federico II, Via Cintia 21, I-80126 Naples, Italy; elipizzo@unina.it

3 Istituto Nazionale di Biostrutture e Biosistemi (INBB), I-00136 Rome, Italy

* Correspondence: anarciel@unina.it

Abstract: Chronic respiratory infections are the main cause of morbidity and mortality in cystic fibrosis (CF) patients, and are characterized by the development of multidrug resistance (MDR) phenotype and biofilm formation, generally recalcitrant to treatment with conventional antibiotics. Hence, novel effective strategies are urgently needed. Antimicrobial peptides represent new promising therapeutic agents. Here, we analyze for the first time the efficacy of three versions of a cryptide identified in human apolipoprotein B (ApoB, residues 887-922) towards bacterial strains clinically isolated from CF patients. Antimicrobial and anti-biofilm properties of ApoB-derived cryptides have been analyzed by broth microdilution assays, crystal violet assays, confocal laser scanning microscopy and scanning electron microscopy. Cell proliferation assays have been performed to test cryptide effects on human host cells. ApoB-derived cryptides have been found to be endowed with significant antimicrobial and anti-biofilm properties towards *Pseudomonas* and *Burkholderia* strains clinically isolated from CF patients. Peptides have been also found to be able to act in combination with the antibiotic ciprofloxacin, and they are harmless when tested on human bronchial epithelial mesothelial cells. These findings open interesting perspectives to cryptide applicability in the treatment of chronic lung infections associated with CF disease.

Keywords: antibiotic resistance; cystic fibrosis; antimicrobial peptides; host defense peptides; cryptides; anti-biofilm peptides; synergistic effects

---

1. Introduction

Cystic fibrosis (CF) is a rare autosomal recessive disease affecting 1 in 2500 newborns in Europe [1]. More than 2000 mutations have been identified in the Cystic Fibrosis Transmembrane conductance Regulator (CFTR) gene and have been associated with the disease. CFTR gene encodes a chloride ion channel whose malfunctioning causes the production of viscous secretions coating the airway epithelia [2,3]. This phenomenon is responsible for the accumulation of trapped microbes, including *Pseudomonas aeruginosa*, with consequent deterioration of lung tissue and impairment of respiratory functions [4]. Indeed, chronic respiratory infections and inflammation are the main causes of death in CF [5]. Despite aggressive antibiotic treatments, *Pseudomonas* strains often grow in CF lungs and lead to chronic and recalcitrant infections characterized by a robust host inflammatory response [6,7]. Pulmonary infections due to the Gram-negative *P. aeruginosa* strain are the main cause of lung decline and death in patients suffering from CF [8–10]. *P. aeruginosa* colonization of host tissues is mediated by an initial attachment of bacteria to epithelial cells [11,12], followed by internalization into cells [13–16]. This phenomenon protects bacteria from host defense mechanisms and from the killing action of conventional antibiotics that hardly enter epithelial cells [17]. This is generally responsible for systemic diffusion of bacteria and for the consequent chronic nature of *P. aeruginosa* lung infections [18]. Moreover, chronic inflammation and mucus provide an environment favorable to the development of resistance phenotype for bacteria in biofilms, thus hampering antibiotic efficacy [19]. *Burkholderia* species also cause serious challenges in CF patients, even if infections associated with these strains are relatively rare [20]. Indeed, a main post-transplant complication is represented by infections caused by multidrug resistant (MDR) bacteria, with the *Burkholderia* species recognized as significant contributors to CF morbidity and mortality associated with increased post-transplant death rate [21,22]. Conventional antibiotics generally appear ineffective and their prolonged use is responsible for the development of the MDR phenotype. The concomitant decrease in the pharmaceutical industry research pipeline for novel antimicrobial agents during the last three decades has, thus, resulted in an urgent need for the discovery of novel effective antimicrobial strategies [23]. In this scenario, naturally occurring antimicrobial peptides (AMPs), or their derivatives, represent an appealing source for the generation of new therapeutic agents able to treat chronic MDR bacterial infections [24,25]. AMPs are produced by all living organisms as the first line of defense against invading microorganisms, and the majority of them are characterized by net positive charge at neutral pH and by the tendency to form amphipathic structures in a hydrophobic environment [26,27]. So far, hundreds of naturally occurring AMPs have been isolated and characterized as highly efficacious, safe, and tolerable antimicrobials [28,29]. Being able to selectively interact with bacterial cytoplasmic membranes in a manner not dependent upon specific receptors, AMPs are generally endowed with broad-spectrum antimicrobial activity [30,31], and several of them have been reported to combat biofilms because of their potent bactericidal activity and their ability to first penetrate and then to disorganize biofilm structures [32]. Furthermore, AMPs frequently synergize with antimicrobial compounds to repress molecular pathways leading to biofilm development [32]. Here, we analyze for the first time the antimicrobial and anti-biofilm properties of two recently characterized AMPs [33] towards *Pseudomonas* and *Burkholderia* strains clinically isolated from CF patients. AMPs under test have been identified in human apolipoprotein B (ApoB) by using a bioinformatic method developed by our research group [33–41]. Indeed, it is increasingly evident that eukaryotic proteins, with functions not necessarily related to host defense, act as sources of "cryptic" bioactive peptides released upon proteolytic processing by bacterial and/or host proteases [42–44]. We previously characterized two variants of the cryptide identified in human ApoB (residues 887–922), i.e., peptides ApoB887–923 and ApoB887–911 [33]. These two host defense peptides (HDPs), recombinantly produced in bacterial cells, have been here named r(P)ApoB$_L^{Pro}$ and r(P)ApoB$_S^{Pro}$ because of the presence of a Pro residue becoming the N-terminus of the peptides released by the acidic cleavage of an Asp-Pro bond [33,36]. Here, we also characterized a further peptide, i.e., a version of the longest peptide characterized by the presence of an Ala residue instead of a Pro residue in position six of peptide sequence, here named r(P)ApoB$_L^{Ala}$. Peptides r(P)ApoB$_L^{Pro}$ and r(P)ApoB$_S^{Pro}$ have been previously found to be endowed with antimicrobial, anti-biofilm, wound healing and immunomodulatory properties, and are able to synergistically act in combination with either conventional antibiotics or EDTA [33]. On the other hand, peptides have been found to be neither toxic nor hemolytic towards mammalian cells [33]. It has been also demonstrated that electrostatic interactions between negatively charged bacterial membranes and positively charged ApoB-derived AMPs play a key role in mediating peptide toxicity, although they are strongly influenced by the composition of negatively charged bacterial surfaces and by defined extracellular microenvironments [35]. Here, we demonstrate that the three ApoB-derived cryptides exert significant antimicrobial and anti-biofilm effects towards *Pseudomonas* and *Burkholderia* strains clinically isolated from CF patients and that they are able to act in combination with the ciprofloxacin antibiotic, widely used to treat chronic lung infections in CF patients [45]. Furthermore, ApoB-derived cryptides have been found to be not toxic when tested on human bronchial epithelial mesothelial cells. Altogether, these findings open interesting perspectives to peptide applicability, suggesting the possibility to develop in the future successful combinatorial therapeutic approaches, based on the concomitant administration of AMPs and conventional antibiotics, with a consequently very low potential to induce a resistance phenotype.

2. Results

2.1. *Evaluation of ApoB-Derived Peptide Effects on Clinically Isolated Baterial Strains*

In order to evaluate the ApoB-derived peptide ability to counteract microbial infections in CF, their effects were tested on six clinically isolated bacterial strains, i.e., *P. aeruginosa* RP 73, *P. aeruginosa* KK 27, *P. aeruginosa* 14, *P. aeruginosa* AA2, *Burkholderia multivorans* LMG 17582, and *Burkholderia cenocepacia* LMG 18863. To this purpose, the susceptibility of planktonic bacteria to ApoB-derived peptides was examined by using broth microdilution method [33] that allows the measurement of minimum inhibitory concentration (MIC) values. As reported in Table 1, the three ApoB-derived peptides under test were found to exert antimicrobial effects on three out of six bacterial strains tested. In particular, bacterial strains *P. aeruginosa* RP 73, *P. aeruginosa* KK 27, and *B. multivorans* LMG 17582 were found to be susceptible to ApoB-derived peptide antimicrobial activity, with MIC_{100} values ranging from 5 to 40 μM (Table 1). Peptide r(P)ApoB$_L^{Ala}$ was found to be the most active in directly killing bacterial cells (Table 1).

Table 1. Minimum inhibitory concentration (MIC) values determined for r(P)ApoB$_L^{Pro}$, r(P)ApoB$_L^{Ala}$ and r(P)ApoB$_S^{Pro}$ tested on clinically isolated bacterial strains.

	MIC_{100} (μM)		
	r(P)ApoB$_L^{Pro}$	r(P)ApoB$_L^{Ala}$	r(P)ApoB$_S^{Pro}$
P. aeruginosa RP 73	10–20	5–10	20–40
P. aeruginosa 14	>40	>40	>40
P. aeruginosa AA2	>40	>40	>40
P. aeruginosa KK 27	20–40	10–20	20–40
Burkholderia cenocepacia LMG 18863	>40	>40	>40
Burkholderia multivorans LMG 17582	10–20	10–20	20–40

2.2. *Evaluation of ApoB-Derived Peptide Anti-biofilm Activity on Clinically Isolated Baterial Strains*

2.2.1. Evaluation of ApoB-Derived Peptide Anti-Biofilm Activity by Microtiter Plate Assay

To evaluate whether recombinant ApoB-derived peptides are endowed with anti-biofilm activity, analyses were performed on clinically isolated bacterial strains *P. aeruginosa* RP 73, *P. aeruginosa* KK 27, *P. aeruginosa* 14, *P. aeruginosa* AA2, *B. multivorans* LMG 17582, and *B. cenocepacia* LMG 18863 in 0.5X Mueller Hinton Broth (MHB). By following different experimental approaches, peptide effects were tested on the three main stages of biofilm development, such as attachment, formation and detachment. To test peptide effects on biofilm attachment, following overnight growth, a bacterial culture was diluted into MHB medium containing increasing concentrations of the peptide under test (0–40 μM), and incubated for 4 h at 37 °C [33]. When, instead, peptide effects were tested on biofilm formation, the experimental procedure described above was followed with the only exception that bacterial cells were incubated with increasing concentrations of peptides for 24 h at 37 °C [33]. Finally, the effects of ApoB-derived peptides were tested on biofilm detachment [33]. In each case, following incubation with peptides, biofilm was analyzed by staining with crystal violet. As shown in Figure 1, ApoB-derived peptides have been found to be effective on biofilm attachment, with the greatest effects obtained in the case of *P. aeruginosa* KK 27 and *P. aeruginosa* 14 bacterial strains for all the three peptides under test. In the case of biofilm formation, the greatest effects were found to be exerted by r(P)ApoB$_L$^{Ala} and r(P)ApoB$_S$^{Pro} on *P. aeruginosa* 14 (~50% inhibition) (Figure 1). Even more interestingly, about 30%–40% biofilm eradication was observed in the case of *B. cenocepacia* LMG 18863 upon treatment with 2.5 μM r(P)ApoB$_L$^{Ala} (Figure 1). A similar effect was obtained upon treatment of *P. aeruginosa* KK 27 preformed biofilm with 2.5 μM r(P)ApoB$_S$^{Pro} (Figure 1). Moreover, about 20% biofilm eradication was observed upon treatment of *P. aeruginosa* RP 73 with very low concentrations (1.25 μM) of r(P)ApoB$_S$^{Pro}.

Altogether, obtained data indicate that peptides exert anti-biofilm effects even on bacterial strains not sensitive to their direct antimicrobial activity. In most of the cases, significant anti-biofilm effects were detected at peptide concentrations (1.25–2.5 μM) lower than those required to directly kill planktonic cells (Table 1 and Figure 1). Data reported in Figure 1 represent the mean ± standard deviation (SD) of at least three independent experiments.

2.2.2. Evaluation of ApoB-Derived Peptides Anti-Biofilm Activity by Laser Scanning Confocal Microscopy

In order to further investigate anti-biofilm properties of ApoB-derived peptides, analyses were also performed by confocal laser scanning microscopy (CLSM). For this approach, we selected two bacterial strains not responsive to ApoB-derived peptides direct antimicrobial activity, such as *B. cenocepacia* LMG 18863 and *P. aeruginosa* 14. Peptide effects on biofilm attachment, formation and detachment were evaluated upon sample staining with LIVE/DEAD BacLight bacterial viability kit. Analyses revealed that all three peptides are able to affect biofilm attachment and formation in the case of *B. cenocepacia* LMG 18863 (Figure 2). Even more interestingly, peptides are able to affect pre-formed biofilm with the strongest effects observed in the presence of r(P)ApoB$_L$^{Ala} (Figure 2). By staining bacterial biofilm with SYPRO® ruby dye, which is able to specifically stain biofilm extracellular matrix, the appearance of highly fluorescent aggregates is clearly evident upon treatment with peptides (Figure 2), thus indicating that peptides induce strong alterations of biofilm matrix architecture, as previously reported for different anti-biofilm agents [46]. Similar results were obtained also in the case of *P. aeruginosa* 14 (Figure 3). These findings are also supported by biofilm biovolume determinations by CLSM reported in Figure 4, that indicate a strong and significant effect of r(P)ApoB$_S$^{Pro} peptide on biofilm eradication in the case of both bacterial strains (Figure 4c,f). Furthermore, peptides have been found to exert significant effects on biofilm biovolume when attachment is tested (Figure 4a,d), except for r(P)ApoB$_L$^{Ala} for which no significant reduction in biovolume is observed, although a disaggregating effect is clearly evident (Figures 2 and 3). This might be due to the fact that, upon treatment with r(P)ApoB$_L$^{Ala} peptide, planktonic cells escape from biofilm by floating, with a consequent significant contribution to biovolume. Altogether, these findings confirm that peptides are able to exert significant anti-biofilm effects even on bacterial strains not sensitive to their direct antimicrobial activity.

2.2.3. Evaluation of ApoB-Derived Peptides Anti-Biofilm Activity by Scanning Electron Microscopy

To analyze morphological modifications of bacterial biofilm upon treatment with peptides, scanning electron microscopy (SEM) analyses were also performed on bacterial strains not responsive to peptide direct antimicrobial activity, such as *B. cenocepacia* LMG 18863 and *P. aeruginosa* 14. In untreated samples, bacteria present smooth and intact surfaces and appear embedded into the extracellular biofilm matrix in the case of both bacterial strains (Figure 5). When bacteria are treated with peptides, instead, a significant decrease or disappearance of biofilm matrix is clearly evident with a concomitant decrease of cell density.

		P. aeruginosa RP 73						*P. aeruginosa* KK 27					
		$r(P)ApoB_L^{Pro}$		$r(P)ApoB_L^{Ala}$		$r(P)ApoB_S^{Pro}$		$r(P)ApoB_L^{Pro}$		$r(P)ApoB_L^{Ala}$		$r(P)ApoB_S^{Pro}$	
	Peptide (µM)	% of biofilm growth	SD	% of biofilm growth	SD	% of biofilm growth	SD	% of biofilm growth	SD	% of biofilm growth	SD	% of biofilm growth	SD
Attachment	0	100	0	100	0	100	0	100	0	100	0	100	0
	0.612	85	20	77	3	78	3	92	4	95	23	101	23
	1.25	74	16	67	11	72	3	75	10	93	14	85	18
	2.5	71	9	65	12	65	4	74	11	67	24	62	8
	5	71	9	72	15	65	12	53	4	46	4	45	0
	10	74	9	65	17	66	8	22	8	20	2	20	4
	20	73	7	64	13	66	8	18	6	21	3	14	4
	40	72	10	75	18	65	17	20	9	20	1	17	7
	Peptide (µM)	% of biofilm growth	SD	% of biofilm growth	SD	% of biofilm growth	SD	% of biofilm growth	SD	% of biofilm growth	SD	% of biofilm growth	SD
Formation	0	100	0	100	0	100	0	100	0	100	0	100	0
	0.612	72	6	94	14	75	2	81	4	93	5	84	10
	1.25	73	7	95	19	77	8	75	13	84	18	80	11
	2.5	68	0	90	1	85	9	70	18	80	17	74	11
	5	82	5	100	1	78	4	72	8	79	14	80	4
	10	77	10	95	5	89	6	64	13	69	25	74	21
	20	82	7	93	10	89	5	58	15	67	13	71	6
	40	36	5	37	11	79	10	64	3	29	7	27	3
	Peptide (µM)	% of biofilm growth	SD	% of biofilm growth	SD	% of biofilm growth	SD	% of biofilm growth	SD	% of biofilm growth	SD	% of biofilm growth	SD
Detachment	0	100	0	100	0	100	0	100	0	100	0	100	0
	0.612	85	4	95	0	76	10	87	3	91	3	87	9
	1.25	82	6	84	7	75	3	80	15	87	14	78	1
	2.5	76	17	82	1	66	11	88	5	88	9	75	7
	5	89	2	92	4	80	16	80	11	87	8	80	13
	10	98	5	84	3	71	13	79	18	83	7	71	16
	20	99	1	88	8	70	25						
	40	95	4	83	12	69	14						

		P. aeruginosa 14						*P. aeruginosa* AA2					
	Peptide (µM)	% of biofilm growth	SD	% of biofilm growth	SD	% of biofilm growth	SD	% of biofilm growth	SD	% of biofilm growth	SD	% of biofilm growth	SD
Attachment	0	100	0	100	0	100	0	100	0	100	0	100	0
	0.612	77	12	98	5	98	5	94	12	95	10	91	13
	1.25	73	20	83	8	83	8	95	11	93	12	88	14
	2.5	75	14	85	5	85	5	99	3	92	14	89	14
	5	70	20	69	17	69	17	98	7	90	16	88	11
	10	55	19	50	18	50	18	97	5	88	19	78	21
	20	40	20	37	12	37	12	94	12	87	19	83	17
	40	33	17	29	8	29	8	87	22	68	21	75	17
	Peptide (µM)	% of biofilm growth	SD	% of biofilm growth	SD	% of biofilm growth	SD	% of biofilm growth	SD	% of biofilm growth	SD	% of biofilm growth	SD
Formation	0	100	0	100	0	100	0	100	0	100	0	100	0
	0.612	75	8	81	14	81	14	90	12	88	10	94	5
	1.25	74	7	75	20	75	20	85	10	79	12	94	12
	2.5	71	7	71	26	71	26	86	15	85	2	95	5
	5	76	18	66	28	66	28	84	15	77	11	89	17
	10	62	20	54	28	54	28	85	16	89	6	90	7
	20	33	13	54	32	54	32	87	12	86	9	90	9
	40	35	15	46	26	46	26	100	7	91	0	95	3
	Peptide (µM)	% of biofilm growth	SD	% of biofilm growth	SD	% of biofilm growth	SD	% of biofilm growth	SD	% of biofilm growth	SD	% of biofilm growth	SD
Detachment	0	100	0	100	0	100	0	100	0	100	0	100	0
	0.612	94	8	96	6	96	6	103	7	103	2	100	1
	1.25	96	5	95	6	95	6	102	12	100	1	96	5
	2.5	93	4	86	13	86	13	93	1	92	7	96	1
	5	100	1	93	2	93	2	104	8	97	2	97	3
	10	95	7	92	8	92	8	96	3	91	6	94	1
	20	105	13	85	17	85	17	100	4	99	11	102	4
	40	94	3	107	10	107	10	100	3	95	13	101	6

		Burkholderia multivorans LMG 17582						*Burkholderia cenocepacia* LMG 18863					
	Peptide (µM)	% of biofilm growth	SD	% of biofilm growth	SD	% of biofilm growth	SD	% of biofilm growth	SD	% of biofilm growth	SD	% of biofilm growth	SD
Attachment	0	100	0	100	0	100	0	100	0	100	0	100	0
	0.612	86	8	86	12	80	6	71	7	63	2	85	4
	1.25	74	5	80	20	76	2	65	5	61	9	64	8
	2.5	79	2	77	25	75	5	67	13	61	11	68	15
	5	79	2	77	22	73	5	71	11	66	7	73	15
	10	77	3	80	23	71	11	75	2	78	17	69	14
	20	82	1	79	22	65	11	69	13	73	5	68	18
	40	82	6	81	19	68	7	69	12	78	3	69	12
	Peptide (µM)	% of biofilm growth	SD	% of biofilm growth	SD	% of biofilm growth	SD	% of biofilm growth	SD	% of biofilm growth	SD	% of biofilm growth	SD
Formation	0	100	0	100	0	100	0	100	0	100	0	100	0
	0.612	77	16	79	9	77	6	74	14	68	13	73	8
	1.25	67	13	75	7	68	9	68	13	75	1	66	8
	2.5	65	18	75	10	71	17	71	18	61	6	66	11
	5	68	18	73	11	66	19	78	13	74	0	64	13
	10	69	17	75	14	74	21	74	15	83	6	63	15
	20	71	11	77	16	75	19	73	13	83	3	78	10
	40	80	5	83	13	78	11	67	8	78	11	79	15
	Peptide (µM)	% of biofilm growth	SD	% of biofilm growth	SD	% of biofilm growth	SD	% of biofilm growth	SD	% of biofilm growth	SD	% of biofilm growth	SD
Detachment	0	100	0	100	0	100	0	100	0	100	0	100	0
	0.612	85	23	86	21	85	25	92	10	89	15	94	9
	1.25	88	17	91	15	82	31	87	18	87	18	98	3
	2.5	100	2	96	7	84	29	90	8	75	10	105	15
	5	92	12	96	7	89	17	89	17	84	14	89	7
	10	93	8	104	6	94	8	101	2	94	5	89	5
	20	93	4	101	4	95	4	91	7	85	18	86	13
	40	93	9	92	9	92	7	108	17	104	14	84	10

Figure 1. Anti-biofilm activity of $r(P)ApoB_L^{Pro}$, $r(P)ApoB_L^{Ala}$, and $r(P)ApoB_S^{Pro}$ peptides on *P. aeruginosa* RP 73, *P. aeruginosa* KK 27, *P. aeruginosa* 14, *P. aeruginosa* AA2, *B. multivorans* LMG 17582, and *B. cenocepacia* LMG 18863 in MHB medium.

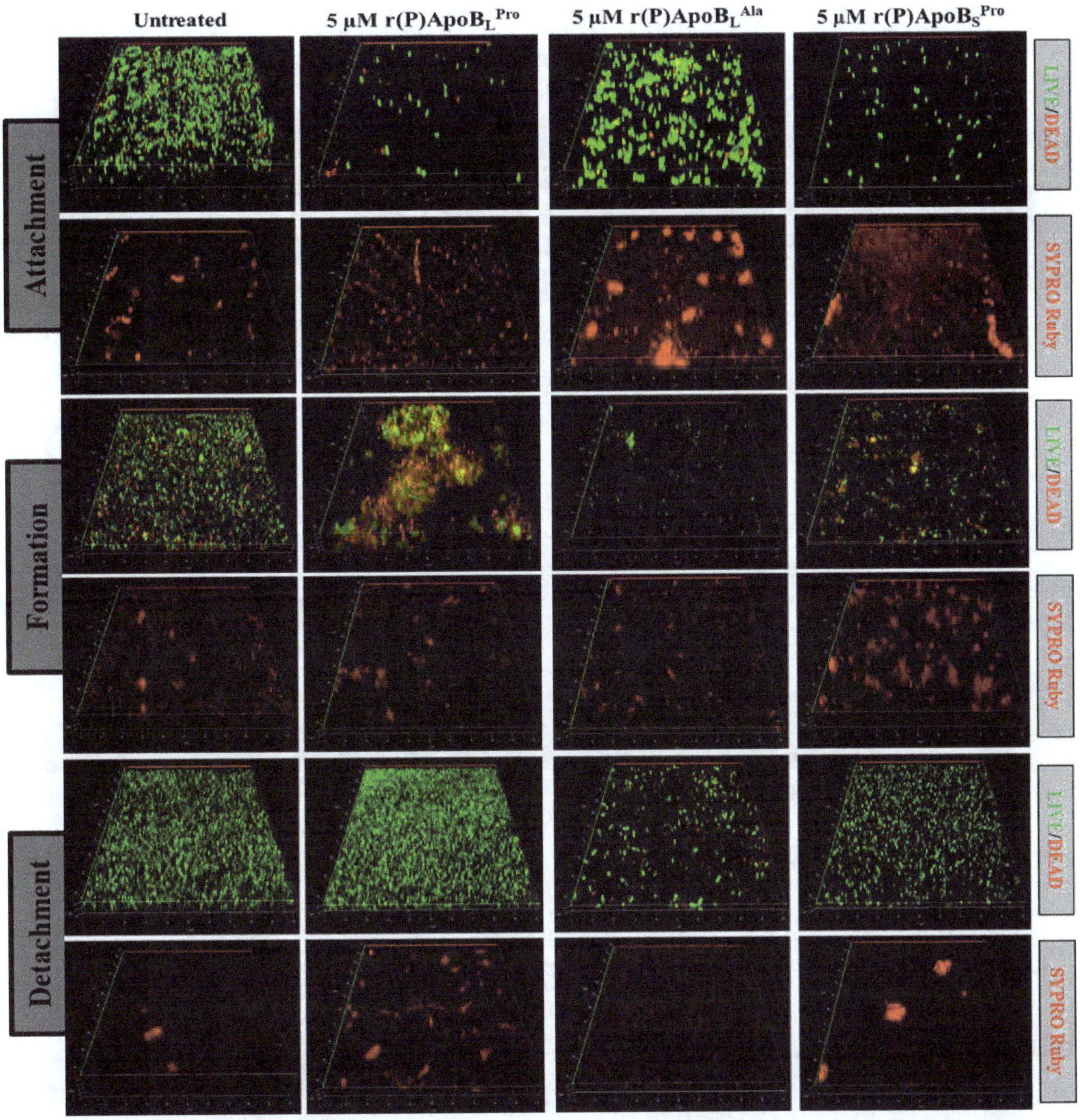

Figure 2. Effects of r(P)ApoB$_L$^{Pro}, r(P)ApoB$_L$^{Ala}, and r(P)ApoB$_S$^{Pro} peptides on *B. cenocepacia* LMG 18863 biofilm attachment, formation and detachment. Biofilm cells were stained by using LIVE/DEAD BacLight bacterial viability kit (Molecular Probes, Eugene, OR, USA) containing 1:1 ratio of Syto-9 (green fluorescence, all cells) and propidium iodide (PI, red fluorescence, dead cells) and FilmTracer™ SYPRO® Ruby biofilm matrix staining (Invitrogen™, F10318). Images are 3D projections of biofilm structure obtained by laser scanning confocal z-stack using Zen Lite 2.3 software. All images were taken under identical conditions.

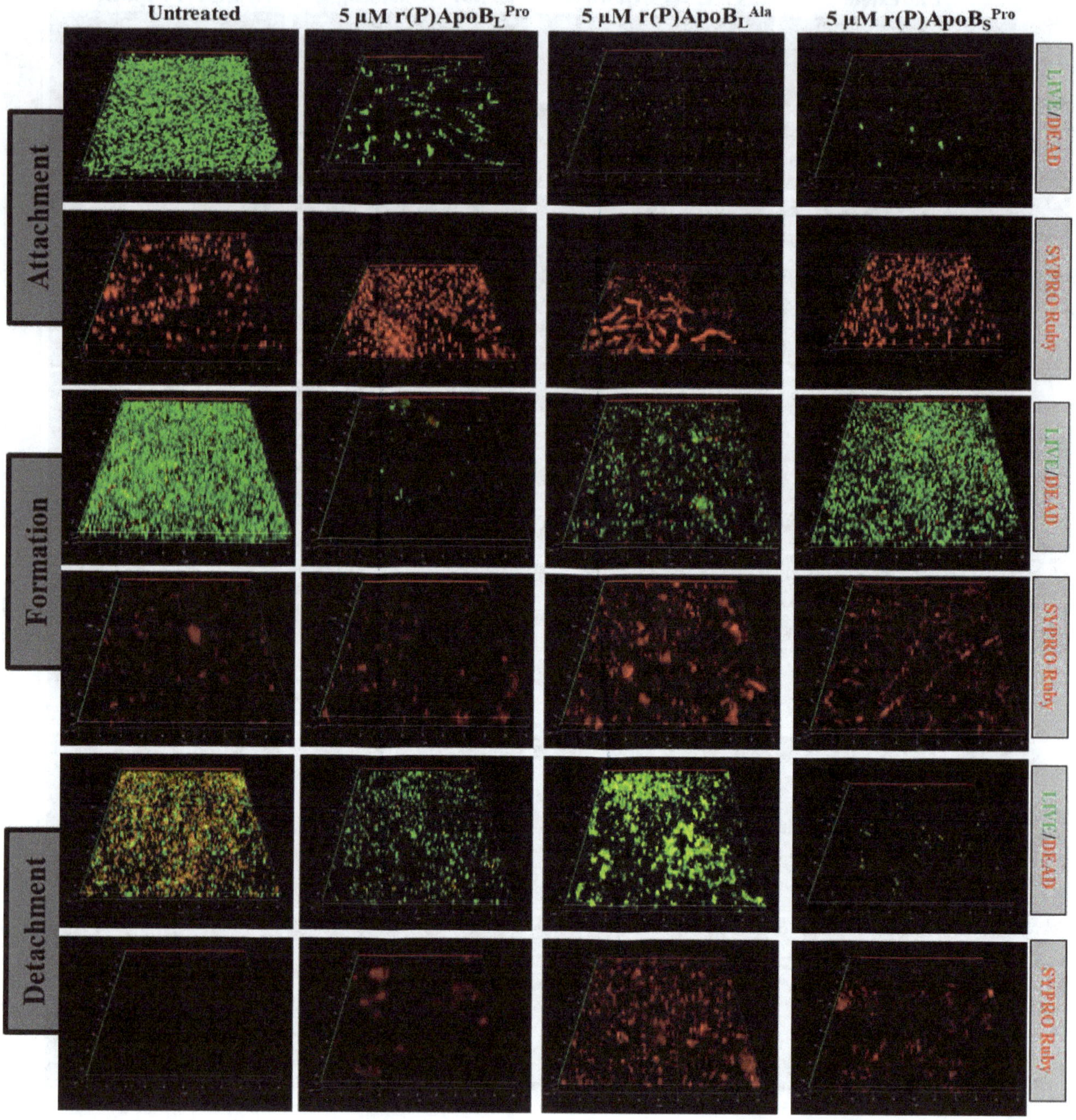

Figure 3. Effects of r(P)ApoB$_L$^{Pro}, r(P)ApoB$_L$^{Ala} and r(P)ApoB$_S$^{Pro} peptides on *P. aeruginosa* 14 biofilm attachment, formation and detachment. Biofilm cells were stained by using LIVE/DEAD BacLight bacterial viability kit (Molecular Probes, Eugene, OR, USA) containing 1:1 ratio of Syto-9 (green fluorescence, all cells) and propidium iodide (PI, red fluorescence, dead cells) and FilmTracer™ SYPRO® Ruby biofilm matrix staining (Invitrogen™, F10318). Images are 3D projections of biofilm structure obtained by laser scanning confocal z-stack using Zen Lite 2.3 software. All images were taken under identical conditions.

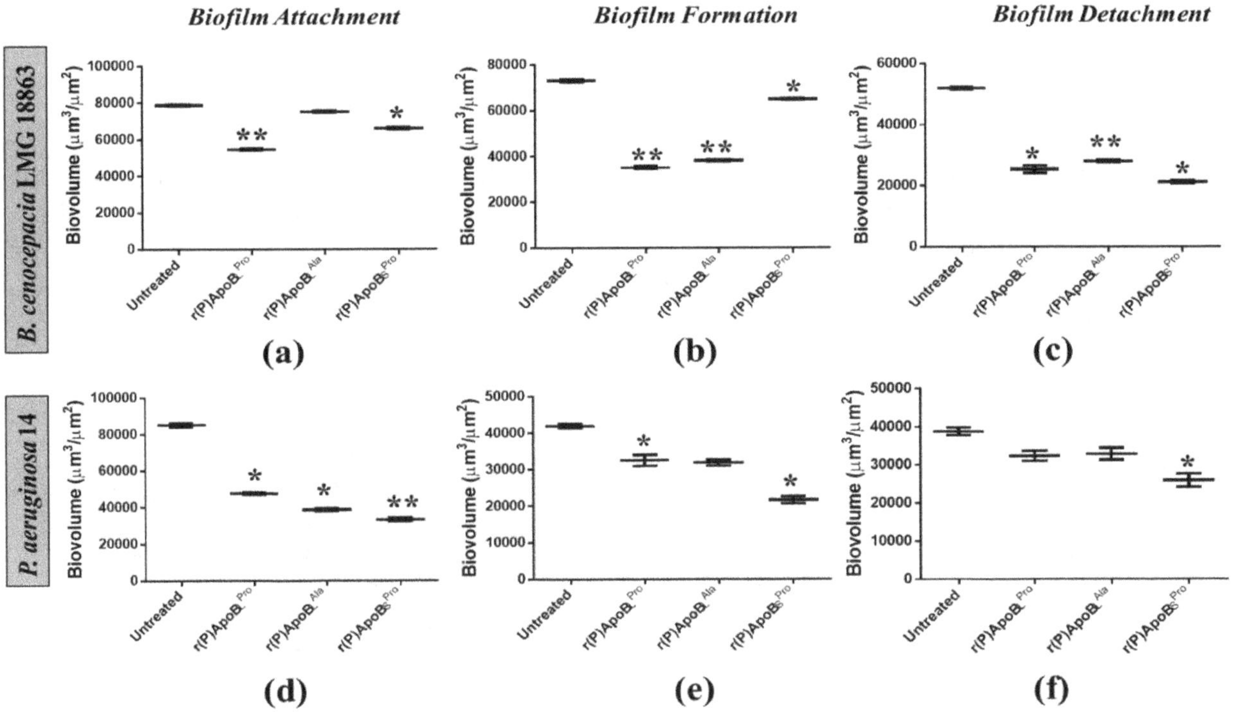

Figure 4. Analysis of the effects of r(P)ApoB$_L$^{Pro}, r(P)ApoB$_L$^{Ala} and r(P)ApoB$_S$^{Pro} peptides on biofilm attachment (**a**,**d**), formation (**b**,**e**) and detachment (**c**,**f**) in the case of *B. cenocepacia* LMG 18863 (**a**–**c**) and *P. aeruginosa* 14 (**d**– **f**). Biovolume (μm^3/μm^2) was measured by using Zen Lite 2.3 software. Significant differences were indicated as * $p < 0.05$ or ** $p < 0.01$ for treated versus control samples.

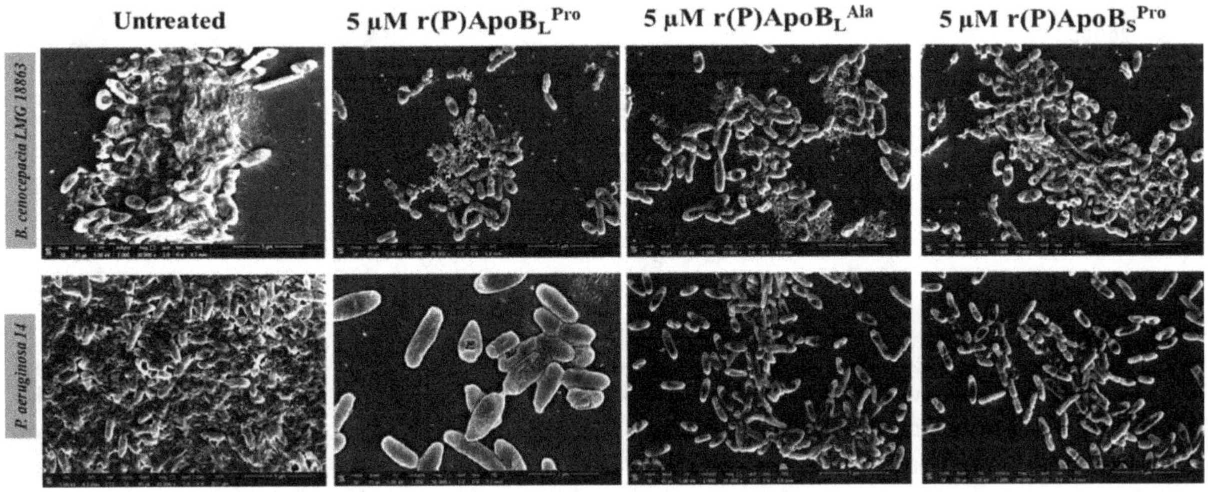

Figure 5. Morphological analyses of *B. cenocepacia* LMG 18863 (top panel) and *P. aeruginosa* 14 (lower panel) preformed biofilms by SEM. Representative images are shown upon treatment of bacterial biofilm with 5 μM r(P)ApoB$_L$^{Pro}, r(P)ApoB$_L$^{Ala}, and r(P)ApoB$_S$^{Pro}. Bars 5 μm.

2.3. Combinatorial Therapeutic Approach

To verify whether ApoB-derived peptides are able to synergistically act in combination with conventional antibiotics to counteract bacterial infections associated with biofilm in CF, CLSM analyses were performed to evaluate the effects of combinations of r(P)ApoB$_L$^{Pro} or r(P)ApoB$_L$^{Ala} and ciprofloxacin on preformed biofilm. Analyses were performed on *B. cenocepacia* LMG 18863 bacterial strain, since chronic lung infections associated with this strain strongly contribute to CF morbidity and mortality and are generally recalcitrant to conventional antibiotics [21,22]. Effects of r(P)ApoB$_L$^{Pro} or r(P)ApoB$_L$^{Ala} peptide in combination with ciprofloxacin were tested on preformed biofilm, in order to better simulate clinical conditions.

As shown in Figure 6, by comparing the effects of combinations of r(P)ApoB$_L$^{Pro} and ciprofloxacin with the effects of single agents on preformed biofilm, a significantly greater reduction of biofilm biovolume is observed in the case of the sample treated with the compound mixture together with a concomitant increase of the number of dead cells embedded into the biofilm matrix (Figure 6). Similarly, about the effects of combinations of r(P)ApoB$_L$^{Ala} and ciprofloxacin on preformed biofilm, a significantly greater reduction of biofilm biovolume is observed in the presence of compounds combination (Figure 7).

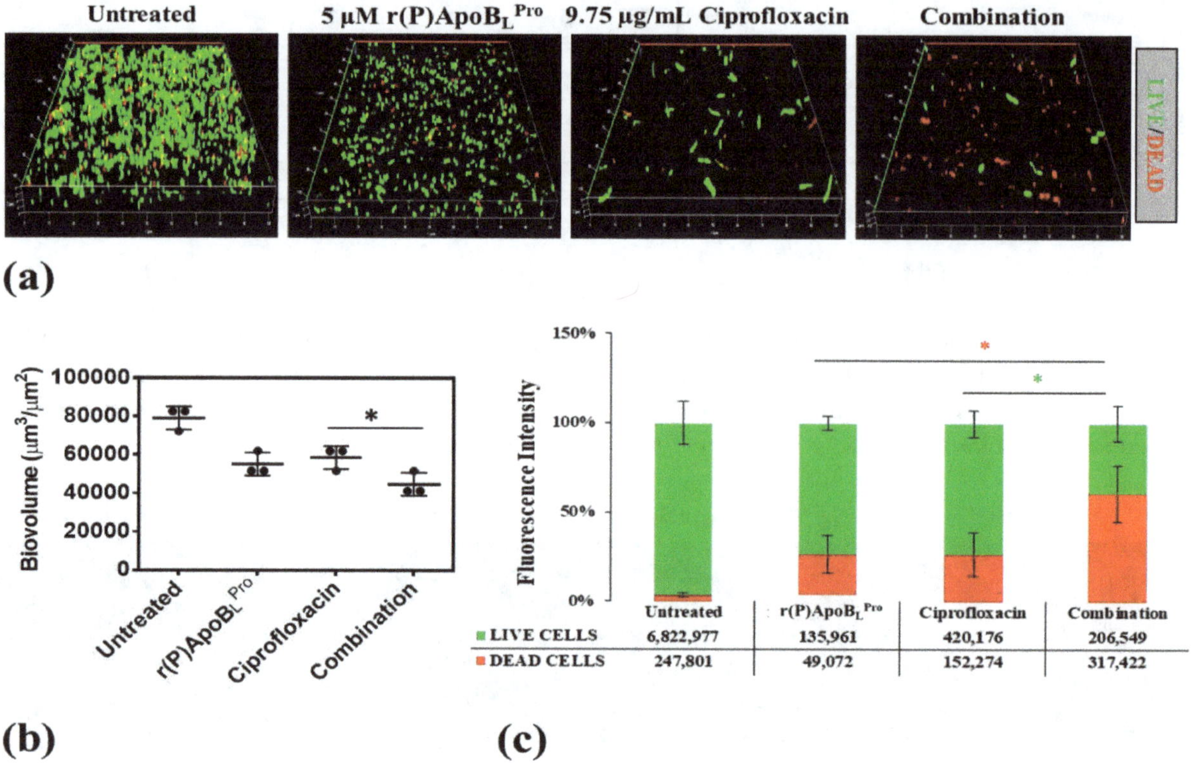

Figure 6. Effects of r(P)ApoB$_{LPro}$, ciprofloxacin and a combination of the two compounds on preformed biofilm (**a**). Biofilm cells were stained by using LIVE/DEAD BacLight bacterial viability kit (Molecular Probes, Eugene, OR) containing 1:1 ratio of Syto-9 (green fluorescence, all cells) and propidium iodide (PI, red fluorescence, dead cells). Images are 3D projections of biofilm structure obtained by laser scanning confocal z-stack using Zen Lite 2.3 software. All images were taken under identical conditions. Biovolume (μm^3/μm^2) was measured by using Zen Lite 2.3 software. Significant differences were indicated as * $p < 0.05$ for treated versus control samples (**b**). Numbers of live and dead cells were evaluated by using Zen Lite 2.3 software (**c**).

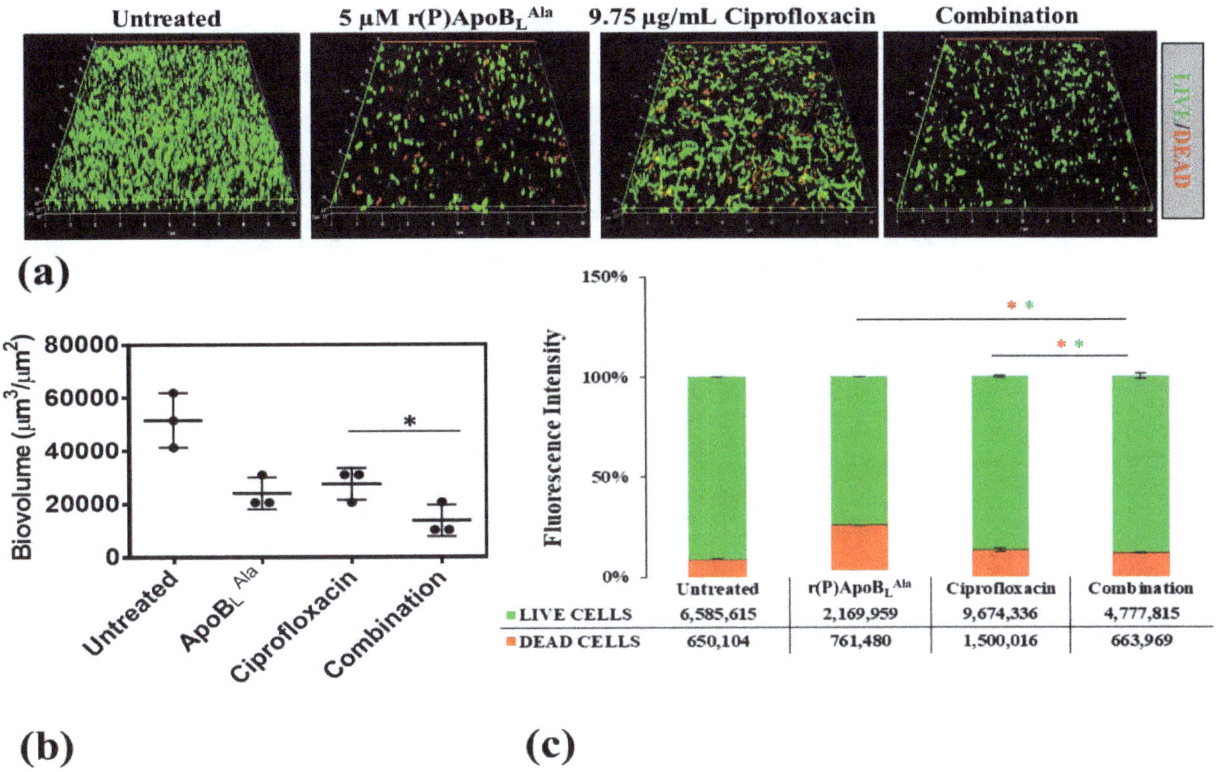

Figure 7. Effects of r(P)ApoB$_L$^{Ala}, ciprofloxacin and a combination of the two compounds on preformed biofilm (**a**). Biofilm cells were stained by using LIVE/DEAD BacLight bacterial viability kit (Molecular Probes, Eugene, OR) containing 1:1 ratio of Syto-9 (green fluorescence, all cells) and propidium iodide (PI, red fluorescence, dead cells). Images are 3D projections of biofilm structure obtained by laser scanning confocal z-stack using Zen Lite 2.3 software. All images were taken under identical conditions. Biovolume (μm^3/μm^2) was measured by using Zen Lite 2.3 software. Significant differences were indicated as * $p < 0.05$ for treated versus control samples (**b**). Numbers of live and dead cells were evaluated by using Zen Lite 2.3 software (**c**).

2.4. Evaluation of Peptide Biocompatibility

Peptide applicability in therapeutic approaches aimed at counteracting bacterial infections associated with CF is strongly dependent on the absence of any toxic effect towards host cells. For this reason, biocompatibility assays were performed to test ApoB-derived peptide effects on immortalized human bronchial epithelial mesothelial (BEAS) cells. As shown in Figure 8, only slight toxic effects were detected and the most biocompatible peptide was found to be r(P)ApoB$_L$^{Ala}. Indeed, in the presence of this peptide, only slight toxic effects were detected upon 72 h treatment and at the highest peptide concentrations tested (Figure 8).

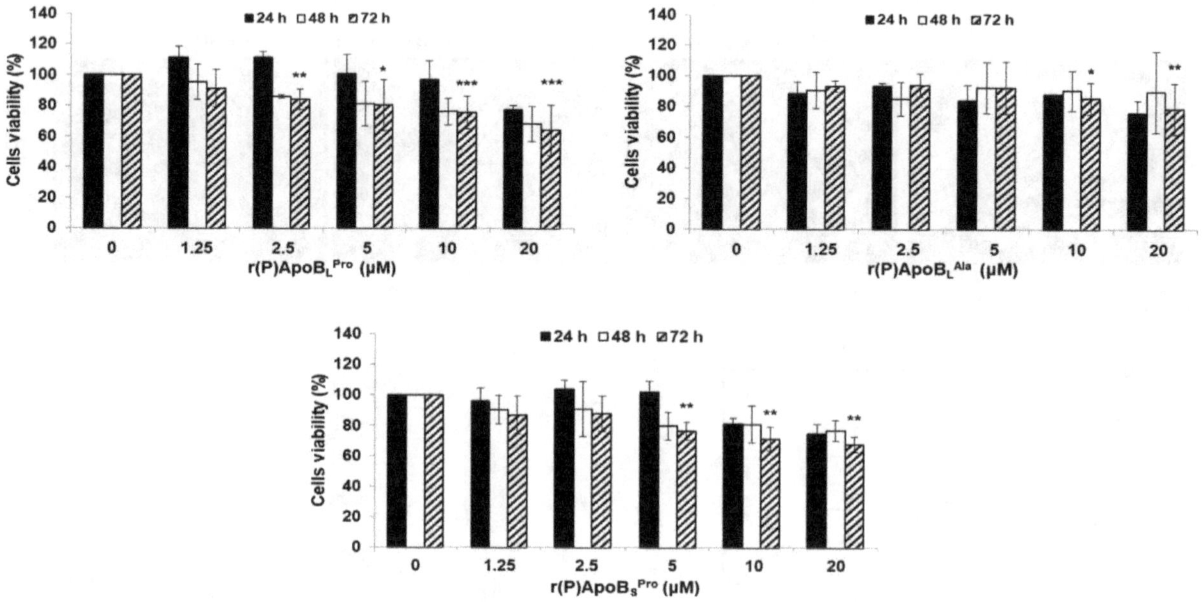

Figure 8. Effects of r(P)$ApoB_L{}^{Pro}$, r(P)$ApoB_L{}^{Ala}$ and r(P)$ApoB_S{}^{Pro}$ peptides on the viability of BEAS cells. Cell viability was assessed by MTT assays, and expressed as the percentage of viable cells with respect to controls (untreated cells). Error bars indicate standard deviations obtained from at least three independent experiments, each one carried out with triplicate determinations. Significant differences were indicated as * $p < 0.05$, ** $p < 0.01$ or *** $p < 0.001$ for treated versus control samples.

3. Discussion

AMPs represent novel promising effective alternative agents to counteract chronic bacterial infections affecting CF patients. Indeed, as these infections are generally recalcitrant to conventional antibiotics because of the development of the MDR phenotype and of biofilm formation, the development of novel therapeutic strategies is strongly necessary. To this purpose, three versions of a cryptide identified in human ApoB [33,35] have been here tested towards six bacterial strains clinically isolated from CF patients, such as *P. aeruginosa* RP 73, *P. aeruginosa* KK 27, *P. aeruginosa* 14, *P. aeruginosa* AA2, *B. multivorans* LMG 17582, and *B. cenocepacia* LMG 18863. ApoB-derived cryptides have been found to exert direct antimicrobial activity towards three out of six bacterial strains tested. Indeed, ApoB-derived AMPs have been found to be active on *P. aeruginosa* RP 73, *P. aeruginosa* KK 27, and *B. multivorans* LMG 17582, with MIC_{100} values ranging from 5 to 40 µM. This is in agreement with recent findings indicating that ApoB-derived cryptides direct antimicrobial activity, although mediated by electrostatic interactions between cationic peptides and negatively charged bacterial membranes, is strongly influenced by chemical composition of LPS molecules exposed on the surface of different strains of *P. aeruginosa* [35]. Indeed, although several bacterial resistance components against antimicrobial peptides have been reported [47], LPS chemical composition has been proposed to play a key role in the case of ApoB-derived cryptide antimicrobial activity [35]. It has been reported that different *Burkholderia* strains present different LPS chemotypes, such as rough, partial rough, or smooth [48]. In particular, in the case of *B. cenocepacia* LMG 18863, the LPS chemotype has been identified as smooth [48]. These differences in LPS chemotype might be responsible for the different susceptibility of *Burkholderia* strains to ApoB-derived cryptides' direct antimicrobial activity. It also has to be highlighted that several *B. cenocepacia* strains have been reported to be naturally resistant to different classes of antibiotics and even to several antimicrobial peptides [49]. This is probably due to the ability of *B. cenocepacia* strains to acquire a resistance phenotype by modifying the LPS chemical composition by substituting a phosphate group with a cationic charged residue of 4-amino-4-deoxy-L-arabinose (L-Ara4N), with a consequent reduction in membrane negative potential, that plays a key role in the interaction between bacterial membranes and antimicrobial peptides [50,51]. Based on these observations, ApoB-derived cryptides direct antimicrobial activity towards *B. multivorans* LMG 17582 appears to be really interesting. It also has to be considered that, in the case of chronic infections affecting CF patients, the mucus phenotype favors bacterial biofilm formation [20]. Bacteria embedded into biofilm matrix are more resistant to conventional antibiotics for several reasons: i) low antibiotic diffusion rate inside biofilm matrix; ii) bacteria metabolic changes due to nutrients missing, with a consequently lower susceptibility to antibiotics; and iii) appearance of persisted cells recalcitrant to conventional antibiotics and playing a key role in long-term infections [52]. Anti-biofilm cationic amphipathic peptides represent an alternative promising approach to treat infections associated with biofilm formation, since peptides act on biofilm specific targets, such as matrix components and/or highly conserved regulatory mechanisms [53]. Here, we tested the ability of r(P)ApoB$_L$^{Pro}, r(P)ApoB$_L$^{Ala} and r(P)ApoB$_S$^{Pro} to affect the biofilm of bacterial strains clinically isolated from CF patients. In particular, we analyzed the ability of ApoB-derived cryptides to interfere with the three main stages of biofilm development, i.e., attachment, formation and detachment [33]. We found that all the three ApoB-derived cryptides are able to exert significant effects on biofilm attachment and formation. Even more interestingly, ApoB-derived cryptides have been found to exert significant anti-biofilm effects even on bacterial strains not sensitive to their direct antimicrobial activity. In particular, ApoB-derived AMPs have been found to affect *P. aeruginosa* 14 biofilm attachment and formation and *B. cenocepacia* LMG 18863 preformed biofilm at a very low concentration (2.5 μM). As reported for different AMPs, obtained data allow us to exclude any correlation between peptide direct antimicrobial activity and their anti-biofilm properties. Indeed, peptide IDR-1018 has been reported to be endowed with strong anti-biofilm activity towards a pool of *P. aeruginosa* and *Burkholderia* strains in the absence of any direct antimicrobial effect [54]. To deeply characterize ApoB-derived cryptides anti-biofilm activity, we also performed analyses by confocal laser scanning microscopy (CLSM) and scanning electron microscopy (SEM) on *P. aeruginosa 14* and *B. cenocepacia* LMG 18863, two strains not sensitive to ApoB-derived AMP's direct antimicrobial activity. CLSM analyses revealed the ability of ApoB-derived cryptides to alter biofilm architecture, as indicated by the appearance of highly fluorescent aggregates only in treated samples upon staining with SYPRO® Ruby, a dye able to specifically label biofilm extracellular matrix. Accordingly, a significant reduction in biofilm biovolume has been evaluated in the case of samples treated with ApoB-derived cryptides. Furthermore, scanning electron microscopy analyses clearly indicate the ability of ApoB-derived cryptides to disrupt the biofilm matrix of bacterial strains not responsive to the peptides' direct antimicrobial activity. These observations are in perfect agreement with data reported for peptide 6K-F17, which is able to strongly affect *P. aeruginosa* biofilm by disrupting the extracellular matrix, thus determining a significant decrease of biofilm biovolume [55]. However, CLSM and SEM analyses indicate only a slight increase of bacterial cells death upon treatment with 6K-F17 [55]. Based on obtained results, we also evaluated the possibility to set up effective combinatorial therapeutic approaches by concomitantly administrating ApoB-derived cryptides and conventional antibiotics to bacterial cells. To this purpose, we analyzed the anti-biofilm properties of combinations of r(P)ApoB$_L$^{Pro} or r(P)ApoB$_L$^{Ala} and the antibiotic ciprofloxacin, which is widely used to treat bacterial infections in CF patients [45]. The effects of compound mixtures have been tested on *P. aeruginosa 14* or *B. cenocepacia* LMG 18863 preformed biofilm. Effects of combinations of r(P)ApoB$_L$^{Pro} or r(P)ApoB$_L$^{Ala} and ciprofloxacin on preformed biofilm have been found to be stronger than those of single agents, with more severe effects on biofilm biovolume. It has been previously reported that, upon biofilm treatment with the ciprofloxacin antibiotic, a deep alteration of the matrix structure and a strong decrease of biofilm biovolume are immediately observed, probably associated with a high killing rate of bacterial cells embedded into the biofilm matrix [56]. However, upon a prolonged exposure to ciprofloxacin, the activation of specific mechanisms leading to a variation of biofilm phenotype makes the antibiotic ineffective [56]. This phenomenon might be overcome by the development of successful combinatorial therapeutic approaches, which present several advantages over conventional therapeutic treatments based on the administration of single agents. Indeed, several anti-biofilm peptides have been reported to be able to act in synergism with a broad range of conventional antibiotics [57]. This allows us to significantly reduce the effective dose of antibiotics up to 64-fold, with a consequent lower possibility to induce MDR phenotype and to simultaneously reduce effective peptide concentrations [57]. In the case of CAMA peptides, synergism with the conventional antibiotics tobramycin, ciprofloxacin and colistin has been demonstrated in the treatment of *P. aeruginosa* biofilm, with the consequent possibility of reducing antibiotics doses up to 8-fold and peptide concentrations up to 10-fold [58]. Since one of the bottlenecks for the development of successful peptide-based therapies is peptide cytotoxicity, we also tested ApoB-derived cryptides effects on immortalized human bronchial epithelial mesothelial (BEAS) cells, and found that peptides are biocompatible, since slight toxic effects are detected only upon 72 h cell treatment and at the highest peptide concentrations tested. Altogether, obtained findings open interesting perspectives to the applicability of ApoB-derived cryptides in the treatment of bacterial chronic infections associated with biofilm formation and characterized by MDR phenotype, such as those affecting CF patients, and to the development in the future of successful combinatorial therapeutic approaches based on the concomitant administration of peptides and conventional antibiotics.

4. Materials and Methods

4.1. Materials

All the reagents were purchase from Sigma-Aldrich (Milan, Italy), unless differently specified.

4.2. Recombinant Production of ApoB-Derived Peptides

Expression and isolation of recombinant ApoB-derived peptides was carried out as previously described [33,35]. Pro → Ala substitution in position six of the longest peptide was obtained by QuikChange II site-directed mutagenesis performed by using the following primers: primer forward 5′-CATTTACCCGCTTTCAGCGCAACATGCGGGTG-3′ and primer reverse 5′-GATCCGCATGTTGCGCTGAAAGCGGGTAAACTG-3′.

4.3. Bacterial Strains and Growth Conditions

Bacterial strains *P. aeruginosa* RP 73, *P. aeruginosa* KK 27, *P. aeruginosa* 14, *P. aeruginosa* AA2, *B. multivorans* LMG 17582, and *B. cenocepacia* LMG 18863 were kindly provided by Dr. Alessandra Bragonzi (Infection and CF Unit, San Raffaele Scientific Institute, Milan, Italy). Bacterial strains were grown in MHB (Becton Dickinson Difco, Franklin Lakes, NJ, USA) and on Tryptic Soy Agar (TSA; Oxoid Ltd., Hampshire, UK). In all the experiments, bacteria were inoculated and grown overnight in MHB at 37 °C.

4.4. Eukaryotic Cells and Growth Conditions

Immortalized human bronchial epithelial mesothelial cells (BEAS) were cultured in high-glucose Dulbecco's modified Eagle's medium (DMEM) supplemented with 10% fetal bovine serum and 1% penicillin-streptomycin at 37 °C in the presence of 5% carbon dioxide (CO_2).

4.5. Cell Viability Assays

Peptide effects on eukaryotic cell viability was evaluated by seeding cells in 96-well plates (100 μL/well) at a density of 3×10^3 cells/well. Upon 24 h, cells were incubated with increasing peptide concentrations (0–40 μM), for 24, 48 and 72 h. At the end of the treatment, cell viability was assessed by the 3-(4,5-dimethylthiazol-2-yl)-2,5-diphenyltetrazolium bromide (MTT) assay. MTT reagent, dissolved in DMEM without phenol red, was added to the cells (100 μL/well) at a final concentration of 0.5 mg/mL. After 4 h at 37 °C, the culture medium was removed and the resulting formazan salts were dissolved by the addition of isopropanol containing 0.1 N HCl (100 μL/well) [41]. Absorbance values of blue formazan were determined at 570 nm by using an automatic plate reader (Synergy™ H4 Hybrid Microplate Reader, BioTek Instruments, Inc., Winooski, VT, USA). Cell survival was expressed as the percentage of viable cells in the presence of the peptide under test, with respect to control cells grown in the absence of the peptide.

4.6. Antimicrobial Activity Assays

To test the antimicrobial activity of ApoB-derived peptides, a previously described experimental procedure was used [33]. MIC_{100} values correspond to the lowest concentration of peptide associated with no detectable bacterial growth.

4.7. Anti-Biofilm Activity by Crystal Violet Assay

ApoB-derived peptides effects on biofilm attachment, formation and detachment were evaluated as previously described [33]. Optical densities at 595 nm of biofilm stained biomasses were measured by using a microtiter plate reader (Synergy™ H4 Hybrid Microplate Reader, BioTek Instruments, Inc., Winooski, VT, USA).

4.8. Anti-Biofilm Activity by CLSM Analyses

Bacterial biofilm was grown on glass cover slips in 24-well plates in 0.5X MHB in static conditions. In particular, bacterial cells from an overnight culture were diluted to about 1×10^8 CFU/mL and then seeded into wells for 4 or 24 h at 37 °C in the presence of the peptide under test, in order to evaluate biofilm attachment and formation, respectively. When effects on preformed biofilm were evaluated, bacterial biofilms were formed for 24 h at 37 °C, and then treated with peptides under test for further 24 h to evaluate their ability to eradicate preformed biofilm. Afterwards, non-adherent bacteria were removed by gently washing samples with sterile phosphate buffer and viability of cells embedded into biofilm structure was determined by sample staining with LIVE/DEAD® BacLight™ Bacterial Viability kit (Molecular Probes, Thermo Fisher Scientific, Waltham, MA, USA), while FilmTracer™ SYPRO® Ruby biofilm matrix dye has been used to stain matrices of biofilms (Invitrogen, Carlsbad, CA, USA). Staining was performed accordingly to manufacturer instructions. Biofilm images were captured by using a confocal laser scanning microscopy (Zeiss LSM 710, Zeiss, Germany) and a 63X objective oil immersion system. Biofilm architecture was analyzed by using the Zen Lite 2.3 software package (Zeiss, Germany). Each experiment was performed in triplicate. All images were taken under identical conditions.

4.9. Anti-Biofilm Activity by Scanning Electron Microscopy

To perform scanning electron microscopy (SEM) analyses, *B. cenocepacia* LMG 18863 and *P. aeruginosa 14* cells were incubated with 5 μM r(P)$ApoB_L^{Pro}$, r(P)$ApoB_L^{Ala}$ or r(P)$ApoB_S^{Pro}$ peptides for 24 h at 37 °C. Following incubation, bacterial biofilms were fixed in 2.5% glutaraldehyde. Following overnight incubation, bacterial biofilms were washed three times in distilled water and then dehydrated with a graded ethanol series: 25% ethanol (1 × 10 min); 50% ethanol (1 × 10 min); 75% ethanol (1 × 10 min); 95% ethanol (1 × 10 min); 100% anhydrous ethanol (3 × 30 min). Bacterial biofilms deposited onto glass substrate were sputter coated with a thin layer of Au-Pd (Sputter Coater Denton Vacuum DeskV) to allow subsequent morphological characterization using a FEI Nova NanoSEM 450 at an accelerating voltage of 5 kV with Everhart Thornley Detector (ETD) and Through Lens Detector (TLD) at high magnification.

4.10. Statistical Analysis

Statistical analysis was performed using a Student's t-test. Significant differences were indicated as * $p < 0.05$, ** $p < 0.01$ or *** $p < 0.001$.

Author Contributions: Conceptualization, R.G. and A.A.; methodology, R.G., A.C., E.D.O., L.T. and R.D.G.; validation, R.G.; formal analysis, R.G.; investigation, R.G., A.C., E.D.O. and R.D.G.; resources, E.P. and A.A.; data curation, R.G., A.C., L.T. and E.D.O.; writing—original draft preparation, R.G., A.C., E.D.O. and A.A.;

writing—review & editing, all authors; supervision, A.A.; project administration, A.A.; funding acquisition, E.P. and A.A. All authors have read and agreed to the published version of the manuscript.

Abbreviations

CF	Cystic Fibrosis
MDR	Multidrug Resistance
ApoB	Apolipoprotein B
HDPs	Host Defense Peptides
CFTR	Cystic fibrosis transmembrane conductance regulator
AMPs	Antimicrobial peptides
MIC	Minimum inhibitory concentration
MHB	Mueller Hinton Broth
CLSM	Confocal laser scanning microscopy
SEM	Scanning electron microscopy
PI	Propidium iodide
LPS	Lipopolysaccharide

References

1. Farrell, P.M. The prevalence of cystic fibrosis in the European Union. *J. Cyst. Fibros.* **2008**, *7*, 450–453. [CrossRef]
2. Evans, C.M.; Koo, J.S. Airway mucus: The good, the bad, the sticky. *Pharmacol Ther.* **2009**, *121*, 332–348. [CrossRef]
3. Chace, K.V.; Flux, M.; Sachdev, G.P. Comparison of physicochemical properties of purified mucus glycoproteins isolated from respiratory secretions of cystic fibrosis and asthmatic patients. *Biochemistry* **1985**, *24*, 7334–7341. [CrossRef] [PubMed]
4. Knowles, M.R.; Durie, P.R. What is cystic fibrosis? *N. Engl. J. Med.* **2002**, *347*, 439–442. [CrossRef] [PubMed]
5. Ciofu, O.; Hansen, C.R.; Høiby, N. Respiratory bacterial infections in cystic fibrosis. *Curr. Opin. Pulm. Med.* **2013**, *19*, 251–258. [CrossRef] [PubMed]
6. Rudkjøbing, V.B.; Thomsen, T.R.; Alhede, M.; Kragh, K.N.; Nielsen, P.H.; Johansen, U.R.; Givskov, M.; Høiby, N.; Bjarnsholt, T. The microorganisms in chronically infected end-stage and non-end-stage cystic fibrosis patients. *FEMS Immunol. Med. Microbiol.* **2012**, *65*, 236–244. [CrossRef]
7. Bjarnsholt, T.; Jensen, P.Ø.; Fiandaca, M.J.; Pedersen, J.; Hansen, C.R.; Andersen, C.B.; Pressler, T.; Givskov, M.; Høiby, N. Pseudomonas aeruginosa biofilms in the respiratory tract of cystic fibrosis patients. *Pediatr. Pulmonol.* **2009**, *44*, 547–558. [CrossRef] [PubMed]
8. Parker, D.; Ahn, D.; Cohen, T.; Prince, A. Innate Immune Signaling Activated by MDR Bacteria in the Airway. *Physio. Rev.* **2016**, *96*, 19–53. [CrossRef]
9. Blanc, D.S.; Petignat, C.; Janin, B.; Bille, J.; Francioli, P. Frequency and molecular diversity of *Pseudomonas aeruginosa* upon admission and during hospitalization: A prospective epidemiologic study. *Clin. Microbiol. Infect.* **1998**, *4*, 242–247. [CrossRef]
10. Sadikot, R.T.; Blackwell, T.S.; Christman, J.W.; Prince, A.S. Pathogen–host interactions in *Pseudomonas aeruginosa* pneumonia. *Am. J. Respir. Crit. Care Med.* **2005**, *171*, 1209–1223. [CrossRef]
11. Larrosa, M.; Truchado, P.; Espin, J.C.; Tomas-Barberan, F.A.; Allende, A.; Garcia-Conesa, M.T. Evaluation of Pseudomonas aeruginosa (PAO1) adhesion to human alveolar epithelial cells A549 using SYTO 9 dye. *Mol. Cell Probes* **2012**, *26*, 121–126. [CrossRef] [PubMed]
12. Hirakata, Y.; Izumikawa, K.; Yamaguchi, T.; Igimi, S.; Furuya, N.; Maesaki, S.; Tomono, K.; Yamada, Y.; Kohno, S.; Yamaguchi, K.; et al. Adherence to and penetration of human intestinal Caco-2 epithelial cell monolayers by Pseudomonas aeruginosa. *Infect. Immun.* **1998**, *66*, 1748–1751. [CrossRef]
13. Pier, G.B.; Grout, M.; Zaidi, T.S. Cystic fibrosis transmembrane conductance regulator is an epithelial cell receptor for clearance of Pseudomonas aeruginosa from the lung. *Proc. Natl. Acad. Sci. USA* **1997**, *94*, 12088–12093. [CrossRef] [PubMed]

14. Pier, G.B.; Grout, M.; Zaidi, T.S.; Olsen, J.C.; Johnson, L.G.; Yankaskas, J.R.; Goldberg, J.B. Role of mutant CFTR in hypersusceptibility of cystic fibrosis patients to lung infections. *Science* **1996**, *271*, 64–67. [CrossRef]
15. Esen, M.; Grassme, H.; Riethmuller, J.; Riehle, A.; Fassbender, K.; Gulbins, E. Invasion of human epithelial cells by Pseudomonas aeruginosa involves src-like tyrosine kinases p60Src and p59Fyn. *Infect. Immun.* **2001**, *69*, 281–287. [CrossRef] [PubMed]
16. Darling, K.E.; Evans, T.J. Effects of nitric oxide on Pseudomonas aeruginosa infection of epithelial cells from a human respiratory cell line derived from a patient with cystic fibrosis. *Infect. Immun.* **2003**, *71*, 2341–2349. [CrossRef]
17. Brinch, K.S.; Frimodt-Moller, N.; Hoiby, N.; Kristensen, H.H. Influence of antidrug antibodies on plectasin efficacy and pharmacokinetics. *Antimicrob. Agents Chemother.* **2009**, *53*, 4794–4800. [CrossRef]
18. Chi, E.; Mehl, T.; Nunn, D.; Lory, S. Interaction of Pseudomonas aeruginosa with A549 pneumocyte cells. *Infect. Immun.* **1991**, *59*, 822–828. [CrossRef]
19. Drenkard, E.; Ausubel, F.M. Pseudomonas biofilm formation and antibiotic resistance are linked to phenotypic variation. *Nature* **2002**, *416*, 740–743. [CrossRef]
20. Scoffone, V.C.; Chiarelli, L.R.; Trespidi, G.; Mentasti, M.; Riccardi, G.; Buroni, S. Burkholderia cenocepacia Infections in Cystic Fibrosis Patients: Drug Resistance and Therapeutic Approaches. *Front. Microbiol.* **2017**, *8*, 1592. [CrossRef]
21. Alexander, B.D.; Petzold, E.W.; Reller, L.B.; Palmer, S.M.; Davis, R.D.; Woods, C.W.; Lipuma, J.J. Survival after lung transplantation of cystic fibrosis patients infected with Burkholderia cepacia complex. *Am. J. Transplant.* **2008**, *8*, 1025–1030. [CrossRef] [PubMed]
22. Chaparro, C.; Keshavjee, S. Lung transplantation for cystic fibrosis: An update. *Expert Rev. Respir. Med.* **2016**, *10*, 1269–1280. [CrossRef] [PubMed]
23. Mercer, D.K.; O'Neil, D.A. Peptides as the next generation of anti-infectives. *Future Med. Chem.* **2013**, *5*, 315–337. [CrossRef] [PubMed]
24. Haney, E.F.; Hancock, R.B. Peptide design for antimicrobial and immunomodulatory applications. *Biopolymers* **2013**, *100*, 572–583. [CrossRef]
25. Cruz, J.; Ortiz, C.; Guzman, F.; Fernandez-Lafuente, R.; Torres, R. Antimicrobial peptides: Promising compounds against pathogenic microorganisms. *Curr. Med. Chem.* **2014**, *21*, 2299–2321. [CrossRef]
26. Epand, R.M.; Vogel, H.J. Diversity of antimicrobial peptides and their mechanisms of action. *Biochim. Biophys. Acta* **1999**, *1462*, 11–28. [CrossRef]
27. Shai, Y. Mode of action of membrane active antimicrobial peptides. *Biopolymers* **2002**, *66*, 236–248. [CrossRef]
28. Cao, H.; Ke, T.; Liu, R.; Yu, J.; Dong, C.; Cheng, M.; Huang, J.; Liu, S. Identification of a Novel Proline-Rich Antimicrobial Peptide from Brassica napus. *PLoS ONE* **2015**, *10*, e0137414. [CrossRef]
29. Fosgerau, K.; Hoffmann, T. Peptide therapeutics: Current status and future directions. *Drug Discov. Today* **2015**, *20*, 122–128. [CrossRef]
30. Yeaman, M.R.; Yount, N.Y. Mechanisms of antimicrobial peptide action and resistance. *Pharmacol. Rev.* **2003**, *55*, 27–55. [CrossRef]
31. Vineeth Kumar, T.V.; Sanil, G. A Review of the Mechanism of Action of Amphibian Antimicrobial Peptides Focusing on Peptide-Membrane Interaction and Membrane Curvature. *Curr. Protein. Pept. Sci.* **2017**, *18*, 1263–1272. [PubMed]
32. Shahrour, H.; Ferrer-Espada, R.; Dandache, I.; Bárcena-Varela, S.; Sánchez-Gómez, S.; Chokr, A.; Martinez-de-Tejada, G. AMPs as Anti-biofilm Agents for Human Therapy and Prophylaxis. *Adv. Exp. Med. Biol.* **2019**, *1117*, 257–279. [PubMed]
33. Gaglione, R.; Dell'Olmo, E.; Bosso, A.; Chino, M.; Pane, K.; Ascione, F.; Itri, F.; Caserta, S.; Amoresano, A.; Lombardi, A.; et al. Novel human bioactive peptides identified in Apolipoprotein B: Evaluation of their therapeutic potential. *Biochem. Pharmacol.* **2017**, *130*, 34–50. [CrossRef] [PubMed]
34. Pane, K.; Durante, L.; Crescenzi, O.; Cafaro, V.; Pizzo, E.; Varcamonti, M.; Zanfardino, A.; Izzo, V.; Di Donato, A.; Notomista, E. Antimicrobial potency of cationic antimicrobial peptides can be predicted from their amino acid composition: Application to the detection of "cryptic" antimicrobial peptides. *J. Theor. Biol.* **2017**, *419*, 254–265. [CrossRef]
35. Gaglione, R.; Cesaro, A.; Dell'Olmo, E.; Della Ventura, B.; Casillo, A.; Di Girolamo, R.; Velotta, R.; Notomista, E.; Veldhuizen, E.J.A.; Corsaro, M.M.; et al. Effects of human antimicrobial cryptides identified in apolipoprotein B depend on specific features of bacterial strains. *Sci. Rep.* **2019**, *9*, 6728. [CrossRef]

36. Gaglione, R.; Pane, K.; Dell'Olmo, E.; Cafaro, V.; Pizzo, E.; Olivieri, G.; Notomista, E.; Arciello, A. Cost-effective production of recombinant peptides in Escherichia coli. *N. Biotechnol.* **2019**, *51*, 39–48. [CrossRef]
37. Pane, K.; Cafaro, V.; Avitabile, A.; Torres, M.T.; Vollaro, A.; De Gregorio, E.; Catania, M.R.; Di Maro, A.; Bosso, A.; Gallo, G.; et al. Identification of Novel Cryptic Multifunctional Antimicrobial Peptides from the Human Stomach Enabled by a Computational-Experimental Platform. *ACS Synth. Biol.* **2018**, *7*, 2105–2115. [CrossRef]
38. Zanfardino, A.; Bosso, A.; Gallo, G.; Pistorio, V.; Di Napoli, M.; Gaglione, R.; Dell'Olmo, E.; Varcamonti, M.; Notomista, E.; Arciello, A.; et al. Human apolipoprotein E as a reservoir of cryptic bioactive peptides: The case of ApoE 133-167. *J. Pept. Sci.* **2018**, *24*, e3095. [CrossRef]
39. Pizzo, E.; Pane, K.; Bosso, A.; Landi, N.; Ragucci, S.; Russo, R.; Gaglione, R.; Torres, M.D.T.; de la Fuente-Nunez, C.; Arciello, A.; et al. Novel bioactive peptides from PD-L1/2, a type 1 ribosome inactivating protein from Phytolacca dioica L. Evaluation of their antimicrobial properties and anti-biofilm activities. *Biochim. Biophys. Acta Biomembr.* **2018**, *1860*, 1425–1435. [CrossRef]
40. Pizzo, E.; Cafaro, V.; Di Donato, A.; Notomista, E. Cryptic Antimicrobial Peptides: Identification Methods and Current Knowledge of their Immunomodulatory Properties. *Curr. Pharm. Des.* **2018**, *24*, 1054–1066. [CrossRef]
41. Gaglione, R.; Pirone, L.; Farina, B.; Fusco, S.; Smaldone, G.; Aulitto, M.; Dell'Olmo, E.; Roscetto, E.; Del Gatto, A.; Fattorusso, R.; et al. Insights into the anticancer properties of the first antimicrobial peptide from Archaea. *Biochim. Biophys. Acta Gen. Subj.* **2017**, *1861*, 2155–2164. [CrossRef] [PubMed]
42. Kasetty, G.; Papareddy, P.; Kalle, M.; Rydengård, V.; Walse, B.; Svensson, B.; Mörgelin, M.; Malmsten, M.; Schmidtchen, A. The C-terminal sequence of several human serine proteases encodes host defense functions. *J. Innate Immun.* **2011**, *3*, 471–482. [CrossRef] [PubMed]
43. Lee, D.Y.; Huang, C.M.; Nakatsuji, T.; Thiboutot, D.; Kang, S.A.; Monestier, M.; Gallo, R.L. Histone H4 is a major component of the antimicrobial action of human sebocytes. *J. Invest. Dermatol.* **2009**, *129*, 2489–2496. [CrossRef] [PubMed]
44. Beck, W.H.; Adams, C.P.; Biglang-Awa, I.M.; Patel, A.B.; Vincent, H.; Haas-Stapleton, E.J.; Weers, P.M. Apolipoprotein A-I binding to anionic vesicles and lipopolysaccharides: Role for lysine residues in antimicrobial properties. *Biochim. Biophys. Acta* **2013**, *1828*, 1503–1510. [CrossRef] [PubMed]
45. Langton Hewer, S.C.; Smyth, A.R. Antibiotic strategies for eradicating Pseudomonas aeruginosa in people with cystic fibrosis. *Cochrane Database Syst. Rev.* **2014**, *11*, CD004197.
46. Sanchez, Z.; Tani, A.; Kimbara, K. Extensive reduction of cell viability and enhanced matrix production in Pseudomonas aeruginosa PAO1 flow biofilms treated with a D-amino acid mixture. *Appl. Environ. Microbiol.* **2013**, *79*, 1396–1399. [CrossRef]
47. Bechinger, B.; Gorr, S.U. Antimicrobial Peptides: Mechanisms of Action and Resistance. *J. Dent. Res.* **2017**, *96*, 254–260. [CrossRef]
48. De Soyza, A.; Ellis, C.D.; Khan, C.M.A.; Corris, P.A.; Demarco De Hormaeche, R. Burkholderia cenocepacia lipopolysaccharide, lipid A, and proinflammatory activity. *Am. J. Respir. Crit. Care Med.* **2004**, *170*, 70–77. [CrossRef]
49. Mahenthiralingam, E.; Urban, T.A.; Goldberg, J.B. The multifarious, multireplicon Burkholderia cepacia complex. *Nat. Rev. Microbiol.* **2005**, *3*, 144–156. [CrossRef]
50. Raetz, C.R.H.; Reynolds, C.M.; Trent, M.S.; Bishop, R.E. Lipid A Modification Systems in Gram-Negative Bacteria. *Annu. Rev. Biochem.* **2007**, *76*, 295–329. [CrossRef]
51. Olaitan, A.O.; Morand, S.; Rolain, J.M. Mechanisms of polymyxin resistance: Acquired and intrinsic resistance in bacteria. *Front. Microbiol.* **2014**, *5*, 29–30. [CrossRef] [PubMed]
52. Mulcahy, L.R.; Burns, J.L.; Lory, S.; Lewis, K. Emergence of Pseudomonas aeruginosa strains producing high levels of persister cells in patients with cystic fibrosis. *J. Bacteriol.* **2010**, *192*, 6191–6199. [CrossRef] [PubMed]
53. Pletzer, D.; Hancock, R.E.W. Antibiofilm peptides: Potential as broadspectrum agents. *J. Bacteriol.* **2016**, *198*, 2572–2578. [CrossRef] [PubMed]
54. Mansour, S.C.; de la Fuente-Núñez, C.; Hancock, R.E. Peptide IDR-1018: Modulating the immune system and targeting bacterial biofilms to treat antibiotic-resistant bacterial infections. *J. Pept. Sci.* **2015**, *21*, 323–329. [CrossRef] [PubMed]

55. Beaudoin, T.; Stone, T.A.; Glibowicka, M.; Adams, C.; Yau, Y.; Ahmadi, S.; Bear, C.E.; Grasemann, H.; Waters, V.; Deber, C.M. Activity of a novel antimicrobial peptide against Pseudomonas aeruginosa biofilms. *Sci. Rep.* **2018**, *8*, 14728. [CrossRef] [PubMed]
56. Soares, A.; Roussel, V.; Pestel-Caron, M.; Barreau, M.; Caron, F.; Bouffartigues, E.; Chevalier, S.; Etienne, M. Understanding Ciprofloxacin Failure in *Pseudomonas aeruginosa* Biofilm: Persister Cells Survive Matrix Disruption. *Front. Microbiol.* **2019**, *10*, 2603. [CrossRef]
57. Reffuveille, F.; De La Fuente-Núñez, C.; Mansour, S.; Hancock, R.E.W. A broad-spectrum antibiofilm peptide enhances antibiotic action against bacterial biofilms. *Antimicrob. Agents Chemother.* **2014**, *58*, 5363–5371. [CrossRef]
58. Dosler, S.; Karaaslan, E. Inhibition and destruction of Pseudomonas aeruginosa biofilms by antibiotics and antimicrobial peptides. *Peptides* **2014**, *62*, 32–37. [CrossRef]

3

Dendritic Cell-Airway Epithelial Cell Cross-Talk Changes with Age and Contributes to Chronic Lung Inflammatory Diseases in the Elderly

Anshu Agrawal

Division of Basic and Clinical Immunology, Department of Medicine, University of California Irvine, Irvine, CA 92697, USA; aagrawal@uci.edu

Academic Editor: Monica De la Fuente

Abstract: Age-associated dysregulated immune and inflammatory responses are one of the major factors responsible for the prevalence of chronic respiratory diseases in the older population. Pulmonary dendritic cells (DCs) are present below the airway epithelial cells (AECs) and are critical in initiating effective immune responses to harmful pathogens while maintaining tolerance against harmless antigens. The interaction between DCs and AECs plays a crucial role in lung immunity at homeostasis and during infections. The functions of both DCs and AECs are impacted with age. The present report reviews how the potential crosstalk between pulmonary DCs and AECs is dysregulated in the elderly impairing the capacity to maintain tolerance at the respiratory surfaces, which results in severe and chronic respiratory inflammatory diseases. We also discuss how such DC-AECs crosstalk will provide insight into the mechanisms underlying the increased susceptibility of the elderly to pulmonary inflammatory diseases.

Keywords: dendritic cells; airway epithelial cells; age; inflammation; human; crosstalk

---

1. Introduction

Chronic respiratory diseases are a major cause of health concern in the elderly [1–4]. In the US, alone, close to 24 million adults are estimated to have evidence of impaired lung function, indicative of chronic obstructive pulmonary disease (COPD), with most patients being 65 years or older [5]. An estimated 10 million others are diagnosed with chronic bronchitis, with the highest rate detected in people aged 65 years or older [6,7]. Furthermore, nearly 90% of the 4.7 million diagnosed with emphysema are 50 years or older [8]. The incidence of cancer and idiopathic pulmonary fibrosis is also significantly higher in older adults [3,9]. Respiratory infections in the aged population are also often severe and frequently require hospitalization [10]. The prevalence of chronic respiratory diseases is expected to double in the coming decades because of increased life expectancy in developed countries. Since the underlying pathological mechanisms of chronic respiratory diseases are not well understood, current therapies are neither specific nor effective. Airway immune cells are equipped to respond, and distinguish between, innocuous and pathogenic inhalants. One of the most important innate immune cells are dendritic cells (DCs), which act as initiators and regulators of the immune response [11]. DCs are present below the epithelial cell layer and survey the airway via extension of dendrites [12]. Emerging evidence indicates that airway DCs play a pivotal role in mediating airway tolerance against harmless antigens while mounting inflammatory responses against harmful pathogens [13–15]. This review focuses on the role of the interactions between DCs and airway epithelial cells (AECs) in chronic respiratory diseases of the elderly.

2. Age-Associated Deterioration and/or Dysregulation of Human Dendritic Cell Functions

Ageing has a significant impact on DC functions [16–24]. Several reports suggest that phagocytosis, migration, and cytokine secretion are impaired in DCs isolated from aged individuals (60–90 years of age) compared to DCs from young individuals (20–40 years of age) [25]. Moreover, we [17,26] and others [27] have shown that, even in the absence of infection, DCs from aged individuals exist in a semi-activated state that is characterized by an increase in the basal-level of Nuclear factor kappa B (NFκB) activation and pro-inflammatory cytokines production. We have also found that peripheral blood-derived DCs from aged individuals produce relatively higher basal levels of pro-inflammatory cytokines/chemokines Interleukin-6 (IL-6), C-X-C Motif Chemokine Ligand-8 (CXCL-8), CXCL-10, and Tumor necrosis factor-alpha (TNF-α), compared to young individuals [26]. In addition, DCs from aged individuals also produce high levels of metalloproteinases (known as ADAMs, or A Disintegrin And Metalloproteinase) as compared to DC from young individuals [26]. The ADAMs play an important role in tissue remodeling [28,29], via degradation of the structural proteins. This semi-activated state of aged DCs results in increased sensitivity to self-antigens, such as human DNA, and in the erosion of peripheral tolerance [17]. Furthermore, DCs from aged individuals, but not from young individuals, display an intrinsic defect in the production of interleukin-10 (IL-10), a potent anti-inflammatory cytokine that controls excessive production of pro-inflammatory mediators [20]. In addition, the secretion of protective cytokines in response to infections is impaired with aged DCs; DCs from aged individuals secrete reduced levels of Type-I-Interferons (IFNs) and Type III IFNs [18,19] in response to influenza and *Chlamydia pneumoniae* [30]. Other studies have also reported reduced secretion of type I IFNs by plasmacytoid dendritic cells (pDCs) and myeloid dendritic cells (mDCs) in response to viral infections [24,31–33]. While the role of type-I IFNs in viral protection is well established, emerging evidence indicates that type-III IFNs may play a more significant role in controlling the infections of the respiratory tract [34]. Respiratory viruses, such as influenza and respiratory syncytial virus, were reported to be more pathogenic and replicated to higher titers in the lungs of mice lacking receptors for both type-I and type-III IFNs compared to mice deficient in only type-I IFN receptor [35]. This is because receptors for type-I IFN, Interferon alpha receptor 1 (IFNAR1), and Interferon alpha receptor 2 (IFNAR2) are expressed on almost all tissues of the body while Interferon lambda receptor 1IFNLR1, one of the chains of the receptor for type-III IFNs, is expressed primarily on epithelial cells of the mucosa [34]. Impaired type-III IFN production against respiratory infections also enhances acute exacerbations, which are a major cause of morbidity and mortality in chronic respiratory diseases such as COPD [36]. The capacity of influenza-infected DCs from aged individuals to prime CD4+and CD8+ effector T cells is also significantly reduced, as compared to influenza-infected DCs from young individuals [18]. Deterioration and dysregulation of DCs' function could contribute to age-associated elevated mucosal inflammation seen in the elderly.

3. Age-Associated Changes in Airway Epithelial Cell (AEC) Functions

Ageing affects not only DC functions as outlined above, but also the functions of the AECs. One study reports that nasal epithelial tissue from aged subjects without respiratory disease displayed microtubular disarrangements and a significant reduction in ciliary beat frequency [37]. Ageing also decreased clearance of Teflon particles in small airways from older adults [38]. Furthermore, secretion of mucus by AECs is also affected with age. Mucus secretion, as measured by periodic acid-Schiff (PAS) staining and mRNA expression of mucin-5 subtype A and C (MUC-5AC), was found to be increased in older mice challenged intra-tracheally with ovalbumin [39]. A decrease in responses to oxidative stress was also observed in older AECs [40]. Age-associated changes in lung extracellular matrix components were also reported to affect the function of AECs. The expression of laminin α3, tissue factor, and N-cadherin was observed to be decreased in human bronchial epithelial cells incubated in old versus young lung matrix [41]. In a study of patients with chronic rhinosinusitis, age-associated reduced production of S100A8/9 proteins was observed in the elderly. S100A8/9 proteins or calprotectin are produced during infections and serve as chemoattractants for neutrophils and monocytes [42].

In summary, these studies suggest that AEC functions are significantly impacted with age and, thus, may play a major role in age-associated chronic respiratory diseases.

4. Immunological Cross-Talk between Airway Epithelial Cells (AECs) and Dendritic Cells (DCs) in Health and Disease

The epithelial cells lining the airways and nasal passages not only act as a barrier to prevent entry of the pathogens, but also play an active role in regulating immune responses. The close proximity of DCs to AECs results in continuous interaction and modulation of functions between the two cell types. For example, during viral infections DCs secrete pro-inflammatory cytokines, such as type I and type III interferons, which upregulate the expression of class I major histocompatibility complex (MHC) on AECs to enhance the antiviral responses [43]. The pro-inflammatory cytokines produced by DCs also act on tight junction proteins of the epithelial cell barrier to enhance the permeability and allow infiltration of immune cells to the site of infection [44]. As DCs influence epithelial cell functions, AECs can also affect the function of DCs [14,45]. AECs line the respiratory tract constituting the primary cellular barrier, expressing PRRs (pathogen recognition receptors) as well as receptors for allergens; this enables AECs to respond to antigens and allergens, thereby initiating the first step in the host-pathogen interaction [46].

Recent evidences suggest that local microenvironment defines the type of immune response elicited by the host [47]. Hammad et al. demonstrated that TLR4 signaling on AECs is responsible for the migration of mouse lung DCs to the mediastinal nodes in response to LPS inhalation [14]. In addition, viral infection of AECs also leads to the production of type I and III interferons, which activate DCs. Similarly activation of AECs by HDM (house dust mite) induces the release of various chemokines, such as C-C Motif Chemokine Ligand 2 (CCL2) and CCL20, which can attract immature DCs or monocytic precursors to the lung in mice [48,49]. DC-AEC interactions have also been demonstrated to play an important role in inducing Th2 responses against allergens [49]. Murine studies have indicated that activation of AECs by allergens induces the secretion of IL-25, IL-33, and thymic stromal lymphopoietin (TSLP). All of these act on DCs to enhance Th2 responses via OX40-OX40L interactions [49]. Recently, IL-25 has also been demonstrated to act on murine DCs to induce the secretion of CCL-17 which attracts Th9 cells during allergic inflammation [50]. However, in vitro human studies suggest that AECs may also prevent Th2 responses by enhancing the Th1 polarizing capacity of DCs since differentiation of monocytes in the presence of activated AECs leads to increased secretion of IL-12, IL-6, and TNF-α [51]. In addition to chemokines and cytokines produced by AECs, damage associated molecules or alarmins released during epithelial injury or death can also affect DC function. The concentration of alarmins, such as high mobility group box 1 protein (HM-GB1), Adenosine tri phosphate (ATP), and uric acid, are reported to be increased in the airways of asthmatic subjects. These molecules which are believed to be the products of dying epithelial cells can activate DCs to enhance inflammation [49].

In addition to affecting DC functions during infections, AECs also modulate DC function at homeostasis. The airways are constantly exposed to harmless, inhaled antigens and to prevent an immune response against them, the immune cells, such as DCs, have been reported to exist in a suppressed state, at least in mice [52]. AECs secrete retinoic acid (RA), Transforming growth factor-beta (TGF-β), and granulocyte macrophage colony stimulating factor (GM-CSF) in a steady state (in the absence of stimulation), rendering DCs and alveolar macrophages tolerogenic and prevent inflammation in the airways in murine studies [53–55]. Emerging evidence from human studies indicates airway monocytes have a more tolerant phenotype compared to blood monocytes, while lung CD1c+ DCs are more activated [56–58]. Baharom et al. [56] examined the phenotype of lung CD1c+ DCs in the airways and blood on samples from the airways via bronchial washing and broncho-alveolar lavage as well as mucosal tissue (endobronchial biopsies) from 20 healthy subjects with ages ranging from 18–40 years. They observed increased maturation of the CD1c+ DCs in the airway compared to blood and endobronchial biopsies. Another recent, comprehensive study by Granot et al. [58] has compared the myeloid DC subset distribution, maturation, and migration in mucosal tissues (lungs, intestines) and draining lymph nodes from 78 human organ donors with ages ranging from less than one year to 93 years. Their results suggest that highest numbers of CD1c+ DCs with migratory and mature phenotype are present in the lung draining lymph nodes. Furthermore, in another detailed study from 72 human lungs, pulmonary CD1c+ DCs were reported to be able to activate T cells in the mixed lymphocyte reaction [57]. In keeping with these observations, AECs have been shown to affect the immune surveillance function of DCs in a steady state. Using a 2D model system of monocyte-derived DCs and AECs, Rate et al. [59] observed an increased upregulation of several chemokine and TLR genes in DCs cultured with AECs at homeostasis. Our recent study also supports this data as we also observed upregulation of several pathogen recognition receptors (PRRs) and chemokine genes using a model of human myeloid DC (CD1c+ and CD141+) and AEC co-culture [60]. Furthermore, our study suggests that the CD1c+ subset of mDC was the major subset displaying the upregulation of PRR function while the CD141+ mDC subset was not affected. The above-mentioned studies with human lung [56–58] also did not report increased activation of the CD141+ mDC subset. Thus, it may be possible that there exists a division of labor between DC subsets with CD141+ mDC subset playing a role in tolerance and the CD1c+ mDC subset in immune surveillance. This suggests a scenario where AECs secrete factors to upregulate the immune surveillance function of CD1c+ DCs so that their response to infections is not compromised because of immunosuppressive environment of the airways. Collectively, these findings suggest that efficient interaction between the AECs and DCs contributes to respiratory health. Age-associated changes in the function of both AECs and DCs, thus, can prove detrimental to respiratory health.

5. Age-Associated Alterations in the Crosstalk between Airway Epithelial Cells and Dendritic Cells: Effect of DCs on AECs

While most studies have focused on murine models due the problems in obtaining lung tissue from humans, particularly from healthy aged subjects, few studies have examined the effect of age on mucosal DCs [61–63]. Biopsy of the lung is not a routine procedure and broncho-alveolar lavage (BAL) in the elderly is also not common. Furthermore, the numbers of DCs in the BAL are too few to perform mechanistic and functional studies. However, a very recent study by Granot et al. [58] has compared the DC populations in various organs including the lung, as a function of age. Though the authors did not observe a significant decline in DC numbers with age in all tissues, including the lungs, they did observe increased maturation of CD1c+ DCs in the mesenteric lymph nodes of older adults. Since ageing induces changes in the function of blood DCs, which also populate the lung, DC-AECs crosstalk may be affected. At homeostasis, virtually no information on the effect of DCs on AECs exists. To examine this and to simulate the airway mucosa, where DCs are in close contact with the epithelial cell barrier, we have developed a two-dimensional (2D) model where AECs are cultured on a transwell membrane insert and purified DCs from the blood are added to the bottom chamber. Such 2D culture systems are increasingly being used to replicate the lung environment and to study DC-epithelial crosstalk in humans [64,65]. As mentioned earlier, circulatory and monocyte-derived DCs from aged subjects displayed an enhanced basal state of activation [16,27]. The pro-inflammatory nature of DCs from aged subjects induced the activation of AECs in the absence of an acute insult (Figure 1) [26]. The barrier function of AECs was also compromised due to an increase in permeability. Furthermore, DCs from aged subjects induced significant upregulation of CXCL-10, CCL-20, and CCL-26 chemokines in AECs compared to DCs from young individuals. All three chemokines are involved in inflammation of the lung. CCL-20 (MIP3-β) is upregulated in the airways of patients with obstructive airway diseases [66], binding to CCR-6 expressed on epithelial cells and inducing the secretion of mucus. It also acts as a major chemoattractant for DCs [67]. CCL-26 (Eotaxin-3) attracts eosinophils, which are major players in lung inflammation [68]. CXCL-10 (IP-10) attracts T cells [69] and IP-10 levels are substantially increased in COPD patients [70,71]. The major factor responsible for the activation of AECs by DCs from aged individuals was the chronic, low-level TNF-α secretion. Altogether, this study suggests that aged DCs induce secretion of chemokines from AECs in the absence of any stimulation, attracting pro-inflammatory cells into airways of the elderly (Figure 1). Infiltration of immune cells in the airway will enhance inflammation. Furthermore, DCs from aged subjects also secrete increased levels of ADAMs, which are metalloproteases that can degrade the extracellular matrix components. In this context, ageing is associated with alterations to two extracellular matrix proteins: collagen and elastin [40,41].

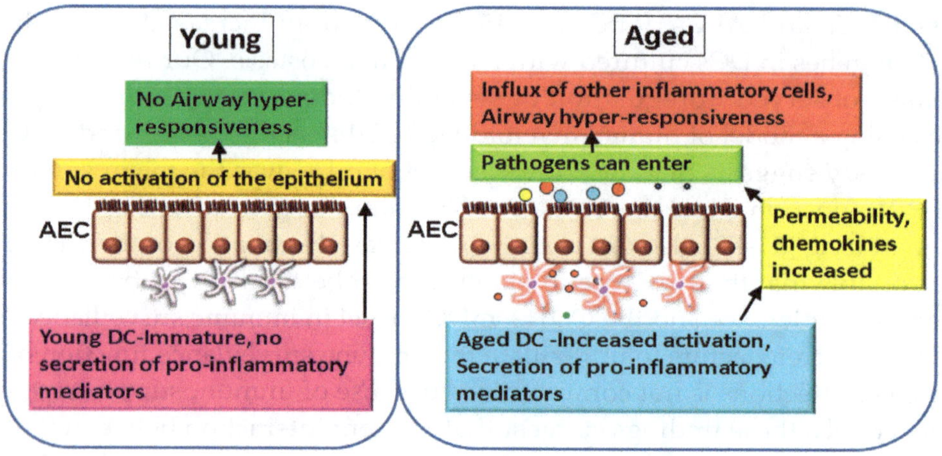

Figure 1. Altered DC-airway epithelial cell (AECs) crosstalk leads to impaired mucosal tolerance and inflammation in the elderly. In normal healthy lung from young subjects, dendritic cells (DCs) do not activate the epithelium at homeostasis and there is no inflammation and hyper-responsiveness (**left**). In contrast, in the aged lung, DCs secrete low levels of chronic inflammatory mediators, such as TNF-α and IL-6, which modulate the functions of AECs. The permeability, as well as secretion of chemokines (colored circles) by epithelium, are increased which allows infiltration of cells to the airways and leads to airway hyper-responsiveness. Permeability to infections is also increased (**right**).

6. Age-Associated Alterations in the Crosstalk between Airway Epithelial Cells and Dendritic Cells: Effect of AECs on DCs

Airways are constantly exposed to harmless inhaled antigens. The DCs and macrophages in the airways exist in a state of immune suppression or tolerance to prevent immune response to the harmless antigens. Retinoic acid and other factors secreted by AECs play a crucial role in maintaining tolerance at these surfaces [72]. RA is a lipophilic molecule that controls the activity of a constellation of genes via binding to nuclear receptors [73–75]. Vitamin A is derived from the diet, and the liver constitutes a large reservoir of vitamin A in the form of retinal esters. Retinal esters are hydrolyzed to retinol and released into the blood [76]. Once retinol enters cells expressing appropriate enzymes, it is converted successively into retinal and RA [77]. The first step of the conversion is catalyzed by alcohol dehydrogenases and by microsomal retinol dehydrogenases (RDH) that are expressed by most cells, including DCs. The second step consists of the oxidation of retinal into RA and is catalyzed by three aldehyde dehydrogenases (ALDHs), known as retinaldehyde dehydrogenase 1 (RALDH1), RALDH2, and RALDH3, encoded by the *Aldh1a1*, *-2*, and *-3* genes, respectively [78]. RALDH expression is limited to certain cell types and, despite the widespread availability of retinol, only cells expressing one of the RALDHs can oxidize retinaldehyde to RA [73,74,79,80]. DCs, alveolar macrophages, and AECs at the mucosa are the three cell types that express RALDHs and can convert retinal to RA [45,80,81]. RA is essential for maintaining epithelial health and it also acts on DCs to render them tolerogenic and induce Foxp3^{+} regulatory T cells [73]. RA production and action by mucosa-associated DCs has been proposed to maintain the balance between effector T cells (Th1 and Th17 cells) and Foxp3+ regulatory T cells in the respiratory tract and to constitute a major mechanism underlying airway mucosal tolerance [81–84]. Ageing lung has been reported to display increased secretion of pro-inflammatory cytokines (IL-1β, IL-6, and TNF-α) at homeostasis suggesting a loss of mucosal tolerance [85]. Murine studies also indicate the presence of low grade chronic inflammation in the tracheas of older mice [86]. Insight into the possible mechanisms was obtained when the response of DCs from aged (>60 years) and young (20–40 years) subjects was examined for their response to RA. DCs from aged individuals displayed an impaired response to RA [87]. The induction of T regulatory cells was reduced by RA-treated DCs from aged subjects. The upregulation of two surface markers, CD141 and GARP (glycopherin associated regulatory protein) on DCs by RA was found to be essential for induction of T regulatory cells. The expression of both these surface receptors was reduced on the RA-treated DCs from aged individuals versus the young controls. Defective response to RA by aged DCs can, thus, enhance inflammation in the airways of the elderly (Figure 2). The status of production of RA by DCs and AECs during ageing has not been studied though age-associated decrease of vitamin A concentrations is well documented. Decreases in retinoid metabolism and signaling are also a characteristic of age-related disorders [88]. Thus, it is possible that reduced production, as well as decreased response of DCs to RA, impairs tolerance at the airways to enhance inflammation. In light of recent human studies mentioned earlier [56–58], it will be more interesting to determine the effect and production of RA on different mDC subsets especially since CD141+ mDCs are considered the human equivalent of CD103+ murine DCs, which is the subset most responsive to RA [53,89,90]. In addition to DCs, the response of alveolar macrophages to RA should also be examined as a murine study suggests that alveolar macrophages are the primary cells responding to RA and inducing regulatory T cells [81]. Furthermore, as mentioned, AECs also enhance the immune-surveillance function of DCs [59]; since DCs functions are compromised in the elderly, impaired surveillance may be the reason behind the age-associated increased susceptibility to respiratory infections. In addition, it will be important to determine the age-associated alterations in the status of IL-25, IL-33, and TSLP secretion by AECs as these may also play a significant role in COPD and asthma in the older adults. Virtually no information exists about these mediators in the elderly.

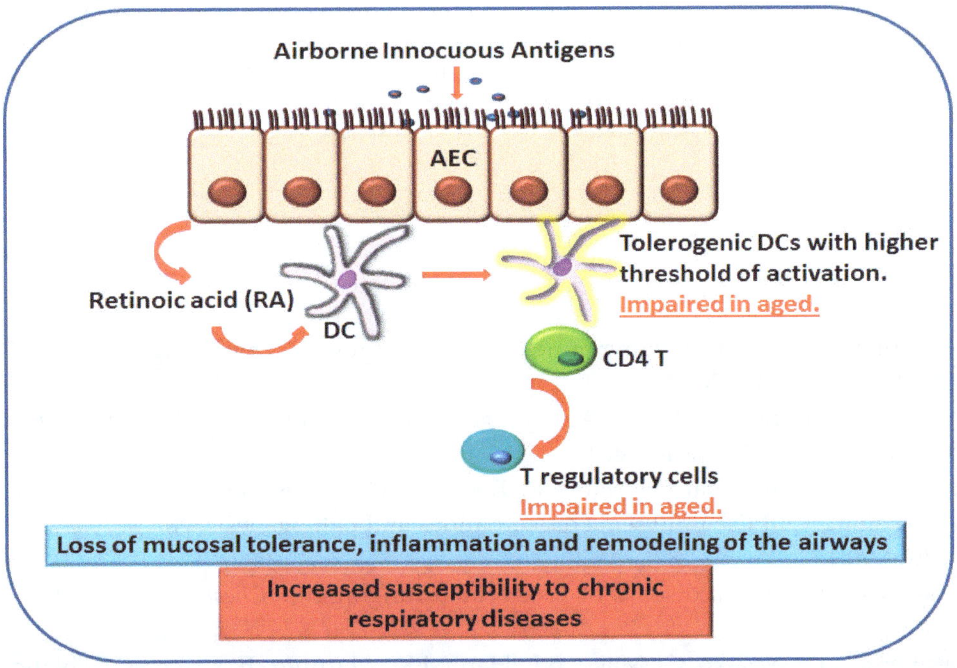

Figure 2. Impaired response of DCs from elderly to retinoic acid (RA) results in a loss of mucosal tolerance and inflammation. Retinoic acid produced by AECs (arrow 1, top) acts on DCs (arrow 2, middle) to induce T regulatory cells (arrow 3, bottom) and mucosal tolerance to prevent immune response to harmless inhaled antigens. DCs from aged subjects display reduced response to RA which leads to impaired induction of T regulatory cells and mucosal tolerance. This enhances inflammation and leads to airway hyper-responsiveness.

7. Microbial Metabolites and DC Function in the Airways

In addition to AECs and DCs, the microbiome of the oral/airway can also affect DC and AEC function. Microbes secrete a number of metabolites that can act on cells to modulate their functions. For example, butyric acid produced by microbiota has also been demonstrated to play a major role in controlling inflammation in the gut [91]. In this respect, we have recently demonstrated that different microbes present in oral microbiome produce unique metabolites, which have a differential effect on the DC activation and T cell priming [92]. For instance, the *Pseudomonas* spp. secretes putrescine and glucose, which activate an inflammatory response in DCs, while *Streptococci* secrete 2,3-butanediol, which does not activate DCs. Interestingly, as people age, microbial communities in the oropharynx and anterior nares become more analogous, suggesting that ageing disrupts the ability to maintain distinct microbial communities at different sites [93]. Changes in the microbiome can affect the concentration of secreted metabolites which, in turn, can modulate the functions of immune cells to enhance inflammation. Alternatively, DCs from aged subjects may also display increased inflammatory responses to the microbial metabolites. Further studies are necessary to confirm these unanswered, interesting questions.

8. Concluding Remarks

It is clear that DC-AEC interactions change with age at homeostasis. These changes can enhance airway inflammation by affecting the permeability and activation of the epithelial barrier. Furthermore, DCs from aged subjects also display a defect in responding to signals from epithelial cells, particularly RA which is essential for induction and maintenance of mucosal tolerance. This can further increase inflammation and remodeling in the airways. The aged airways may, therefore, be more permissible to cellular infiltrations as well as infections. Defects in DC-AEC crosstalk may, therefore, contribute to the age-associated increase in chronic respiratory diseases in the elderly.

Acknowledgments: The project described was supported by AG045216 to AA and National Center for Research Resources and the National Center for Advancing Translational Sciences, National Institutes of Health, through grant UL1 TR000153. The content is solely the responsibility of the authors and does not necessarily represent the official views of the NIH.

References

1. Brandenberger, C.; Muhlfeld, C. Mechanisms of lung aging. *Cell Tissue Res.* **2017**, *367*, 469–480. [CrossRef] [PubMed]
2. Campisi, J. Cellular Senescence and Lung Function during Aging. Yin and Yang. *Ann. Am. Thorac. Soc.* **2016**, *13*, S402–S406. [CrossRef] [PubMed]
3. Pardo, A.; Selman, M. Lung Fibroblasts, Aging, and Idiopathic Pulmonary Fibrosis. *Ann. Am. Thorac. Soc.* **2016**, *13*, S417–S421. [CrossRef] [PubMed]
4. Vij, N.; Chandramani, P.; Westphal, C.V.; Hole, R.; Bodas, M. Cigarette smoke induced autophagy-impairment accelerates lung aging, COPD-emphysema exacerbations and pathogenesis. *Am. J. Physiol. Cell Physiol.* **2016**. [CrossRef] [PubMed]
5. Ito, K.; Barnes, P.J. COPD as a disease of accelerated lung aging. *Chest* **2009**, *135*, 173–180. [CrossRef] [PubMed]
6. Kim, V.; Sternberg, A.L.; Washko, G.; Make, B.J.; Han, M.K.; Martinez, F.; Criner, G.J.; National Emphysema Treatment Trial Research Group. Severe chronic bronchitis in advanced emphysema increases mortality and hospitalizations. *COPD* **2013**, *10*, 667–678.
7. Lange, P.; Parner, J.; Prescott, E.; Vestbo, J. Chronic bronchitis in an elderly population. *Age Ageing* **2003**, *32*, 636–642. [CrossRef] [PubMed]
8. Gelb, A.F.; Yamamoto, A.; Mauad, T.; Kollin, J.; Schein, M.J.; Nadel, J.A. Unsuspected mild emphysema in nonsmoking patients with chronic asthma with persistent airway obstruction. *J. Allergy Clin. Immunol.* **2014**, *133*, 263–265. [CrossRef] [PubMed]

9. Chilosi, M.; Carloni, A.; Rossi, A.; Poletti, V. Premature lung aging and cellular senescence in the pathogenesis of idiopathic pulmonary fibrosis and COPD/emphysema. *Transl. Res.* **2013**, *162*, 156–173. [CrossRef] [PubMed]
10. Yanagi, S.; Tsubouchi, H.; Miura, A.; Matsuo, A.; Matsumoto, N.; Nakazato, M. The Impacts of Cellular Senescence in Elderly Pneumonia and in Age-Related Lung Diseases that Increase the Risk of Respiratory Infections. *Int. J. Mol. Sci.* **2017**, *18*, 503. [CrossRef] [PubMed]
11. Ullrich, S.E. Two-way traffic on the bridge from innate to adaptive immunity. *J. Investig. Dermatol.* **2010**, *130*, 1773–1775. [CrossRef] [PubMed]
12. Lambrecht, B.N.; Hammad, H. Lung dendritic cells in respiratory viral infection and asthma: From protection to immunopathology. *Annu. Rev. Immunol.* **2012**, *30*, 243–270. [CrossRef] [PubMed]
13. Lambrecht, B.N.; Hammad, H. Taking our breath away: Dendritic cells in the pathogenesis of asthma. *Nat. Rev. Immunol.* **2003**, *3*, 994–1003. [CrossRef] [PubMed]
14. Hammad, H.; Chieppa, M.; Perros, F.; Willart, M.A.; Germain, R.N.; Lambrecht, B.N. House dust mite allergen induces asthma via Toll-like receptor 4 triggering of airway structural cells. *Nat. Med.* **2009**, *15*, 410–416. [CrossRef] [PubMed]
15. Sertl, K.; Takemura, T.; Tschachler, E.; Ferrans, V.J.; Kaliner, M.A.; Shevach, E.M. Dendritic cells with antigen-presenting capability reside in airway epithelium, lung parenchyma, and visceral pleura. *J. Exp. Med.* **1986**, *163*, 436–451. [CrossRef] [PubMed]
16. Agrawal, A.; Agrawal, S.; Cao, J.N.; Su, H.; Osann, K.; Gupta, S. Altered innate immune functioning of dendritic cells in elderly humans: A role of phosphoinositide 3-kinase-signaling pathway. *J. Immunol.* **2007**, *178*, 6912–6922. [CrossRef] [PubMed]
17. Agrawal, A.; Tay, J.; Ton, S.; Agrawal, S.; Gupta, S. Increased reactivity of dendritic cells from aged subjects to self-antigen, the human DNA. *J. Immunol.* **2009**, *182*, 1138–1145. [CrossRef] [PubMed]
18. Sridharan, A.; Esposo, M.; Kaushal, K.; Tay, J.; Osann, K.; Agrawal, S.; Gupta, S.; Agrawal, A. Age-associated impaired plasmacytoid dendritic cell functions lead to decreased CD4 and CD8 T cell immunity. *Age* **2011**, *33*, 363–376. [CrossRef] [PubMed]
19. Prakash, S.; Agrawal, S.; Cao, J.N.; Gupta, S.; Agrawal, A. Impaired secretion of interferons by dendritic cells from aged subjects to influenza: Role of histone modifications. *Age* **2013**, *35*, 1785–1797. [CrossRef] [PubMed]
20. Agrawal, S.; Gollapudi, S.; Gupta, S.; Agrawal, A. Dendritic cells from the elderly display an intrinsic defect in the production of IL-10 in response to lithium chloride. *Exp. Gerontol.* **2013**, *48*, 1285–1292. [CrossRef] [PubMed]
21. Agrawal, A. Mechanisms and implications of age-associated impaired innate interferon secretion by dendritic cells: A mini-review. *Gerontology* **2013**, *59*, 421–426. [CrossRef] [PubMed]
22. Cao, J.; Agrawal, A.; Jia, Z.; Sherman, E.; Gupta, S. Alterations in Gene Array Patterns in Dendritic Cells from Aged Humans. *PLoS ONE* **2014**, *9*, e106471. [CrossRef] [PubMed]
23. Della Bella, S.; Clerici, M.; Villa, M.L. Disarming dendritic cells: A tumor strategy to escape from immune control? *Expert Rev. Clin. Immunol.* **2007**, *3*, 411–422. [CrossRef] [PubMed]
24. Jing, Y.; Shaheen, E.; Drake, R.R.; Chen, N.; Gravenstein, S.; Deng, Y. Aging is associated with a numerical and functional decline in plasmacytoid dendritic cells, whereas myeloid dendritic cells are relatively unaltered in human peripheral blood. *Hum. Immunol.* **2009**, *70*, 777–784. [CrossRef] [PubMed]
25. Agrawal, A.; Gupta, S. Impact of aging on dendritic cell functions in humans. *Ageing Res. Rev.* **2011**, *10*, 336–345. [CrossRef] [PubMed]
26. Prakash, S.; Agrawal, S.; Vahed, H.; Ngyuen, M.; Benmohamad, L.; Gupta, S.; Agrawal, A. Dendritic cells from aged subjects contribute to chronic airway inflammation by activating bronchial epithelial cells under steady state. *Mucosal Immunol.* **2014**, *7*, 1386–1394. [CrossRef] [PubMed]
27. Panda, A.; Qian, F.; Mohanty, S.; van Duin, D.; Newman, F.K.; Zhang, L.; Chen, S.; Towle, V.; Belshe, R.B.; Fikrig, E.; et al. Age-associated decrease in TLR function in primary human dendritic cells predicts influenza vaccine response. *J. Immunol.* **2010**, *184*, 2518–2527. [CrossRef] [PubMed]
28. Khokha, R.; Murthy, A.; Weiss, A. Metalloproteinases and their natural inhibitors in inflammation and immunity. *Nat. Rev. Immunol.* **2013**, *13*, 649–665. [CrossRef] [PubMed]
29. Manicone, A.M.; McGuire, J.K. Matrix metalloproteinases as modulators of inflammation. *Semin. Cell Dev. Biol.* **2008**, *19*, 34–41. [CrossRef] [PubMed]

30. Prakash, S.; Agrawal, S.; Ma, D.; Gupta, S.; Peterson, E.M.; Agrawal, A. Dendritic cells from aged subjects display enhanced inflammatory responses to Chlamydophila pneumoniae. *Mediat. Inflamm.* **2014**, *2014*, 436438. [CrossRef] [PubMed]
31. Garbe, K.; Bratke, K.; Wagner, S.; Virchow, J.C.; Lommatzsch, M. Plasmacytoid dendritic cells and their Toll-like receptor 9 expression selectively decrease with age. *Hum. Immunol.* **2012**, *73*, 493–497. [CrossRef] [PubMed]
32. Stout-Delgado, H.W.; Yang, X.; Walker, W.E.; Tesar, B.M.; Goldstein, D.R. Aging impairs IFN regulatory factor 7 up-regulation in plasmacytoid dendritic cells during TLR9 activation. *J. Immunol.* **2008**, *181*, 6747–6756. [CrossRef] [PubMed]
33. Qian, F.; Wang, X.; Zhang, L.; Lin, A.; Zhao, H.; Fikrig, E.; Montgomery, R.R. Impaired interferon signaling in dendritic cells from older donors infected in vitro with West Nile virus. *J. Infect. Dis.* **2011**, *203*, 1415–1424. [CrossRef] [PubMed]
34. Hermant, P.; Michiels, T. Interferon-lambda in the context of viral infections: Production, response and therapeutic implications. *J. Innate Immun.* **2014**, *6*, 563–574. [CrossRef] [PubMed]
35. Mordstein, M.; Neugebauer, E.; Ditt, V.; Jessen, B.; Rieger, T.; Falcone, V.; Sorgeloos, F.; Ehl, S.; Mayer, D.; Kochs, G.; et al. Lambda interferon renders epithelial cells of the respiratory and gastrointestinal tracts resistant to viral infections. *J. Virol.* **2010**, *84*, 5670–5677. [CrossRef] [PubMed]
36. Miller, E.K.; Hernandez, J.Z.; Wimmenauer, V.; Shepherd, B.E.; Hijano, D.; Libster, R.; Serra, M.E.; Bhat, N.; Batalle, J.P.; Mohamed, Y.; et al. A mechanistic role for type III IFN-lambda1 in asthma exacerbations mediated by human rhinoviruses. *Am. J. Respir. Crit. Care Med.* **2012**, *185*, 508–516. [CrossRef] [PubMed]
37. Ho, J.C.; Chan, K.N.; Hu, W.H.; Lam, W.K.; Zheng, L.; Tipoe, G.L.; Sun, J.; Leung, R.; Tsang, K.W. The effect of aging on nasal mucociliary clearance, beat frequency, and ultrastructure of respiratory cilia. *Am. J. Respir. Crit. Care Med.* **2001**, *163*, 983–988. [CrossRef] [PubMed]
38. Svartengren, M.; Falk, R.; Philipson, K. Long-term clearance from small airways decreases with age. *Eur. Respir. J.* **2005**, *26*, 609–615. [CrossRef] [PubMed]
39. Busse, P.J.; Zhang, T.F.; Srivastava, K.; Schofield, B.; Li, X.M. Effect of ageing on pulmonary inflammation, airway hyperresponsiveness and T and B cell responses in antigen-sensitized and -challenged mice. *Clin. Exp. Allergy* **2007**, *37*, 1392–1403. [CrossRef] [PubMed]
40. Busse, P.J.; Mathur, S.K. Age-related changes in immune function: Effect on airway inflammation. *J. Allergy Clin. Immunol.* **2010**, *126*, 690–699. [CrossRef] [PubMed]
41. Godin, L.M.; Sandri, B.J.; Wagner, D.E.; Meyer, C.M.; Price, A.P.; Akinnola, I.; Weiss, D.J.; Panoskaltsis-Mortari, A. Decreased Laminin Expression by Human Lung Epithelial Cells and Fibroblasts Cultured in Acellular Lung Scaffolds from Aged Mice. *PLoS ONE* **2016**, *11*, e0150966. [CrossRef] [PubMed]
42. Tieu, D.D.; Kern, R.C.; Schleimer, R.P. Alterations in epithelial barrier function and host defense responses in chronic rhinosinusitis. *J. Allergy Clin. Immunol.* **2009**, *124*, 37–42. [CrossRef] [PubMed]
43. Ank, N.; Paludan, S.R. Type III IFNs: New layers of complexity in innate antiviral immunity. *BioFactors* **2009**, *35*, 82–87. [CrossRef] [PubMed]
44. Martin, L.D.; Rochelle, L.G.; Fischer, B.M.; Krunkosky, T.M.; Adler, K.B. Airway epithelium as an effector of inflammation: Molecular regulation of secondary mediators. *Eur. Respir. J.* **1997**, *10*, 2139–2146. [CrossRef] [PubMed]
45. Hammad, H.; Lambrecht, B.N. Dendritic cells and epithelial cells: Linking innate and adaptive immunity in asthma. *Nat. Rev. Immunol.* **2008**, *8*, 193–204. [CrossRef] [PubMed]
46. Holtzman, M.J.; Byers, D.E.; Alexander-Brett, J.; Wang, X. The role of airway epithelial cells and innate immune cells in chronic respiratory disease. *Nat. Rev. Immunol.* **2014**, *14*, 686–698. [CrossRef] [PubMed]
47. Mayer, A.K.; Bartz, H.; Fey, F.; Schmidt, L.M.; Dalpke, A.H. Airway epithelial cells modify immune responses by inducing an anti-inflammatory microenvironment. *Eur. J. Immunol.* **2008**, *38*, 1689–1699. [CrossRef] [PubMed]
48. Lambrecht, B.N.; Hammad, H. Lung dendritic cells: Targets for therapy in allergic disease. *Chem. Immunol. Allergy* **2008**, *94*, 189–200. [PubMed]
49. Lambrecht, B.N.; Hammad, H. Allergens and the airway epithelium response: Gateway to allergic sensitization. *J. Allergy Clin. Immunol.* **2014**, *134*, 499–507. [CrossRef] [PubMed]

50. Claudio, E.; Tassi, I.; Wang, H.; Tang, W.; Ha, H.L.; Siebenlist, U. Cutting Edge: IL-25 Targets Dendritic Cells To Attract IL-9-Producing T Cells in Acute Allergic Lung Inflammation. *J. Immunol.* **2015**, *195*, 3525–3529. [CrossRef] [PubMed]
51. Rate, A.; Upham, J.W.; Bosco, A.; McKenna, K.L.; Holt, P.G. Airway epithelial cells regulate the functional phenotype of locally differentiating dendritic cells: Implications for the pathogenesis of infectious and allergic airway disease. *J. Immunol.* **2009**, *182*, 72–83. [CrossRef] [PubMed]
52. Duan, W.; Croft, M. Control of regulatory T cells and airway tolerance by lung macrophages and dendritic cells. *Ann. Am. Thorac. Soc.* **2014**, *11* (Suppl. 5), S306–S313. [CrossRef] [PubMed]
53. Coombes, J.L.; Siddiqui, K.R.; Arancibia-Carcamo, C.V.; Hall, J.; Sun, C.M.; Belkaid, Y.; Powrie, F. A functionally specialized population of mucosal CD103+ DCs induces Foxp3+ regulatory T cells via a TGF-beta and retinoic acid-dependent mechanism. *J. Exp. Med.* **2007**, *204*, 1757–1764. [CrossRef] [PubMed]
54. Leepiyasakulchai, C.; Ignatowicz, L.; Pawlowski, A.; Kallenius, G.; Skold, M. Failure to recruit anti-inflammatory CD103+ dendritic cells and a diminished CD4+ Foxp3+ regulatory T cell pool in mice that display excessive lung inflammation and increased susceptibility to Mycobacterium tuberculosis. *Infect. Immun.* **2012**, *80*, 1128–1139. [CrossRef] [PubMed]
55. Manicassamy, S.; Pulendran, B. Retinoic acid-dependent regulation of immune responses by dendritic cells and macrophages. *Semin. Immunol.* **2009**, *21*, 22–27. [CrossRef] [PubMed]
56. Baharom, F.; Thomas, S.; Rankin, G.; Lepzien, R.; Pourazar, J.; Behndig, A.F.; Ahlm, C.; Blomberg, A.; Smed-Sorensen, A. Dendritic Cells and Monocytes with Distinct Inflammatory Responses Reside in Lung Mucosa of Healthy Humans. *J. Immunol.* **2016**, *196*, 4498–4509. [CrossRef] [PubMed]
57. Desch, A.N.; Gibbings, S.L.; Goyal, R.; Kolde, R.; Bednarek, J.; Bruno, T.; Slansky, J.E.; Jacobelli, J.; Mason, R.; Ito, Y.; et al. Flow Cytometric Analysis of Mononuclear Phagocytes in Nondiseased Human Lung and Lung-Draining Lymph Nodes. *Am. J. Respir. Crit. Care Med.* **2016**, *193*, 614–626. [CrossRef] [PubMed]
58. Granot, T.; Senda, T.; Carpenter, D.J.; Matsuoka, N.; Weiner, J.; Gordon, C.L.; Miron, M.; Kumar, B.V.; Griesemer, A.; Ho, S.H.; et al. Dendritic Cells Display Subset and Tissue-Specific Maturation Dynamics over Human Life. *Immunity* **2017**, *46*, 504–515. [CrossRef] [PubMed]
59. Rate, A.; Bosco, A.; McKenna, K.L.; Holt, P.G.; Upham, J.W. Airway epithelial cells condition dendritic cells to express multiple immune surveillance genes. *PLoS ONE* **2012**, *7*, e44941. [CrossRef] [PubMed]
60. Agrawal, S.; Srivastava, R.; Rahmatpanah, F.; Madiraju, C.; BenMohamed, L.; Agrawal, A. Airway Epithelial Cells Enhance the Immunogenicity of Human Myeloid Dendritic Cells under Steady State. *Clin. Exp. Immunol.* **2017**. [CrossRef] [PubMed]
61. Iwasaki, A. Mucosal dendritic cells. *Annu. Rev. Immunol.* **2007**, *25*, 381–418. [CrossRef] [PubMed]
62. Chang, S.Y.; Ko, H.J.; Kweon, M.N. Mucosal dendritic cells shape mucosal immunity. *Exp. Mol. Med.* **2014**, *46*, e84. [CrossRef] [PubMed]
63. Holt, P.G.; Stumbles, P.A.; McWilliam, A.S. Functional studies on dendritic cells in the respiratory tract and related mucosal tissues. *J. Leukoc. Biol.* **1999**, *66*, 272–275. [PubMed]
64. Rothen-Rutishauser, B.; Mueller, L.; Blank, F.; Brandenberger, C.; Muehlfeld, C.; Gehr, P. A newly developed in vitro model of the human epithelial airway barrier to study the toxic potential of nanoparticles. *Altex* **2008**, *25*, 191–196. [CrossRef] [PubMed]
65. Blank, F.; Wehrli, M.; Lehmann, A.; Baum, O.; Gehr, P.; von Garnier, C.; Rothen-Rutishauser, B.M. Macrophages and dendritic cells express tight junction proteins and exchange particles in an in vitro model of the human airway wall. *Immunobiology* **2011**, *216*, 86–95. [CrossRef] [PubMed]
66. Kim, S.; Lewis, C.; Nadel, J.A. CCL20/CCR6 feedback exaggerates epidermal growth factor receptor-dependent MUC5AC mucin production in human airway epithelial (NCI-H292) cells. *J. Immunol.* **2011**, *186*, 3392–3400. [CrossRef] [PubMed]
67. Haczku, A. The dendritic cell niche in chronic obstructive pulmonary disease. *Respir. Res.* **2012**, *13*, 80. [CrossRef] [PubMed]
68. Abonyo, B.O.; Alexander, M.S.; Heiman, A.S. Autoregulation of CCL26 synthesis and secretion in A549 cells: A possible mechanism by which alveolar epithelial cells modulate airway inflammation. *Am. J. Physiol. Lung Cell. Mol. Physiol.* **2005**, *289*, L478–L488. [CrossRef] [PubMed]
69. Groom, J.R.; Luster, A.D. CXCR3 in T cell function. *Exp. Cell Res.* **2011**, *317*, 620–631. [CrossRef] [PubMed]

70. Wark, P.A.; Bucchieri, F.; Johnston, S.L.; Gibson, P.G.; Hamilton, L.; Mimica, J.; Zummo, G.; Holgate, S.T.; Attia, J.; Thakkinstian, A.; et al. IFN-gamma-induced protein 10 is a novel biomarker of rhinovirus-induced asthma exacerbations. *J. Allergy Clin. Immunol.* **2007**, *120*, 586–593. [CrossRef] [PubMed]
71. Spurrell, J.C.; Wiehler, S.; Zaheer, R.S.; Sanders, S.P.; Proud, D. Human airway epithelial cells produce IP-10 (CXCL10) in vitro and in vivo upon rhinovirus infection. *Am. J. Physiol. Lung Cell. Mol. Physiol.* **2005**, *289*, L85–L95. [CrossRef] [PubMed]
72. Del Rio, M.L.; Bernhardt, G.; Rodriguez-Barbosa, J.I.; Forster, R. Development and functional specialization of CD103+ dendritic cells. *Immunol. Rev.* **2010**, *234*, 268–281. [CrossRef] [PubMed]
73. Guilliams, M.; Crozat, K.; Henri, S.; Tamoutounour, S.; Grenot, P.; Devilard, E.; de Bovis, B.; Alexopoulou, L.; Dalod, M.; Malissen, B. Skin-draining lymph nodes contain dermis-derived CD103(-) dendritic cells that constitutively produce retinoic acid and induce Foxp3(+) regulatory T cells. *Blood* **2010**, *115*, 1958–1968. [CrossRef] [PubMed]
74. Napoli, J.L. Physiological insights into all-trans-retinoic acid biosynthesis. *Biochim. Biophys. Acta* **2012**, *1821*, 152–167. [CrossRef] [PubMed]
75. Blomhoff, R.; Blomhoff, H.K. Overview of retinoid metabolism and function. *J. Neurobiol.* **2006**, *66*, 606–630. [CrossRef] [PubMed]
76. Harrison, E.H. Mechanisms of digestion and absorption of dietary vitamin A. *Annu. Rev. Nutr.* **2005**, *25*, 87–103. [CrossRef] [PubMed]
77. Gudas, L.J. Emerging roles for retinoids in regeneration and differentiation in normal and disease states. *Biochim. Biophys. Acta* **2012**, *1821*, 213–221. [CrossRef] [PubMed]
78. Bchini, R.; Vasiliou, V.; Branlant, G.; Talfournier, F.; Rahuel-Clermont, S. Retinoic acid biosynthesis catalyzed by retinal dehydrogenases relies on a rate-limiting conformational transition associated with substrate recognition. *Chem. Biol. Interact.* **2013**, *202*, 78–84. [CrossRef] [PubMed]
79. Theodosiou, M.; Laudet, V.; Schubert, M. From carrot to clinic: An overview of the retinoic acid signaling pathway. *Cell. Mol. Life Sci.* **2010**, *67*, 1423–1445. [CrossRef] [PubMed]
80. Pino-Lagos, K.; Benson, M.J.; Noelle, R.J. Retinoic acid in the immune system. *Ann. N. Y. Acad. Sci.* **2008**, *1143*, 170–187. [CrossRef] [PubMed]
81. Soroosh, P.; Doherty, T.A.; Duan, W.; Mehta, A.K.; Choi, H.; Adams, Y.F.; Mikulski, Z.; Khorram, N.; Rosenthal, P.; Broide, D.H.; et al. Lung-resident tissue macrophages generate Foxp3+ regulatory T cells and promote airway tolerance. *J. Exp. Med.* **2013**, *210*, 775–788. [CrossRef] [PubMed]
82. Zhao, J.; Lloyd, C.M.; Noble, A. Th17 responses in chronic allergic airway inflammation abrogate regulatory T-cell-mediated tolerance and contribute to airway remodeling. *Mucosal Immunol.* **2013**, *6*, 335–346. [CrossRef] [PubMed]
83. Martin, H.; Taube, C. Regulatory T cells and regulation of allergic airway disease. *Am. J. Clin. Exp. Immunol.* **2012**, *1*, 166–178. [PubMed]
84. Strickland, D.H.; Wikstrom, M.E.; Turner, D.J.; Holt, P.G. Mucosal regulatory T cells in airway hyperresponsiveness. *Chem. Immunol. Allergy* **2008**, *94*, 40–47. [PubMed]
85. Navarro, S.; Driscoll, B. Regeneration of the Aging Lung: A Mini-Review. *Gerontology* **2016**, *63*, 270–280. [CrossRef] [PubMed]
86. Wansleeben, C.; Bowie, E.; Hotten, D.F.; Yu, Y.R.; Hogan, B.L. Age-related changes in the cellular composition and epithelial organization of the mouse trachea. *PLoS ONE* **2014**, *9*, e93496. [CrossRef] [PubMed]
87. Agrawal, S.; Ganguly, S.; Tran, A.; Sundaram, P.; Agrawal, A. Retinoic acid treated human dendritic cells induce T regulatory cells via the expression of CD141 and GARP which is impaired with age. *Aging* **2016**, *8*, 1223–1235. [CrossRef] [PubMed]
88. Manna, P.R.; Stetson, C.L.; Daugherty, C.; Shimizu, I.; Syapin, P.J.; Garrel, G.; Cohen-Tannoudji, J.; Huhtaniemi, I.; Slominski, A.T.; Pruitt, K.; et al. Up-regulation of steroid biosynthesis by retinoid signaling: Implications for aging. *Mech. Ageing Dev.* **2015**, *150*, 74–82. [CrossRef] [PubMed]
89. Del Rio, M.L.; Rodriguez-Barbosa, J.I.; Kremmer, E.; Forster, R. CD103- and CD103+ bronchial lymph node dendritic cells are specialized in presenting and cross-presenting innocuous antigen to CD4+ and CD8+ T cells. *J. Immunol.* **2007**, *178*, 6861–6866. [CrossRef] [PubMed]
90. Haniffa, M.; Shin, A.; Bigley, V.; McGovern, N.; Teo, P.; See, P.; Wasan, P.S.; Wang, X.N.; Malinarich, F.; Malleret, B.; et al. Human tissues contain CD141hi cross-presenting dendritic cells with functional homology to mouse CD103+ nonlymphoid dendritic cells. *Immunity* **2012**, *37*, 60–73. [CrossRef] [PubMed]

91. Nastasi, C.; Candela, M.; Bonefeld, C.M.; Geisler, C.; Hansen, M.; Krejsgaard, T.; Biagi, E.; Andersen, M.H.; Brigidi, P.; Odum, N.; et al. The effect of short-chain fatty acids on human monocyte-derived dendritic cells. *Sci. Rep.* **2015**, *5*, 16148. [CrossRef] [PubMed]
92. Whiteson, K.; Agrawal, S.; Agrawal, A. Differential responses of human dendritic cells to metabolites from the oral/airway microbiome. *Clin. Exp. Immunol.* **2017**, *188*, 371–379. [CrossRef] [PubMed]
93. Whelan, F.J.; Verschoor, C.P.; Stearns, J.C.; Rossi, L.; Luinstra, K.; Loeb, M.; Smieja, M.; Johnstone, J.; Surette, M.G.; Bowdish, D.M. The loss of topography in the microbial communities of the upper respiratory tract in the elderly. *Ann. Am. Thorac. Soc.* **2014**, *11*, 513–521. [CrossRef] [PubMed]

4

The Lung Microbiome in Idiopathic Pulmonary Fibrosis: A Promising Approach for Targeted Therapies

Aline Fastrès [1,†], Florence Felice [2,†], Elodie Roels [1], Catherine Moermans [2], Jean-Louis Corhay [2], Fabrice Bureau [3], Renaud Louis [2], Cécile Clercx [1] and Julien Guiot [2,*]

1 Department of Clinical Sciences, FARAH, Faculty of Veterinary Medicine, University of Liège, 4000 Liège, Belgium; afastres@uliege.be (F.A.); eroels@uliege.be (R.E.); cclercx@uliege.be (C.C.)
2 Respiratory department, CHU Liège. Domaine universitaire du Sart Tilman, B35, 4000 Liège, Belgium; Florence.Felice@student.uliege.be (F.F.); c.moermans@chu.ulg.ac.be (M.C.); jlcorhay@ulg.ac.be (C.J.-L.), R.Louis@uliege.be (L.R.)
3 Laboratory of Cellular and Molecular Immunology, GIGA Research, University of Liège, 4000 Liège, Belgium; fabrice.bureau@uliege.be
* Correspondence: j.guiot@chu.ulg.ac.be
† These authors contributed equally to this work.

Abstract: This review focuses on the role of the lung microbiome in idiopathic pulmonary fibrosis. Although historically considered sterile, bacterial communities have now been well documented in lungs both in healthy and pathological conditions. Studies in idiopathic pulmonary fibrosis (IPF) suggest that increased bacterial burden and/or abundance of potentially pathogenic bacteria may drive disease progression, acute exacerbations, and mortality. More recent work has highlighted the interaction between the lung microbiome and the innate immune system in IPF, strengthening the argument for the role of both host and environment interaction in disease pathogenesis. Existing published data suggesting that the lung microbiome may represent a therapeutic target, via antibiotic administration, immunization against pathogenic organisms, or treatment directed at gastroesophageal reflux. Taken altogether, published literature suggests that the lung microbiome might serve in the future as a prognostic biomarker, a therapeutic target, and/or provide an explanation for disease pathogenesis in IPF.

Keywords: idiopathic pulmonary fibrosis; IPF; interstitial lung diseases; microbiome; microbiota

---

1. Introduction

Idiopathic pulmonary fibrosis (IPF) is a rare lung disease of unknown origin which leads rapidly to death [1,2]. However, the rate of progression of the disease varies among individuals and is still difficult to predict [3]. The prognosis of IPF is poor with a median survival of three to five years after diagnosis without curative therapies besides lung transplantation. However, two antifibrotic drugs, pirfenidone and nintedanib, are known to be effective in slowing down disease progression and in reducing lung related mortality [4,5]. The factors leading to disease initiation and progression remain incompletely known [1]. The current disease paradigm is that repetitive micro-injury to the alveolar epithelium by unknown environmental triggers (e.g., cigarette smoke, gastric microaspiration, particulate dust, viral infections or lung microbial composition) in genetically susceptible individuals leads to aberrant wound healing resulting in fibrosis rather than normal repair [6]. Numerous epidemiologic and genetic studies illustrate that genetic and environmental factors contribute to the risk of developing IPF [7]. In parallel to the different clinical phenotypes and genotypes discovered, molecular mechanisms promoting disease biology are also heterogeneous, and may involve an extensive array of different pathways and processes including apoptosis [8], oxidative stress [9], intra-alveolar coagulation [10], endoplasmic reticulum stress [9], and telomere shortening [11]. Previous studies have identified several genetic variants both associated with sporadic and familial forms of IPF that confer an individual predisposition to develop the disease [12,13]. Of interest, genes involved in host-bacterial defense, including alpha-defensin, have previously been described as up-regulated in IPF patients compared with control [14]. These studies suggest that genetic susceptibility in innate immune defense may play a role in the pathogenesis of IPF, and lend support to the concept that microbiota, through its interaction with the host immune system, may contribute to the sequence of events that result in fibrosis. Other reasons suggesting that infection by modulating microbial communities might interfere with fibrosis initiation or perpetuation processes are supported by the finding that immunosuppressive therapy decreases the progression-free survival time in IPF patients [6]. Besides these observations, adding antibiotics such as cotrimoxazole to specific anti-fibrotic therapies improves quality of life and reduces mortality [15]. Moreover, it is now widely recognized that despite the ancient dogma, the lungs are not sterile [16]. Culture-independent techniques have permitted to identify numerous micro-organisms coexisting in the lungs, such as bacteria, viruses and fungi [16,17]. This natural community of microorganisms, collectively known as the microbiome, populates our respiratory tract, and its role in healthy lung function is increasingly recognized. Not surprisingly, alterations to this respiratory microbiome are seen in multiple respiratory disorders. In the past few years, studies investigating the lower airway microbiome using these culture-independent techniques have shown an increased bacterial burden and taxonomic differences in IPF compared to healthy subjects [18,19]. Alterations of the microbiome may also drive disease progression or acute exacerbation [20]. While IPF microbiome studies have been able to derive bacterial genus and burden, they have not been able to establish a causal, mechanistic link to disease process or progression. It remains unclear whether the changes in lung microbiome reported in the IPF studies are a cause of the disease, or a consequence either of an underlying immune defense defect or of architectural changes. Therefore, recent studies aimed to investigate how the lung microbial community influences host defenses [21,22].

In this review we are going to approach successively the respiratory microbiome in healthy subjects and the main alterations described in IPF microbiome, during stable disease and during exacerbations, as well as its interaction with the host response. We have performed a systematic search in PubMed by typing the words: ("Microbiota"[Mesh]) and (("Lung Diseases, Interstitial"[Mesh]) or "Idiopathic Pulmonary Fibrosis"[Mesh]) and (microbiome) and (("Lung Diseases, Interstitial"[Mesh]) or "Idiopathic Pulmonary Fibrosis"[Mesh]), and selecting those thought to be relevant. Publications dates of selected papers range from 2010 to 2017.

2. Microbiome in Healthy Lungs

The epithelial surfaces of the respiratory tract, previously thought to be sterile, have been shown, by using culture-independent techniques, to accommodate dynamic microbial communities. High-throughput bacterial 16s-rRNA sequencing has been described to identify bacterial DNA in 95.7% of bronchoalveolar lavage (BAL) specimens compared with conventional culture techniques, which detected bacteria in 39.1% of BAL samples [23].

The bacterial communities of healthy lungs closely resemble those of the mouth [24], while being two to four times lower in terms of bacterial burden. In lung tissues, a range from 10 to 100 bacterial cells per 1000 human cells has been previously reported [25]. It is also interesting to point out that despite differences in pH, temperature and oxygen concentration, the microbiome of healthy subjects is relatively constant between individuals [26,27]. The most four represented phyla in normal airways are Bacteroidetes (including the genus *Prevotella* sp.), Firmicutes (including the genera of *Streptococcus* sp. and *Veillonella* sp.) and, to a lesser extent, Proteobacteria and Actinobacteria [27–29].

The exact composition of the lung microbiota results from three main factors. The first one is microbial immigration due to microaspiration of gastric content, direct mucosal dispersion from the oro-nasal cavities, and to the inhalation of air. The second one is the microbial elimination, which results from the mucociliary clearance, cough and immunity. Finally, the third factor is the local microbial growth environment that includes notably nutrient availability, oxygen tension, pH and temperature. As a consequence of those three factors, the lung microbiota represents a steady state between microbial influx, efflux and reproduction rates, the latest being mostly altered in case of pathological processes. In every lung disease studied to date, the lung microbiome is altered compared with that of healthy subjects [30].

Given the sensitivity of the molecular technologies employed, an obvious concern in many studies is contamination of samples from the upper respiratory tract when sampling, providing a false representation of the true microbiome [18,19]. Although most of the published studies have characterized the lung microbiome of healthy subjects using BAL samples, the potential for oropharyngeal contamination should be addressed [31,32]. Besides, in healthy subjects, variation of the lung microbial community composition at spatially distinct lung sites within individuals have been shown [28], however, it remains lower than intersubject community variation [27]. It has recently been demonstrated that contamination contributes negligibly to microbial communities in bronchoscopically acquired specimens, validating the use of bronchoscopy to investigate the lung microbiome [32]. Bronchoscopy is not the only step where contamination can be introduced in studies of the microbiome. Significant variation has also been found when comparing microbiome data from the same patient samples using different sequencer platforms and methodologies [21,33]. Reagents and extraction kits are also significant sources of contamination and become particularly important with low biomass samples, like those generated from the respiratory tract [34,35]. Moreover, it must be remembered that sequencing DNA from a BAL sample provides a "snapshot" in time of the microbial diversity of the lower airways, but does not evaluate the dynamic changes that may be occurring longitudinally.

Beyond studying the microbiota, a small minority of studies have focused on fungi and viruses. Recent studies have shown that commensal fungi not only affect the host immune system, but can also affect bacterial composition and have a particularly important influence during restoration of the bacterial microbiota after antibiotic treatment [36]. Virome is known to be highly variable in lungs and is thought to be a trigger in multiple lung diseases [37].

3. Microbiota in IPF (Idiopathic Pulmonary Fibrosis)

Even if the exact pathophysiology of IPF is still incompletely understood, the microbiome is suspected to play a role in the pathology [38]. Indeed, bacteria can cause epithelial alveolar injury on their own, but can also activate an immune cascade response due to their presence alone [39], the following pro-inflammatory and pro-fibrotic cascades resulting in alterations of the lung architecture.

The hypothesis that IPF progression is influenced by microbes is supported by the finding that immunosuppression increased the risk of death and hospitalization [6]. Another clue concerning the role of bacteria in IPF pathogenesis is the effect of antibiotics on the natural history of the disease. Sulgina and al. attempted to treat 181 IPF patients with cotrimoxazole for 12 months [15], and showed a decreased mortality rate and an increased quality of life, with a decreased need of oxygenotherapy, however, it did not translate into an improvement of pulmonary function. Respiratory infections were also less frequent among the treated group. Unfortunately, almost one-third of patients receiving cotrimoxazole withdrew from the trial due to side effects, mostly rash and nausea.

The microbiome of IPF patients is distinct from healthy individuals: their bacterial load is overall higher, and the genera *Haemophilus*, *Streptococcus*, *Neisseiria* and *Veillonella* sp. are more abundant in patients with IPF compared to controls [40]. It is also very different from the mouth microbiome in comparison to healthy subjects, which suggests a microbial selection in the lower respiratory tract in chronic lung disease [27], as each disease seems to have its own microbial signature, including a loss of diversity along with dysbiosis [41].

The first exploratory application of a culture-independent molecular technique in IPF studied the microbiome in BAL from 17 IPF patients [42]. Using 16s-rRNA gene polymerase chain reaction (PCR) and degenerating gel electrophoresis (DGGE), the study found organisms often associated with the oropharynx, as well as uncultured bacterial sequences corresponding to the *Streptococcus*, *Neisseria* and *Actinobacterium* sp. genera. Interestingly, bacterial DNA was not detected in five out of eight patients colonized with *Pneumocystis jirovecii*, suggesting this fungus may impair bacterial colonization of the airways [42].

A small study then investigated the upper and lower respiratory tract microbiota in a heterogenous group of 18 patients with interstitial lung disease (ILD), including five with idiopathic interstitial pneumonia (IIP), six patients with pneumocystis associated pneumonia and nine healthy controls [43]. The 16s-rRNA gene sequencing of BAL revealed no significant differences in the microbiome between ILD and healthy controls. There was a signal toward lower bacterial diversity in the IIPs but this was not statistically significant.

Later on, a multicenter cohort study of Correlating Outcomes with biochemical Markers to Estimate Time-progression in idiopathic pulmonary fibrosis (COMET) [19], retrospectively characterized the lung microbiota in 55 IPF patients with no active infection at the time of screening by sequencing the genome of the bacteria found in baseline bronchoalveolar lavage fluid (BALF) samples. The study also followed-up participants prospectively at 16 weeks intervals up to 80 weeks in order to provide longitudinal outcome data. In that study, the most prevalent OTUs (operational taxonomic unit) in IPF patients were *Prevotella*, *Veillonella* and *Cronobacter* sp. Moreover, the presence of a specific *Streptococcus* or *Staphylococcus* OTU (among all *Streptococcus* and *Staphylococcus* OTUs) above a certain threshold was associated with a faster-progressing disease, after adjusting for age, sex, smoking status, respiratory function, six-minute-walk test and the presence of gastro-intestinal reflux [19]. However, those OTUs were only found in less than half of the IPF cohort; their presence is thus insufficient to explain the disease pathogenesis on its own but these findings open the possibilities to use those OTUs as prognostic biomarker for disease progression. A limitation to this study is that 16S rRNA sequencing could not be used for species-level identification. Further work, in the form of either culture-specific or microbe-specific sequencing, is needed to formally identify these bacteria.

A large study published in 2014 investigated 65 well-defined IPF patients and 44 controls which included 27 healthy controls and 17 patients with moderate chronic obstructive pulmonary disease (COPD) [18]. The first notable finding was a twofold higher bacterial load (quantified by 16S rRNA gene/mL BALF) in IPF BALF compared with control subjects ($p < 0.0001$). Secondly, there was a significant association between patients with higher BALF bacterial load and disease progression at six months (defined by a decline in forced vital capacity (FVC) by 10%, or death) compared with controls ($p = 0.02$). Furthermore, it was possible to stratify patients according to bacterial burden in order to predict mortality risk, patients with higher bacterial burden having an increased risk of mortality (hazard ratio: 4.59) compared with patients with low bacterial burden. After logistic regression analysis, the abundance of *Veillonella*, *Neisseria*, *Streptococcus* and *Haemophilus* sp. remained significantly associated with IPF. Moreover, the study found that patients carrying a minor allele at the MUC5B promoter had a lower bacterial burden, providing a mechanistic link between bacterial burden and a mutation known to be relevant in IPF.

4. Host Microbial Interactions in IPF

Today, it is still unclear whether changes in microbiome seen in IPF are a cause or a consequence of the disease. The PANTHER trial [6] has identified an increase in mortality with immunosuppressive therapies, suggesting a role of a deficient host immunity in the pathogenesis of the disease. In addition, acute infection is also associated with a greater mortality rate in IPF patients, highlighting once more the crucial role of the immune system in the natural history of the disease [44]. Consequently, studies investigating whether the lung microbiome influences the host defense in IPF are needed.

Search for associations between alterations in the lung microbial community in IPF and host immune response in IPF have been addressed in recent publications [21,22].

In a study from Molyneaux et al. [21], the authors investigated a cohort of 60 patients with IPF from the Interstitial Lung Disease Unit at the Royal Brompton Hospital, London, and 20 matched healthy controls. All participants underwent BAL and blood sample collection. In IPF patients, BAL was performed at baseline. Moreover, for the longitudinal follow-up of these patients, peripheral blood samples were obtained and pulmonary function was further tested up to 12 months after diagnosis. Researchers analyzed gene expression of the host and found two particular groups of genes whose expression correlated with an IPF diagnosis, with higher bacterial burden in the BALF, and specific OTUs. The genes identified also correlated with an increase of neutrophils in both BAL and blood samples. These groups included genes involved in host defense response (*Nlrc4, Pglyrp1, Mmp9, Defa4*). Additionally, that team found two genes encoding specific antimicrobial peptides (*Slpi* and *Camp*). Several of the identified genes were linked to poor survival and disease progression. These results suggest a host response to alterations of the respiratory microbiome in IPF, suggesting that these microbial changes would possibly trigger a response associated with the damage often observed in IPF patients. As they conclude, "the bacterial communities of the lower airways may act as persistent stimuli for repetitive alveolar injury in IPF" [21].

Another independent study [22] evaluated peripheral blood mononuclear cell (PBMC) gene expression, BALF microbiome and in vitro fibroblast responsiveness to cytosine-phosphate-guanine (CpG) antigenic stimulus in 68 IPF patients. Relative inhibition of several gene signaling pathways was associated with reduced progression-free survival time (PFS); some pathways were involved in immune inflammatory response and pathogen infection-like regulation of autophagy, while others are involved in pattern recognition receptors such as Toll-like receptor signaling pathway for example. The down-regulation of immune response pathways is associated with modifications in the abundance of specific OTUs. Indeed, they showed that the decrease of nucleotide binding oligomerization domain (NOD)-like receptor signaling is associated with increased abundance of *Streptococcus* sp. OTU, and that this phenomenon is correlated with poorer PFS. *Staphylococcus* and *Prevotella* sp. OTUs are also associated with poorer PFS, with decreased expression of immune response pathways genes and with overexpression of TLR-9 in PBMC. Finally, the increased presence of a specific *Veillonella* sp. OTU is correlated with increased CpG fibroblast responsiveness. This study demonstrates that host defense, as assessed by immune pathway gene expression, may be modulated by variations in the lower airway microbiome and that bacteria with increased abundance and decreased diversity are associated with decreased immune pathway genes expression and poorer PFS. This study also demonstrates that host-microbiome interaction may influence immune-mediated fibroblast responsiveness.

On the other hand, Wang et al. [45] have attempted to treat IPF patients with aerosolized interferon-gamma as a single therapy. The diversity of the microbiome was not impacted by the treatment; however, the study established a connection between the composition of the microbiome and the disease phenotype regarding inflammatory and fibrotic markers in the lung mucosa, suggesting once more an interaction between host immunity and microbiome.

5. Microbiome Effect on IPF Prognosis and Exacerbation

The progression of IPF is marked with exacerbations, similar to a number of chronic lung diseases. Acute exacerbations are associated with a particularly poor prognosis. Among patients with acute exacerbations, non-survivors had shorter durations of dyspnea, lower arterial oxygen tension (PaO_2)/inspiratory oxygen fraction (FiO_2) ratios, higher C reactive protein (CRP) levels, higher percentages of neutrophils and lower percentages of lymphocytes in BALF compared with survivors. Amongst those factors only CRP was found to be an independent predictor of survival, suggesting that infection (either bacterial or viral) and/or inflammation can be one of the pathogenic mechanisms contributing to acute exacerbations [46].

An exacerbation is currently defined as "an acute, clinically significant deterioration of unidentifiable cause in a patient with underlying IPF" [44], and it requires formal exclusion of an infection for clinical diagnosis. However, the exact pathogenesis of acute exacerbations remains unknown, and it is currently unclear whether it represents an accelerated phase of an underlying fibroproliferative process or an exaggerated lung injury response to unidentified preceding or coexistent infection [20]. Factors supporting a role for infection in exacerbation include the fact that respiratory tract infections in individuals with IPF confer a mortality risk indistinguishable from that seen with acute exacerbations. Moreover, the definition has been challenged by recent studies of the lung microbiome during IPF exacerbations and its influence on disease progression [18,20]. Such studies show that a high bacterial burden at the time of diagnosis seem to be a biomarker for a more-rapidly progressive disease with an increased risk of mortality [18].

Another study on 20 patients with diagnosed acute exacerbations of IPF and 15 matched controls with stable IPF who underwent bronchoscopy and DNA extraction has shown that IPF patients presented an increased bacterial burden during exacerbations, up to four times higher [20]. Their BALF also contained more neutrophils compared to stable IPF patients. This raises the possibility of bacteria playing a role in exacerbations, regardless of the presence of an active infection. They also analyze 16S rRNA gene qPCR and pyrosequencing in both stable and acute exacerbation group in order to explore changes in the BAL microbiota. In case of acute exacerbation there was a notable change in the microbiota with an increase in two potentially pathogenic Proteobacteria OTUs, *Campylobacter* sp. and *Stenotrophomonas* sp., coupled with a significant decrease in *Veillonella* sp., and *Campylobacter* sp., although best known as a gastrointestinal pathogen, was previously identified in the respiratory microbiota of individuals with severe COPD. Its presence in the respiratory microbiota is likely to arise from silent micro-aspiration of gastric contents [20]. To summarize these observations, this pilot study suggests that bacteria may play a causative role in acute exacerbation of IPF. The apparent translocation of bacteria usually confined to the gastrointestinal tract also suggests a role for micro-aspiration. Results of this study, although requiring a prospective longitudinal study for validation, provide a rationale for clinical trials of prophylactic antibiotics as a strategy to prevent acute exacerbations in individuals with IPF.

6. Conclusions and Perspectives

All of these findings open the possibility of a place for antibiotherapy in IPF patients; in particular, they provide a rationale for clinical trials of long-term antibiotherapy acting as an immunomodulator and an antibioprophylaxis to prevent acute exacerbations. In the future, an improved knowledge of the dynamic alterations of the lung microbiome might help to select appropriate, targeted and more personalized antibiotherapy in the course of the disease, in particular in IPF exacerbations. In this context, more advanced metagenomic analyses are required to elucidate the functional role of individual bacterial genera and communities in IPF progression.

As recent studies demonstrated interactions between host immune response and microbial community in IPF, further studies will probably focus on the exploration of therapeutic approaches targeting modulation, not only of the lung microbial community of patients with IPF, but of specific components of the innate immune system.

Author Contributions: Fastrès Aline, Felice Florence, Clercx Cécile and Guiot Julien wrote the manuscript. Fastrès Aline, Felice Florence, Roels Elodie, Moermans Catherine, Corhay Jean-Louis, Bureau Fabrice, Louis Renaud, Clercx Cécile and Guiot Julien reviewed the final version of the manuscript.

Abbreviations

IPF	Idiopathic pulmonary fibrosis
BAL	Bronchoalveolar lavage
DGGE	Degenerative gel electrophoresis
PCR	Polymerase chain reaction
ILD	Interstitial lung disease
IIP	Idiopathic interstitial pneumonia
COMET	Correlating outcomes with biochemical markers to estimate time-progression
BALF	Bronchoalveolar lavage fluid
OTU	Operational taxonomic unit
COPD	Chronic obstructive pulmonary disease
FVC	Forced vital capacity
PBMC	Peripheral blood mononuclear cell
CpG	Cytosine-phosphate-guanine
PFS	Progression-free survival time
NOD	Nucleotide binding oligomerization domain
PaO_2	Lower arterial oxygen tension
FiO_2	Inspiratory oxygen fraction
CRP	C-reactive protein

References

1. Raghu, G. Idiopathic pulmonary fibrosis: Guidelines for diagnosis and clinical management have advanced from consensus-based in 2000 to evidence-based in 2011. *Eur. Respir. J.* **2011**, *37*, 743–746. [CrossRef] [PubMed]
2. Guiot, J.; Moermans, C.; Henket, M.; Corhay, J.L.; Louis, R. Blood biomarkers in idiopathic pulmonary fibrosis. *Lung* **2017**, *195*, 273–280. [CrossRef] [PubMed]
3. Ley, B.; Ryerson, C.J.; Vittinghoff, E.; Ryu, J.H.; Tomassetti, S.; Lee, J.S.; Poletti, V.; Buccioli, M.; Elicker, B.M.; Jones, K.D.; et al. A multidimensional index and staging system for idiopathic pulmonary fibrosis. *Ann. Intern. Med.* **2012**, *156*, 684. [CrossRef] [PubMed]
4. Nathan, S.D.; Albera, C.; Bradford, W.Z.; Costabel, U.; du Bois, R.M.; Fagan, E.A.; Fishman, R.S.; Glaspole, I.; Glassberg, M.K.; Glasscock, K.F.; et al. Effect of continued treatment with pirfenidone following clinically meaningful declines in forced vital capacity: Analysis of data from three phase 3 trials in patients with idiopathic pulmonary fibrosis. *Thorax* **2016**, *71*, 429–435. [CrossRef] [PubMed]
5. Richeldi, L.; Cottin, V.; du Bois, R.M.; Selman, M.; Kimura, T.; Bailes, Z.; Schlenker-Herceg, R.; Stowasser, S.; Brown, K.K. Nintedanib in patients with idiopathic pulmonary fibrosis: Combined evidence from the TOMORROW and INPULSIS(®) trials. *Respir. Med.* **2016**, *113*, 74–79. [CrossRef] [PubMed]
6. Raghu, G.; Anstrom, K.J.; King, T.E.; Lasky, J.A.; Martinez, F.J. Idiopathic Pulmonary Fibrosis Clinical Research Network, Prednisone, Azathioprine, and *N*-Acetylcysteine for pulmonary fibrosis. *N. Engl. J. Med.* **2012**, *366*, 1968–1977. [CrossRef] [PubMed]
7. Kaur, A.; Mathai, S.K.; Schwartz, D.A. Genetics in idiopathic pulmonary fibrosis pathogenesis, prognosis, and treatment. *Front. Med.* **2017**, *4*, 154. [CrossRef] [PubMed]
8. Matsushima, S.; Ishiyama, J. MicroRNA-29c regulates apoptosis sensitivity via modulation of the cell-surface death receptor, Fas, in lung fibroblasts. *Am. J. Physiol. Lung Cell. Mol. Physiol.* **2016**, *311*, 1050–1061. [CrossRef] [PubMed]
9. Cheresh, P.; Kim, S.J.; Tulasiram, S.K.D. Oxidative stress and pulmonary fibrosis. *Biochim. Biophys. Acta Mol. Basis Dis.* **2013**, *1832*, 1028–1040. [CrossRef] [PubMed]
10. Mercer, P.F.; Chambers, R.C. Coagulation and coagulation signalling in fibrosis. *Biochim. Biophys. Acta Mol. Basis Dis.* **2013**, *1832*, 1018–1027. [CrossRef] [PubMed]
11. Dai, J.; Cai, H.; Li, H.; Zhuang, Y.; Min, H.; Wen, Y.; Yang, J.; Gao, Q.; Shi, Y.; Yi, L. Association between telomere length and survival in patients with idiopathic pulmonary fibrosis. *Respirology* **2015**, *20*, 947–952. [CrossRef] [PubMed]

12. Fingerlin, T.E.; Murphy, E.; Zhang, W.; Peljto, A.L.; Brown, K.K.; Steele, M.P.; Loyd, J.E.; Cosgrove, G.P.; Lynch, D.; Groshong, S.; et al. Genome-wide association study identifies multiple susceptibility loci for pulmonary fibrosis. *Nat. Genet.* **2013**, *45*, 613–620. [CrossRef] [PubMed]
13. Noth, I.; Zhang, Y.; Ma, S.-F.; Flores, C.; Barber, M.; Huang, Y.; Broderick, S.M.; Wade, M.S.; Hysi, P.; Scuirba, J.; et al. Genetic variants associated with idiopathic pulmonary fibrosis susceptibility and mortality: A genome-wide association study. *Lancet Respir. Med.* **2013**, *1*, 309–317. [CrossRef]
14. Yang, I.V.; Fingerlin, T.E.; Evans, C.M.; Schwarz, M.I.; Schwartz, D.A. MUC5B and idiopathic pulmonary fibrosis. *Ann. Am. Thorac. Soc.* **2015**, *12*, 193–199. [CrossRef]
15. Shulgina, L.; Cahn, A.P.; Chilvers, E.R.; Parfrey, H.; Clark, A.B.; Wilson, E.C.F.; Twentyman, O.P.; Davison, A.G.; Curtin, J.J.; et al. Treating idiopathic pulmonary fibrosis with the addition of co-trimoxazole: A randomised controlled trial. *Thorax* **2013**, *68*, 155–162. [CrossRef] [PubMed]
16. Kiley, J.P.; Caler, E.V. The lung microbiome a new frontier in pulmonary medicine. *Ann. Am. Thorac. Soc.* **2014**, *11*, 66–70. [CrossRef] [PubMed]
17. Dickson, R.P.; Erb-Downward, J.R.; Martinez, F.J.; Huffnagle, G.B. The microbiome and the respiratory tract. *Annu. Rev. Physiol.* **2016**, *78*, 481–504. [CrossRef] [PubMed]
18. Molyneaux, P.L.; Cox, M.J.; Willis-Owen, S.A.G.; Mallia, P.; Russell, K.E.; Russell, A.-M.; Murphy, E.; Johnston, S.L.; Schwartz, D.A.; Wells, A.U.; et al. The role of bacteria in the pathogenesis and progression of idiopathic pulmonary fibrosis. *Am. J. Respir. Crit. Care Med.* **2014**, *190*, 906–913. [CrossRef] [PubMed]
19. Han, M.L.K.; Zhou, Y.; Murray, S.; Tayob, N.; Noth, I.; Lama, V.N.; Moore, B.B.; White, E.S.; Flaherty, K.R.; Huffnagle, G.B.; et al. Lung microbiome and disease progression in idiopathic pulmonary fibrosis: An analysis of the COMET study. *Lancet Respir. Med.* **2014**, *2*, 548–556. [CrossRef]
20. Molyneaux, P.L.; Cox, M.J.; Wells, A.U.; Kim, H.C.; Ji, W.; Cookson, W.O.C.; Moffatt, M.F.; Kim, D.S.; Maher, T.M. Changes in the respiratory microbiome during acute exacerbations of idiopathic pulmonary fibrosis. *Respir. Res.* **2017**, *18*, 29. [CrossRef] [PubMed]
21. Molyneaux, P.L.; Willis-Owen, S.A.G.; Cox, M.J.; James, P.; Cowman, S.; Loebinger, M.; Blanchard, A.; Edwards, L.M.; Stock, C.; Daccord, C.; et al. Host-microbial interactions in idiopathic pulmonary fibrosis. *Am. J. Respir. Crit. Care Med.* **2017**, *195*, 1640–1650. [CrossRef] [PubMed]
22. Huang, Y.; Ma, S.-F.; Espindola, M.S.; Vij, R.; Oldham, J.M.; Huffnagle, G.B.; Erb-Downward, J.R.; Flaherty, K.R.; Moore, B.B.; White, E.S.; et al. Microbes are associated with host innate immune response in idiopathic pulmonary fibrosis. *Am. J. Respir. Crit. Care Med.* **2017**, *196*, 208–219. [CrossRef] [PubMed]
23. Dickson, R.P.; Erb-Downward, J.R.; Prescott, H.C.; Martinez, F.J.; Curtis, J.L.; Lama, V.N.; Huffnagle, G.B. Analysis of culture-dependent versus culture-independent techniques for identification of bacteria in clinically obtained bronchoalveolar lavage fluid. *J. Clin. Microbiol.* **2014**, *52*, 3605–3613. [CrossRef] [PubMed]
24. Venkataraman, A.; Bassis, C.M.; Beck, J.M.; Young, V.B.; Curtis, J.L.; Huffnagle, G.B.; Schmidt, T.M. Application of a neutral community model to assess structuring of the human lung microbiome. *MBio* **2015**, *6*, e02284-14. [CrossRef] [PubMed]
25. Sze, M.A.; Dimitriu, P.A.; Hayashi, S.; Elliott, W.M.; McDonough, J.E.; Gosselink, J.V.; Cooper, J.; Sin, D.D.; Mohn, W.W.; Hogg, J.C. The lung tissue microbiome in chronic obstructive pulmonary disease. *Am. J. Respir. Crit. Care Med.* **2012**, *185*, 1073–1080. [CrossRef] [PubMed]
26. Charlson, E.S.; Bittinger, K.; Haas, A.R.; Fitzgerald, A.S.; Frank, I.; Yadav, A.; Bushman, F.D.; Collman, R.G. Topographical continuity of bacterial populations in the healthy human respiratory tract. *Am. J. Respir. Crit. Care Med.* **2011**, *184*, 957–963. [CrossRef] [PubMed]
27. Dickson, R.P.; Erb-Downward, J.R.; Freeman, C.M.; McCloskey, L.; Beck, J.M.; Huffnagle, G.B.; Curtis, J.L. Spatial variation in the healthy human lung microbiome and the adapted island model of lung biogeography. *Ann. Am. Thorac. Soc.* **2015**, *12*, 821–830. [CrossRef] [PubMed]
28. Erb-Downward, J.R.; Thompson, D.L.; Han, M.K.; Freeman, C.M.; McCloskey, L.; Schmidt, L.A.; Young, V.B.; Toews, G.B.; Curtis, J.L.; Sundaram, B.; et al. Analysis of the lung microbiome in the "healthy" smoker and in COPD. *PLoS ONE* **2011**, *6*, e16384. [CrossRef] [PubMed]
29. Morris, A.; Beck, J.M.; Schloss, P.D.; Campbell, T.B.; Crothers, K.; Curtis, J.L.; Flores, S.C.; Fontenot, A.P.; Ghedin, E.; Huang, L.; et al. Comparison of the respiratory microbiome in healthy nonsmokers and smokers. *Am. J. Respir. Crit. Care Med.* **2012**, *187*, 1067–1075. [CrossRef] [PubMed]
30. Dickson, R.P.; Erb-Downward, J.R.; Huffnagle, G.B. Towards an ecology of the lung: New conceptual models of pulmonary microbiology and pneumonia pathogenesis. *Lancet Respir. Med.* **2014**, *2*, 238–246. [CrossRef]

31. Grønseth, R.; Drengenes, C.; Wiker, H.G.; Tangedal, S.; Xue, Y.; Husebø, G.R.; Svanes, Ø.; Lehmann, S.; Aardal, M.; Hoang, T.; et al. Protected sampling is preferable in bronchoscopic studies of the airway microbiome. *ERJ Open Res.* **2017**, *3*, 00019–2017. [CrossRef] [PubMed]
32. Dickson, R.P.; Erb-Downward, J.R.; Freeman, C.M.; McCloskey, L.; Falkowski, N.R.; Huffnagle, G.B.; Curtis, J.L. Bacterial topography of the healthy human lower respiratory tract. *MBio* **2017**, *8*, e02287-16. [CrossRef] [PubMed]
33. Hewitt, R.J.; Molyneaux, P.L. The respiratory microbiome in idiopathic pulmonary fibrosis. *Ann. Transl. Med.* **2017**, *5*, 250. [CrossRef] [PubMed]
34. Salter, S.J.; Cox, M.J.; Turek, E.M.; Calus, S.T.; Cookson, W.O.; Moffatt, M.F.; Turner, P.; Parkhill, J.; Loman, N.J.; Walker, A.W. Reagent and laboratory contamination can critically impact sequence-based microbiome analyses. *BMC Biol.* **2014**, *12*, 87. [CrossRef] [PubMed]
35. Willner, D.; Daly, J.; While, D.; Grimwood, K.; Wainwright, C.E.; Hugenholtz, P. Comparison of DNA extraction methods for microbial community profiling with an application to pediatric bronchoalveolar lavage samples. *PLoS ONE* **2012**, *7*, e34605. [CrossRef] [PubMed]
36. Erb-Downward, J.R.; Falkowski, N.R.; Mason, K.L.; Muraglia, R.; Huffnagle, G.B. Modulation of post-antibiotic bacterial community reassembly and host response by candida albicans. *Sci. Rep.* **2013**, *3*, 2191. [CrossRef] [PubMed]
37. Moradi, P.; Keyvani, H.; Javad, M.S.-A.; Karbalaie, N.M.H.; Esghaei, M.; Bokharaei-Salim, F.; Ataei-Pirkooh, A.; Monavari, S.H. Investigation of viral infection in idiopathic pulmonary fibrosis among Iranian patients in Tehran. *Microb. Pathog.* **2017**, *104*, 171–174. [CrossRef] [PubMed]
38. Maher, T.M.; Wells, A.U.; Laurent, G.J. Idiopathic pulmonary fibrosis: Multiple causes and multiple mechanisms? *Eur. Respir. J.* **2007**, *30*, 835–839. [CrossRef] [PubMed]
39. Molyneaux, P.L.; Maher, T.M. Respiratory microbiome in IPF: Cause, effect, or biomarker? *Lancet Respir. Med.* **2014**, *2*, 511–513. [CrossRef]
40. Molyneaux, P.L.; Maher, T.M.; Maher, T.M. The role of infection in the pathogenesis of idiopathic pulmonary fibrosis. *Eur. Respir. Rev.* **2013**, *22*, 376–381. [CrossRef] [PubMed]
41. Faner, R.; Sibila, O.; Agustí, A.; Bernasconi, E.; Chalmers, J.D.; Huffnagle, G.B.; Manichanh, C.; Molyneaux, P.L.; Paredes, R.; Pérez, B.V.; et al. The microbiome in respiratory medicine: Current challenges and future perspectives. *Eur. Respir. J.* **2017**, *49*, 1602086. [CrossRef] [PubMed]
42. Friaza, V.; la Horra, Cd.; Rodríguez-Domínguez, M.J.; Martín-Juan, J.; Cantón, R.; Calderón, E.J.; del Campo, R. Metagenomic analysis of bronchoalveolar lavage samples from patients with idiopathic interstitial pneumonia and its antagonic relation with Pneumocystis jirovecii colonization. *J. Microbiol. Methods* **2010**, *82*, 98–101. [CrossRef] [PubMed]
43. Garzoni, C.; Brugger, S.D.; Qi, W.; Wasmer, S.; Cusini, A.; Dumont, P.; Gorgievski-Hrisoho, M.; Mühlemann, K.; von Garnier, C.; Hilty, M. Microbial communities in the respiratory tract of patients with interstitial lung disease. *Thorax* **2013**, *68*, 1150–1156. [CrossRef] [PubMed]
44. Collard, H.R.; Moore, B.B.; Flaherty, K.R.; Brown, K.K.; Kaner, R.J.; King, J.T.E.; Lasky, J.A.; Loyd, J.E.; Noth, I.; Olman, M.A.; et al. Acute exacerbations of idiopathic pulmonary fibrosis. *Am. J. Respir. Crit. Care Med.* **2007**, *176*, 636–643. [CrossRef] [PubMed]
45. Wang, J.; Lesko, M.; Badri, M.H.; Kapoor, B.C.; Wu, B.G.; Li, Y.; Smaldone, G.C.; Bonneau, R.; Kurtz, Z.D.; Condos, R.; et al. Lung microbiome and host immune tone in subjects with idiopathic pulmonary fibrosis treated with inhaled interferon-γ. *ERJ Open Res.* **2017**, *3*, 00008-2017. [CrossRef] [PubMed]
46. Song, J.W.; Hong, S.-B.; Lim, C.-M.; Koh, Y.; Kim, D.S. Acute exacerbation of idiopathic pulmonary fibrosis: Incidence, risk factors and outcome. *Eur. Respir. J.* **2011**, *37*, 356–363. [CrossRef] [PubMed]

5

Disrupting the Btk Pathway Suppresses COPD-Like Lung Alterations in Atherosclerosis Prone ApoE$^{-/-}$ Mice Following Regular Exposure to Cigarette Smoke

Jon M. Florence [1], Agnieszka Krupa [1,2], Laela M. Booshehri [1], Adrian L. Gajewski [1,2] and Anna K. Kurdowska [1,*]

1 Department of Cellular and Molecular Biology, University of Texas Health Science Center, Tyler, TX 75708, USA; jon.florence@uthct.edu (J.M.F); agakrupa@yahoo.com (A.K.); laela.booshehri@gmail.com (L.M.B.); gajewski@biol.uni.lodz.pl (A.L.G.)

2 Laboratory of Gastroimmunology, Department of Immunology and Infectious Biology, Faculty of Biology and Environmental Protection, University of Lodz, 90-237 Lodz, Poland

* Correspondence: anna.kurdowska@uthct.edu

Abstract: Chronic obstructive pulmonary disease (COPD) is associated with severe chronic inflammation that promotes irreversible tissue destruction. Moreover, the most broadly accepted cause of COPD is exposure to cigarette smoke. There is no effective cure and significantly, the mechanism behind the development and progression of this disease remains unknown. Our laboratory has demonstrated that Bruton's tyrosine kinase (Btk) is a critical regulator of pro-inflammatory processes in the lungs and that Btk controls expression of matrix metalloproteinase-9 (MMP-9) in the alveolar compartment. For this study apolipoprotein E null (ApoE$^{-/-}$) mice were exposed to SHS to facilitate study in a COPD/atherosclerosis comorbidity model. We applied two types of treatments, animals received either a pharmacological inhibitor of Btk or MMP-9 specific siRNA to minimize MMP-9 expression in endothelial cells or neutrophils. We have shown that these treatments had a protective effect in the lung. We have noted a decrease in alveolar changes related to SHS induced inflammation in treated animals. In summary, we are presenting a novel concept in the field of COPD, i.e., that Btk may be a new drug target for this disease. Moreover, cell specific targeting of MMP-9 may also benefit patients affected by this disease.

Keywords: chronic lung inflammation; emphysema; second hand smoke; Bruton's tyrosine kinase; matrix metalloproteinase-9

---

1. Background

Second hand smoke (SHS) can illicit damage to lung tissue by altering signaling pathways that regulate both inflammatory responses and repair processes in the alveolar compartment. In fact, the induction of abnormal inflammation by SHS is a well-recognized underlying cause of pathogenic features characteristic of chronic obstructive pulmonary disease (COPD) [1]. A substantially enhanced inflammatory immune response in the airways and lungs is a hallmark of COPD. Natural history of the disease classically begins with inflammatory changes in the larger airways (chronic bronchitis). Remodeling and narrowing of the small airways and parenchymal tissue destruction with airspace enlargement (emphysema) are also well-recognized features of COPD [1,2].

Development of novel therapies for COPD would not be possible without animal models that adequately reflect pathophysiology of this disease. Animal models utilizing cigarette smoke exposure display the characteristic features of human COPD including accumulation of inflammatory cells, small airway fibrosis/remodeling, mucus hyper-secretion, lung dysfunction and development of emphysema [3]. In mouse models of COPD, chronic exposure of mice to cigarette smoke triggers typical pathological hallmarks of the disorder, such as pulmonary inflammation, airway remodeling and airspace enlargement caused by the destruction of alveolar walls [3–10].

Novel studies from our laboratory have shown that activation of Bruton's tyrosine kinase (Btk) was significantly increased in lungs during severe inflammation [11,12]. Btk belongs to a family of Tec kinases, non-receptor intracellular tyrosine kinases. Tec kinases typically reside in an inactive form in the cytoplasm, and are translocated to the membrane fraction upon cell stimulation where they initiate downstream signaling cascades [11,13]. We have also noted that Btk may regulate expression of matrix metalloproteinase-9 (MMP-9) in the lung [11,12]. Matrix metalloproteinases (MMPs) are proteolytic enzymes capable of degrading matrix components. This process is beneficial in normal physiological states, but can be harmful in pathological conditions. Significantly, increased levels of MMP-9 have been detected in the lungs of smokers with COPD [14] as well as smoke exposed mice [5,10,15].

It should be stressed that exposure of mice to SHS remains the best animal system for defining, testing, and evaluating novel drug targets for COPD [3]. The model of apolipoprotein E deficient ($ApoE^{-/-}$) mice that we employed in the study mimics systemic co-morbidities of COPD and accurately reflects multiple aspects of the corresponding clinical disease [4–7,15]. We have applied two types of treatments to $ApoE^{-/-}$ mice exposed to SHS. The animals received either a pharmacological inhibitor of Btk or MMP-9 specific siRNA to minimize MMP-9 expression in endothelial cells or neutrophils. We previously reported on the impact of these treatments with respect to the atherosclerotic aspect of this model [16]. Here we show that all treatments resulted in reduction of pulmonary changes related to COPD progression. Targeting Btk or cell specific expression of MMP-9 may be prospective treatments for COPD patients.

2. Results

2.1. *Exposure to SHS Induces Alveolar Destruction and Airspace Enlargement in Lungs of $ApoE^{-/-}$ Mice*

Hart's Elastin stain was used to assess alveolar wall destruction in lungs of $ApoE^{-/-}$ mice on standard rodent chow or "Western Diet" (WD) fed mice with or without SHS exposure. Evaluation of alveolar wall condition was based on observation of airspace elastin, its appearance and continuance. In normal mice airspace elastin appears as thin continuous strands which outline alveolar walls [17,18]. As shown in Figure 1a, alveolar destruction in the SHS exposed animals is visible as a loss of elastic round, intact alveoli. Moreover appearance of elastin nodules is a consequence of alveolar destruction, and result from recoil of severed elastin strands upon loss of tension [19,20]. Black arrows denote possible breaks in elastic fibers in lungs of mice exposed to SHS. Destruction of alveolar walls was assessed by counting numbers of breaks in elastic fibers and the numbers were significantly higher in smoke exposed animals (Figure 1b).

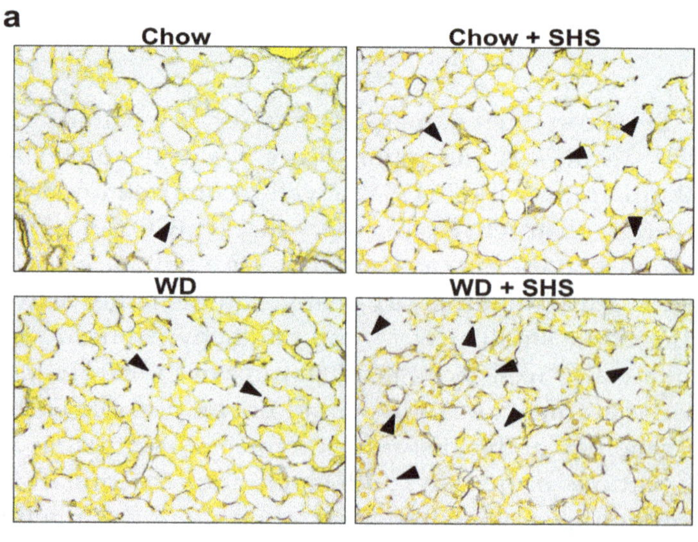

Figure 1. *Cont.*

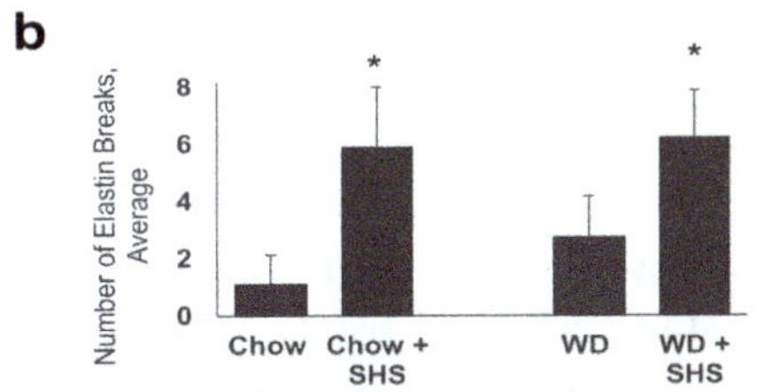

Figure 1. Hart's Elastin stained lung tissue sections from ApoE$^{-/-}$ mice. ApoE$^{-/-}$ mice were fed rodent chow without (Chow) or with second hand smoke exposure (Chow + SHS). Other groups were fed Western Diet without (WD) or with smoke exposure (WD + SHS). (**a**) Representative images are shown. Black arrows point out strand breaks in alveolar walls, 20x objective used. Destruction of alveolar walls was assessed by counting numbers of breaks in elastin fibers (**b**). Groups exposed to SHS scored significantly higher, the Kruskal-Wallis ANOVA on ranks was used to assess statistical significance between groups ($p < 0.001$) followed by post hoc testing with Dunn's multiple comparison test for groups of interest ($p < 0.05$), four to six mice per group were analyzed, * Significant difference detected.

To study the differences in airspace enlargement in lungs of ApoE$^{-/-}$ mice with or without cigarette smoke exposure we calculated the mean linear intercept length (MLI) [21] using Hematoxylin and Eosin stained lung tissue sections. As shown in Figure 2, the MLI was significantly higher in smoke exposed mice fed regular diet (Figure 2B) as well as in mice fed WD and exposed to smoke relative to non-smoking groups (Figure 2B).

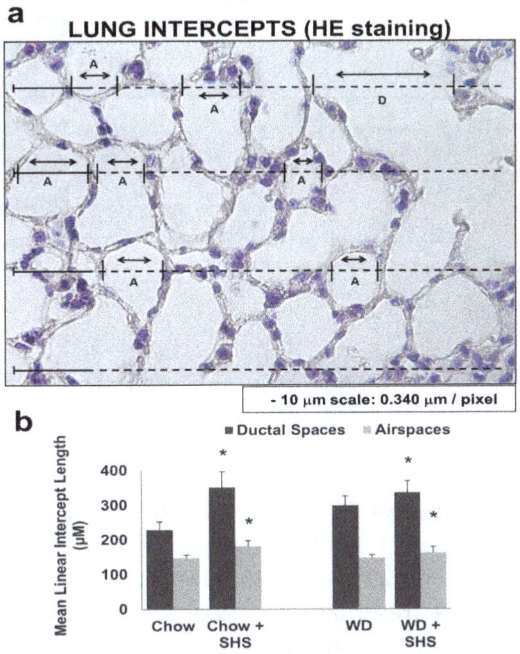

Figure 2. Morphometric analysis of lung sections from ApoE$^{-/-}$ mice fed rodent chow without (Chow) or with second hand smoke exposure (Chow + SHS) or fed Western Diet without (WD) or with smoke exposure (WD + SHS). Representative image of hematoxylin and eosin stained lung tissue section from ApoE$^{-/-}$ mice (Air spaces—A and Ductal spaces—D) (**a**). The MLI calculated using hematoxylin and eosin stained lung sections (**b**). Groups exposed to SHS scored significantly higher. For airspace group scores the Kruskal–Wallis ANOVA on ranks was used to assess statistical significance ($p < 0.001$) followed by post hoc testing with Dunn's multiple comparison test for Chow $\pm$ SHS groups ($p < 0.05$). As Dunn's test did not give a p value for the pairwise comparison of WD $\pm$ SHS groups, the non-parametric Mann-Whitney test with Bonferroni correction for multiple comparisons was used instead ($p = 0.016$). For ductal space group scores one way ANOVA was used ($p < 0.001$) followed by post hoc Fisher's least significant difference tests. Chow $\pm$ SHS ($p < 0.001$), WD $\pm$ SHS ($p = 0.004$), three to five mice per group were evaluated. * Significant difference detected.

2.2. *Exposure to SHS Triggers an Increase in Airway Wall Collagen in Lungs of ApoE$^{-/-}$ Mice*

Picro-Sirius Red stained lung sections were examined under plane polarized light to visualize collagen content of the airway walls. This method is known to have higher specificity for collagen as well as allowing differentiation between thick and fine fibers missed by traditional trichrome methods [22]. When viewed with polarized light the hue of collagen fibers is indicative of collagen fiber thickness with very fine fibers appearing green while thick fibers produce a yellow to orange/red birefringence with respect to increasing thickness [22]. As shown in Figure 3 the layer of airway collagen is wider and comprised much more of thick fibers in smoke exposed and/or western diet fed mice relative to non-smoking chow fed controls as indicated by the shift in birefringence (increased orange/red color). Statistical analysis is presented in Figure 3b.

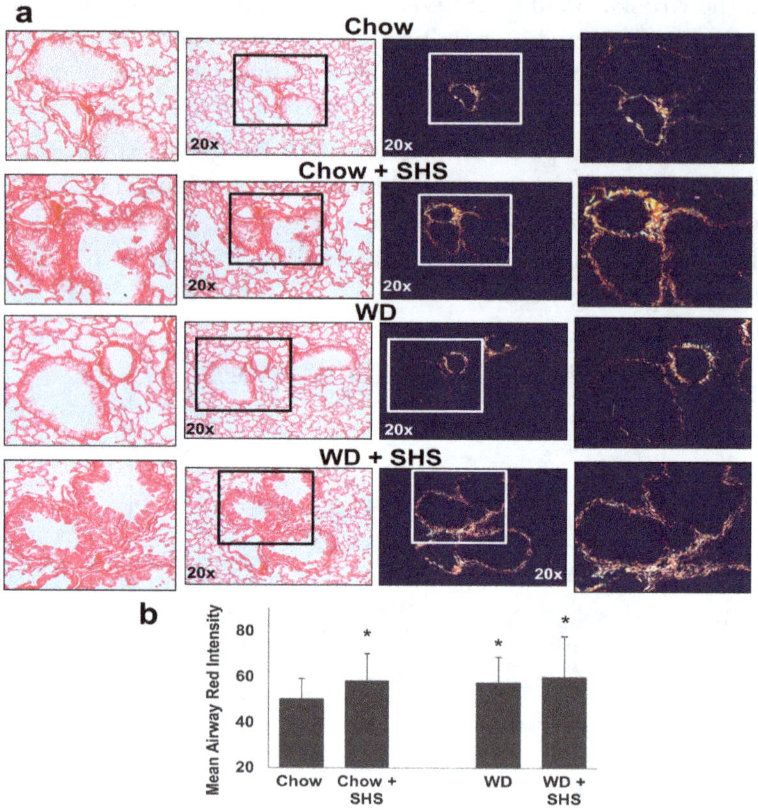

Figure 3. Collagen deposition in lungs of ApoE$^{-/-}$ mice fed rodent chow without (Chow) or with second hand smoke exposure (Chow + SHS) or fed Western Diet without (WD) or with smoke exposure (WD + SHS). Picro-sirius red stained lung tissue sections were viewed under regular light (left panels) or polarized light (right panels). Representative images are shown (**a**). Differences in intensity of red-orange birefringence from Picro-sirius red stained airways were evaluated using ImageJ software. Results were expressed as mean red component intensities (**b**). Groups exposed to SHS and/or WD scored significantly higher than the chow fed, air only group ($p < 0.05$). Kruskal-Wallis ANOVA on ranks was used to assess statistical significance between groups ($p < 0.001$) followed by post hoc testing with Dunn's multiple comparison test for groups of interest, four to five mice per group were evaluated. * Significant difference detected.

2.3. *Treatments with a Pharmacological Inhibitor of Btk or MMP-9 Specific siRNA Targeting Either Endothelial Cells or Neutrophils Causes a Decrease in Alveolar Changes Related to COPD Progression*

We subsequently applied long term treatments to ApoE$^{-/-}$ mice fed WD and exposed to SHS. As these mice had increased lung MMP-9 (Figure S1), treatments were designed to directly or indirectly reduce lung MMP-9 levels (Figure S2). The animals received either a pharmacologic inhibitor of Btk

(PCI-32765) or MMP-9 directed siRNA designed to minimize cell specific MMP-9 expression in endothelial cells or neutrophils. These treatments were protective in ApoE$^{-/-}$ mice fed WD and exposed to SHS.

Hart's Elastin stain was used to analyze airway destruction/strand breaks in alveolar walls of ApoE$^{-/-}$ mice exposed to cigarette smoke and treated with Btk inhibitor, or MMP-9 siRNA targeting endothelial cells and neutrophils. As shown in Figure 4, fewer elastin breaks were observed in lungs of mice treated with Btk inhibitor and with MMP-9 siRNA targeting endothelial cells (Figure 4) or neutrophils (Figure 5).

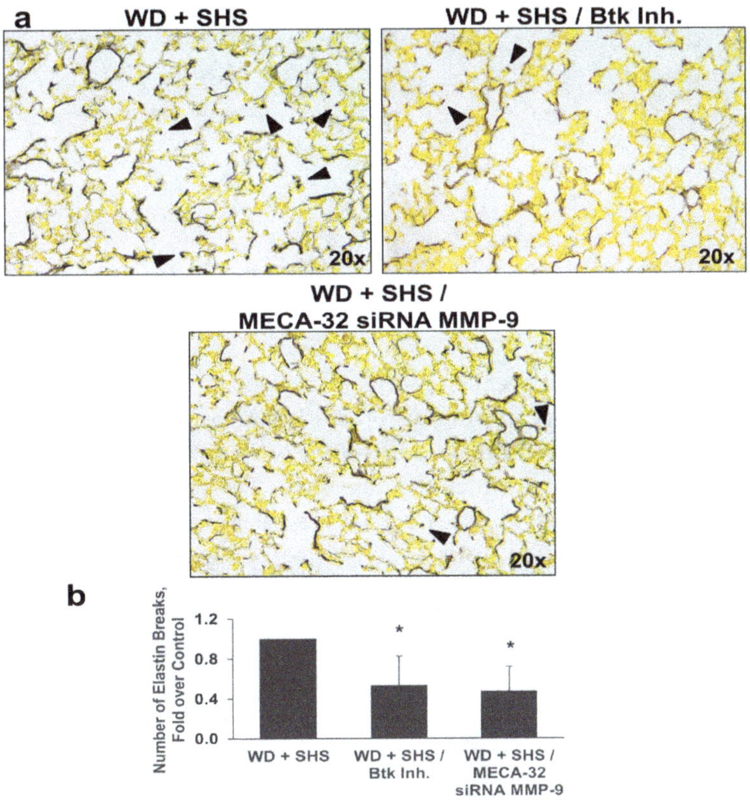

Figure 4. Analysis of alveolar elastin breaks in lungs of ApoE$^{-/-}$ mice fed WD and exposed to SHS only (WD + SHS), with Btk inhibitor treatment (WD + SHS/Btk Inh.), or treated with endothelial cell targeted siRNA for MMP-9 (WD + SHS/MECA-32 siRNA MMP-9). Representative images are shown. Black arrows point out strand breaks in alveolar walls (**a**). Destruction of alveolar walls was assessed by counting numbers of breaks in elastin fibers (**b**). Groups receiving treatment scored significantly lower than the control group ($p < 0.05$). Kruskal–Wallis ANOVA on ranks was used to assess statistical significance between groups ($p < 0.001$) followed by post hoc testing with Dunn's multiple comparison test for groups of interest, four to six mice per group were evaluated. * Significant difference detected.

Hematoxylin and eosin staining was used for morphometric analysis of airspace enlargement and to calculate MLI length which was significantly lower in mice that received the Btk inhibitor and MMP-9 siRNA targeting endothelial cells (Figure 6a), as well as in mice treated with MMP-9 directed siRNA designed to minimize cell specific MMP-9 expression in neutrophils (Figure 6b).

Moreover, we employed Picro-Sirius Red staining to analyze airway collagen deposition in lungs of ApoE$^{-/-}$ mice exposed to smoke and treated with Btk inhibitor or MMP-9 siRNA. As shown in Figure 7 there was a decrease in collagen deposition and less thick collagen fibers in treated animals relative to control mice. Collagen deposition in airways was significantly decreased in mice treated with the Btk inhibitor (Figure 7b). The difference in lung vasculature collagen content did not reach statistical significance for treated mice compared to untreated animals although vascular collagen content was substantially lower in mice that received endothelial cell targeted MMP-9 specific siRNA (Figure 7b).

We also noted a decrease in airway collagen deposition in mice that received neutrophil targeted MMP-9 directed siRNA (Figure 8a,b) and again vascular collagen content was substantially lower in mice that received neutrophil targeted MMP-9 specific siRNA but this difference did not reach statistical significance.

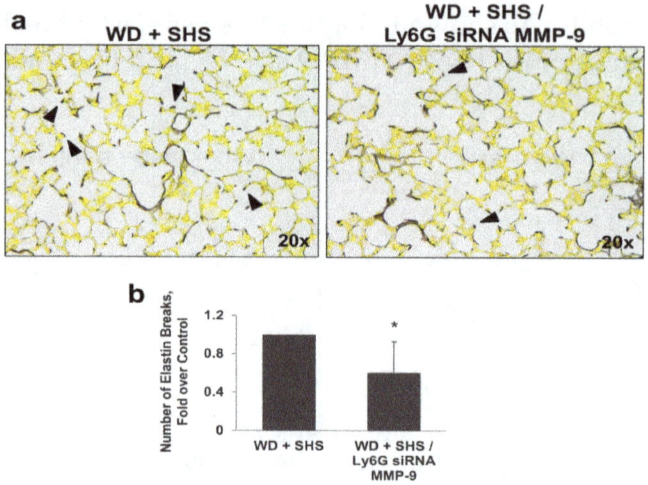

Figure 5. Analysis of alveolar elastin breaks in lungs of ApoE$^{-/-}$ mice fed WD and exposed to SHS only (WD + SHS) or treated with neutrophil targeted siRNA for MMP-9 (WD + SHS/Ly6G siRNA MMP-9). Black arrows point out strand breaks in alveolar walls (**a**). Destruction of alveolar walls was assessed by counting numbers of breaks in elastin fibers (**b**). The treatment group scored significantly lower than the control groups ($p < 0.001$). The non-parametric Mann–Whitney test was used to assess statistical significance between groups, four to five mice per group were analyzed. * Significant difference detected.

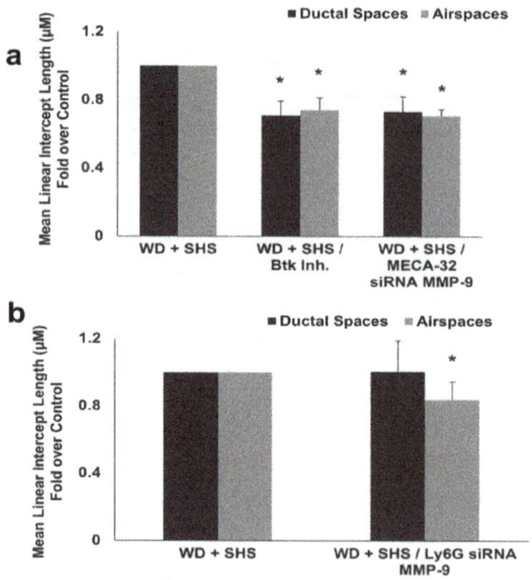

Figure 6. (**a**) Morphometric analysis of lungs from ApoE$^{-/-}$ mice fed WD and exposed to SHS only (WD + SHS), with Btk inhibitor treatment (WD + SHS/Btk Inh.), or treated with endothelial cell targeted siRNA for MMP-9 (WD + SHS/MECA-32 siRNA MMP-9) showed reduced scores in treatment groups ($p < 0.05$). Kruskal-Wallis ANOVA on ranks was used to assess statistical significance between groups ($p < 0.001$) followed by post hoc testing with Dunn's multiple comparison test for groups of interest, four to six animals per group were evaluated, with two groups of control animals combined. (**b**) Analysis of MLI in lungs of ApoE$^{-/-}$ mice fed WD and exposed to SHS or fed WD and exposed to SHS plus treatment with neutrophil targeted siRNA for MMP-9 (WD + SHS/Ly6G siRNA MMP-9) showed reduced scores in the treatment group ($p > 0.001$). Student's t-test was used to assess statistical significance, four mice per group were analyzed. * Significant difference detected.

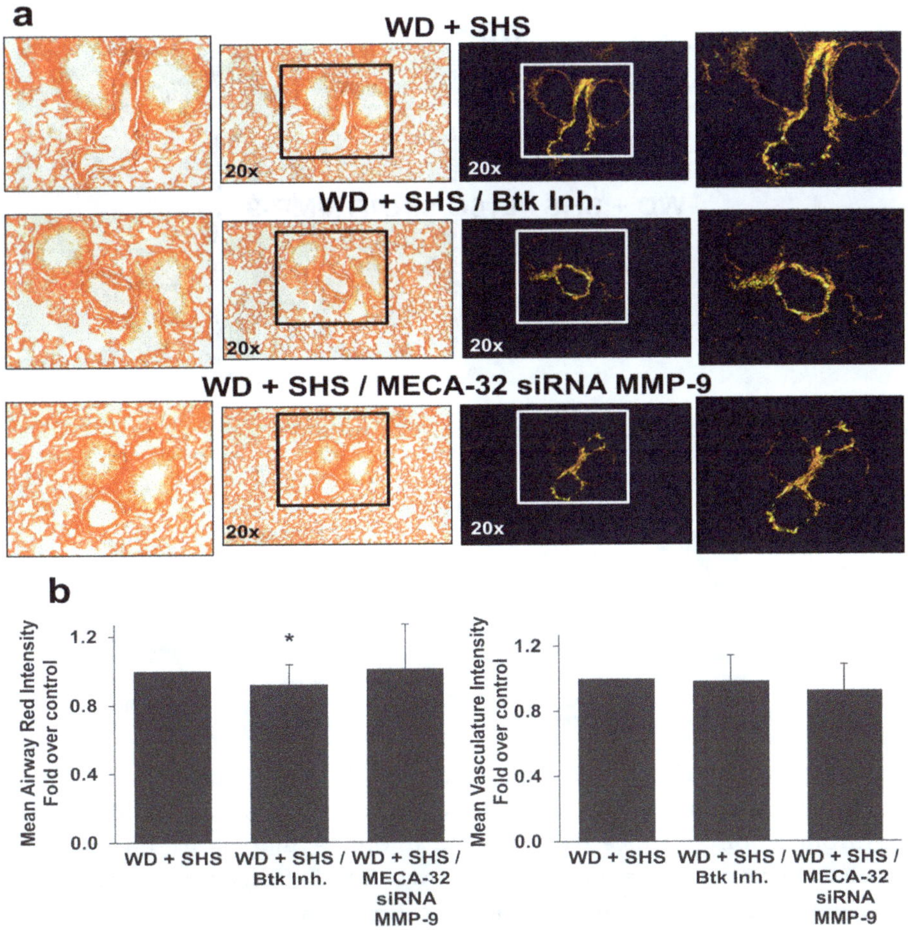

Figure 7. Collagen deposition in lungs of ApoE$^{-/-}$ mice fed WD and exposed to SHS only (WD + SHS), with Btk inhibitor treatment (WD + SHS/Btk Inh.), or treated with endothelial cell targeted siRNA for MMP-9 (WD + SHS/MECA32 siRNA MMP-9). Picro-sirius red stained lung sections from ApoE$^{-/-}$ mice were viewed under regular light (left panels) or polarized light (right panels). Representative images are shown (**a**). Differences in hue of Picro-sirius red stained airways were evaluated using ImageJ software. Results are expressed as mean red component intensities (airway) or mean total intensity (vasculature) (**b**). Btk inhibition or EC targeted MMP-9 specific siRNA impacted collagen deposition in the airways or lung vasculature respectively. Kruskal-Wallis ANOVA on ranks was used to assess statistical significance in red intensity between groups ($p < 0.081$). As Dunn's multiple comparison test was not possible we assessed the reduction observed in the Btk inhibitor treated group using the non-parametric Mann-Whitney test with Bonferroni correction for multiple comparisons ($p = 0.019$). For mean vascular intensity one way ANOVA was used to assess differences between groups ($p = 0.227$) and as Fishers least significant difference test was not possible, we assessed the reduction observed in the MECA-32 siRNA MMP-9 treated group using Student's t-test with Bonferroni correction for multiple comparison ($p = 0.097$), four to six animals per group were evaluated, with two groups of control animals combined. * Significant difference detected.

Finally, we tested the level of MMP-9 in lung homogenates of ApoE$^{-/-}$ mice exposed to smoke and treated with Btk inhibitor and MMP-9 siRNA targeting endothelial cells and neutrophils. Figure 9a and supplemental Figure S3 shows that the level of MMP-9 is reduced in mice that received the Btk inhibitor as well as animals that were treated with MMP-9 directed siRNA targeted to endothelial cells. Reduced lung MMP-9 in animals treated with MMP-9 directed siRNA targeting neutrophils is shown in Figure 9b.

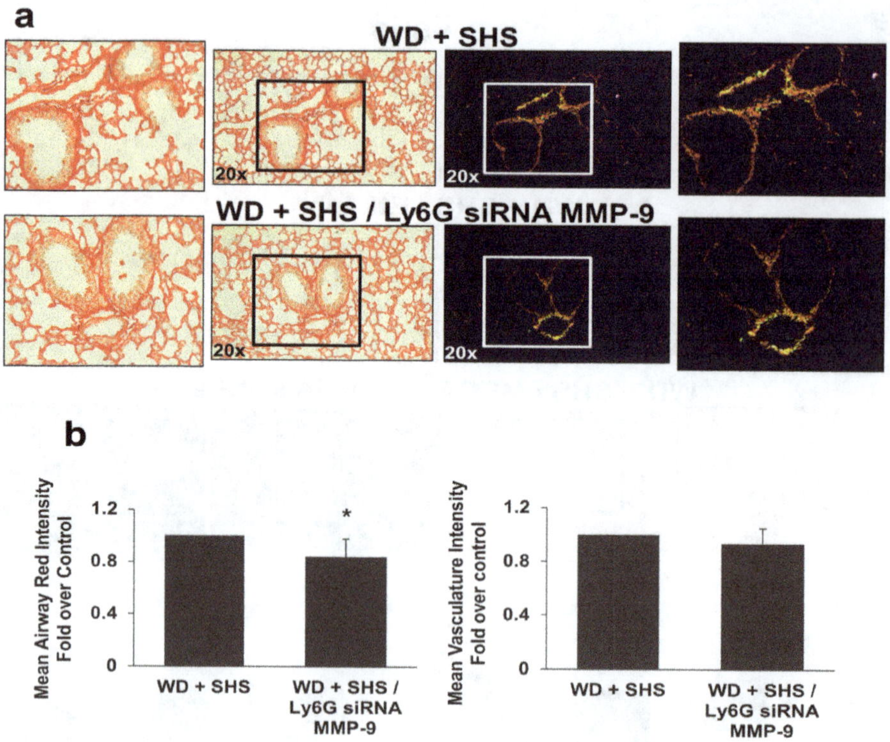

Figure 8. Collagen deposition in lungs of ApoE$^{-/-}$ mice fed WD and exposed to SHS only (WD + SHS), or treated with PMN targeted siRNA for MMP-9 (WD + SHS/Ly6G siRNA MMP-9). Picro-sirius red stained sections from ApoE$^{-/-}$ mice were viewed under regular light (left panels) or polarized light (right panels). Representative images are shown (**a**). Differences in hue of Picro-sirius red stained airways were evaluated using ImageJ software. Results are expressed as mean red component intensities (airway) or mean total intensity (vasculature) (**b**). PMN targeted MMP-9 specific siRNA impacted collagen deposition. The non-parametric Mann-Whitney test (airway, $p > 0.001$) or Student's t-test (vasculature, $p = 0.098$) were used to assess statistical significance between groups as indicated by group normality, five mice per group were evaluated. * Significant difference detected.

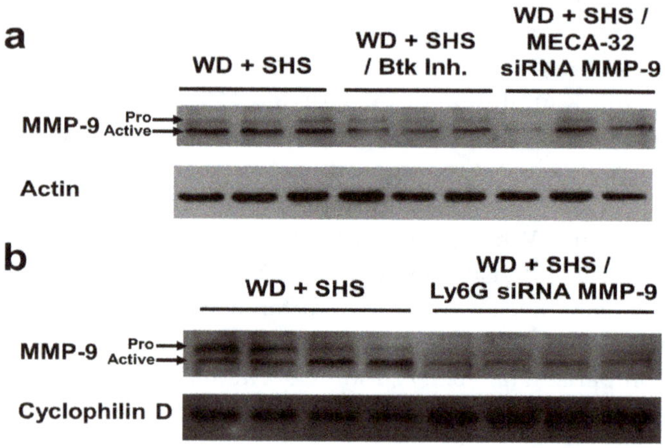

Figure 9. Levels of MMP-9 in lung homogenates (**a**). Western blot from ApoE$^{-/-}$ mice fed WD and exposed to SHS only (WD + SHS), with Btk inhibitor treatment (WD + SHS/Btk Inh.), or treated with endothelial cell targeted siRNA for MMP-9 (WD + SHS/MECA-32 siRNA MMP-9). Three mice per group were analyzed (**b**). Western Blot from ApoE$^{-/-}$ mice fed WD and exposed to SHS only (WD + SHS) or treated with neutrophil targeted siRNA (WD + SHS/Ly6G siRNA MMP-9). Four animals per group were analyzed.

3. Discussion

Emphysema/COPD, a smoking-related complex inflammatory airway disease, is the third leading cause of death in the United States [1,3]. Persistent chronic inflammation associated with COPD eventually triggers irreversible tissue destruction [1]. Current treatments for COPD do not effectively inhibit chronic inflammation or reverse the pathology of disease, and at the same token do not successfully target the factors that initiate and drive the long-term progression of disease. Regrettably treatment options are very limited and mainly focus on improving quality of life [2]. This limitation is due to a lack of understanding for the mechanisms and mediators that drive the induction and progression of chronic inflammation, emphysema and altered lung function. It should be stressed that airflow limitation in COPD is not fully reversible. At present, casual interventions that can stop progression of this disease are not available [1]. There is a clear need for new therapies that can prevent the induction and progression of COPD [3].

Animal models remain essential for the development of novel therapies. Exposure of mice to cigarette smoke triggers characteristic features of human COPD including the accumulation of pro-inflammatory cells and mediators, small airway fibrosis/remodeling, mucus hypersecretion, lung dysfunction, and the development of emphysema. In addition, models that mimic systemic co-morbidities are equally important [3–8]. Moreover, existing treatments for COPD are mainly focused on symptom alleviation (especially dyspnea) and reduction in exacerbations [2,23]. A hallmark of COPD is an enhanced inflammatory immune response in the airway and the lung. Targeting this pathway is a logical approach to the treatment of COPD [2].

Vascular abnormalities are well known as comorbidities of COPD [24,25]. They include endothelial dysfunction, arterial stiffness and atherogenesis. Furthermore pulmonary vascular collagen deposition is observed in patients with mild COPD as well as smokers suggesting it too contributes to the web of comorbidities associated with COPD [26]. Similarly, cardiovascular problems go hand in hand with decline in lung function in smokers. In addition, recent studies indicate that vascular inflammation, endothelial dysfunction and oxidative modification of lipids may contribute to the pathogenesis of COPD [25,27,28]. Therefore, it comes as no surprise that abnormal morphology and a substantial decrease in lung function are found in ApoE$^{-/-}$ mice which are susceptible to cardiovascular issues and are prone to atherosclerosis [4–7,29]. Exposure to cigarette smoke causes premature emphysema, abnormal lung inflammation, and airspace enlargement with altered mechanical properties in lungs of these mice [4–7]. Additionally, deposition of thick collagen fibers around airways in smoke exposed animals, a suspected source of increased airway stiffness and associated airway resistance, was observed as well as vascular deposition. These observations have also been reported in an elastase induced emphysema mouse model [20]. In the study we employed atherosclerosis prone apolipoprotein E deficient (ApoE$^{-/-}$) mice as an animal model which mimics systemic co-morbidities of COPD and accurately reflects the corresponding clinical disease [4–7,15]. Our findings in this emerging comorbidity model revealed reduced alveolar changes associated with COPD progression in cigarette exposed ApoE$^{-/-}$ mice treated with either Btk inhibitor, or siRNA directed to MMP-9. Previous studies have made direct comparisons of lung alterations in ApoE$^{-/-}$ and WT mice are made in the context of smoke exposure and western diet/HFD respectively. In one such study relative to WT mice ApoE$^{-/-}$ mice were shown to have similar if not greater lung macrophage and neutrophil numbers following SHS exposure, as well as higher levels of lipid peroxidation, chemokines (MCP-1 and KC), MMP-9 and MMP-12, greater mean linear intercept, and reduced eNOS activity. Additionally several of these factors were increased significantly in ApoE$^{-/-}$ mice relative to WT mice without smoke exposure [5]. Another study showed ApoE$^{-/-}$ mice fed a high fat/high cholesterol (western) diet for 12 weeks had significantly increased septal thickening and mean linear intercepts relative to WT mice fed western diets and ApoE$^{-/-}$ mice fed a standard chow diet as well as increases in CD68 and TLR4 positive cells in lung tissue. Furthermore ApoE$^{-/-}$ mice fed a western diet had significantly higher BALF TNF-α, IL-4, IL-6, IL-17, and IFN-γ compared to normal chow fed ApoE$^{-/-}$

mice [29]. Additionally, recent reviews contain excellent discussions on the emergence of this model in CVD/COPD comorbidity studies [4,30].

Btk plays a critical role in the pathophysiology of inflammatory lung diseases [11,12]. Therefore, we hypothesized that it may also contribute to alveolar changes related to progression of COPD. Indeed, administration of a specific pharmacological inhibitor of Btk was protective in ApoE$^{-/-}$ mice fed WD and exposed to SHS. Further, MMPs, and specifically MMP-9, have been implicated in pathogenesis of COPD [14]. Brajer et al. showed a correlation between higher concentrations of MMP-9 in serum and increased progression of systematic inflammation in COPD patients [23]. Significantly, recent studies from our laboratory indicate that Btk may regulate expression of MMP-9 in lungs [11,12]. In agreement with this observation, we have noted a decrease in MMP-9 levels in lungs of mice treated with a Btk inhibitor. Moreover, animals that received siRNA specific for MMP-9 targeted to endothelial cells or neutrophils through conjugation with F(ab′)$_2$ fragments of cell specific markers MECA-32 and Ly6G 1A8 respectively displayed diminished alveolar changes related to COPD progression. Meijer et al. also implicated the importance of neutrophil involvement in COPD [31]; interestingly Btk inhibition may moderate neutrophil activity regarding excessive inflammation in the lungs. Both Btk and MMP-9 appear to be attractive targets for alleviation of COPD progression.

One limitation of our current research design involved using a pharmacological inhibitor of Btk which was capable of inhibiting Btk in cell types other than neutrophils. However, silencing Btk specifically in neutrophils is a viable route for future experiments; a method utilizing cell-specific siRNA targeting Btk in neutrophils has been previously established in our laboratory [12]. Further studies with a cell-specific siRNA for Btk may be ideal for targeting desired cell types within the lungs. Furthermore, our study design employed intravenous injection of both the Btk inhibitor and siRNA conjugates. Although this method is known to allow treatments such as ours to enter the lungs [32], an intranasal approach may potentially improve lung specific cell targeting, and therefore be a preferred approach for future studies involving siRNA-based treatments. This study is further limited by the lack of non-specific (scrambled) siRNA control treatment groups. However, in a previous publication from our lab [12] we demonstrated specificity of MMP-9 directed siRNA relative to control (scrambled) siRNA in vivo in neutrophils alongside BTK directed siRNA, additionally the Btk directed siRNA specificity was shown in vitro relative to control siRNA. In the previously employed short duration model fewer treatments were required and including these controls was both necessary for establishing specificity and economically feasible. For an experimental duration such as we used here with a premium modified siRNA product, unfortunately, addition of control siRNA groups was cost prohibitive. The siRNA used in both studies is a very high quality product which we have had great success with, therefore it was felt that addition of this control group would not alter the results obtained under the current design. Additionally, the current study observed silencing of MMP-9 exclusively in endothelial cells and neutrophils. Future studies regarding both Btk and MMP-9 in other cell types such as macrophages are of interest for our lab and perhaps others [33]. Irrespective of the limitations, our findings provide evidence that through Btk signaling MMP-9 may play a significant role in the development of lung inflammation and ultimately the progression of COPD.

4. Methods

4.1. Animal Studies

All studies involving animals were approved by the IACUC (Institutional Animal Care and Use Committee) at the University of Texas Health Science Center at Tyler (protocol 514, initial approval received 04/25/2012), and conform to National Institutes of Health guidelines. Age matched female Murine Pathogen Free ApoE$^{-/-}$ mice were divided into four treatment groups consisting of either animals fed a high fat, high cholesterol Western Diet (WD) (D12079B, Research Diets Inc., New Brunswick, NJ, USA) with and without SHS exposure or animals fed standard rodent chow (PicoLab Rodent Diet 20, LabDiet, St. Louis, MO, USA) with and without SHS exposure. Mice were exposed to passive cigarette smoke using a whole-body smoke exposure system (TE-10B, Teague Enterprises, Woodland, CA, USA), as previously described [16]. Briefly, mice were exposed to a combination of 11% mainstream and 89% side stream smoke from 40 3R4F reference cigarettes twice daily, 5 days a week for up to 11 weeks. Control (nonsmoking) animals were exposed to ambient air only. Treatment animals were injected intravenously [tail vein injection] with either Bruton's tyrosine kinase inhibitor (BTK Inh) PCI-32765 (Selleck Chemicals, Houston, TX, USA) or siRNA specific for MMP-9 (Invitrogen, Carlsbad, CA, USA) conjugated with $F(ab')_2$ fragments of anti-mouse neutrophil antibody (clone Ly-6G 1A8, Bio X Cell, West Lebanon, NH, USA) or anti-mouse endothelial cell antibody (clone MECA-32, Bio X Cell). $F(ab')_2$ fragments were generated with Pierce $F(ab')_2$ Preparation Kit (Thermo Fisher Scientific, Waltham, MA, USA) and conjugated to a siRNA carrier using T3-Max Conjugation Kits (Bioo Scientific, Austin, TX, USA). Treatments began after 7 weeks of WD/SHS exposure and lasted 2 or 4 weeks while continuing regular WD/SHS exposure. Control animals were exposed only to WD/SHS throughout the experiments. Five to six animals per treatment group and four to five animals per control group were used.

Following SHS exposure with/without treatment, mice were euthanized and the thoracic cavity was opened; blood was collected directly from the right ventricle. The renal vein was then cut and excess blood was flushed from the vasculature through the heart with cold PBS. The largest lung lobe was fixed for histology using ExCell Plus (American MasterTech, Lodi, CA, USA) and the remaining lobes were homogenized for further analysis.

4.2. Histochemical Evaluation of Emphysemic Changes

For histochemical analysis, fixed lungs were embedded in paraffin and sectioned for staining. Tissue sections were stained with Hart's Elastin, Picro-Sirius Red (PSR), Hematoxylin and Eosin.

Differences in hue of PSR red stained airways were evaluated using ImageJ software. For airway analysis images were converted to RGB format, then the airway was selected as the region of interest (ROI) and mean intensities of only the red components were measured to exclude background and thin (green) fibers. Results were expressed as red intensity for each ROI. Differences in lung vasculature collagen content were measured in ImageJ by converting color images to gray-scale, selecting vasculature as the ROI, and measuring mean intensities. MLI was calculated to quantify airspace enlargement according to a previously described method [21] using Hematoxylin and Eosin stained lung tissue sections. Hart's Elastin stained lung sections were employed to analyze a destruction of alveolar walls (breaks in elastic fibers) [17–20].

4.3. Western Blotting

Lung homogenates were normalized for equal protein concentration based on Bradford assay results, denatured in reducing Laemmle sample buffer, and then loaded into SDS-PAGE gel. Separated proteins were transferred to a polyvinylidene difluoride membrane (Pall Corp., Port Washington, NY, USA). The membrane was blocked and incubated with anti-MMP-9 antibody (C-20), anti-Actin antibody (I-19), or anti-cyclophilin D antibody (C-14) (Santa Cruz Biotechnology, Dallas, TX, USA) followed by HRP conjugated secondary antibodies (Jackson ImmunoResearch, West Grove, PA, USA). Bound antibodies were detected using enhanced chemiluminescence reagents (Bio-Rad Clarity ECL, Hercules, CA, USA). Finally, the membrane was exposed to X-ray film (HXR0810, Hawkins X-Ray Supply, Oneonta, AL, USA).

4.4. Statistics

Results are expressed as the mean $\pm$ STD. Differences between multiple groups were evaluated by one way ANOVA or the non-parametric Kruskal-Wallis ANOVA on ranks as dictated by variance/normality followed by post hoc analysis with Fisher's least significant difference test or Dunn's multiple comparison test respectively. In cases where Dunn's test was unable to yield a direct evaluation for significance comparisons between groups of interest were performed using the nonparametric

Mann-Whitney test with Bonferroni correction for multiple comparisons. Differences between paired groups were evaluated with Student's *t*-test or the non-parametric Mann-Whitney rank sum test as dictated by variance/normality. The specific analyses used are indicated in individual figure legends. All statistics were performed using SIGMAPLOT 11 (Systat Software Inc., San Jose, CA, USA). Significance was defined as $p < 0.05$.

5. Conclusions

Cell specific targeting of Bruton's tyrosine kinase (Btk) and/or matrix metalloproteinase-9 (MMP-9) may have potential as treatments for COPD in patients. Inhibition of Btk showed promising protective effects in the lungs of our animal model, WD fed, SHS exposed $ApoE^{-/-}$ mice. Similarly, silencing MMP-9 in endothelial cells or neutrophils considerably diminished the progression of COPD characteristics in this animal model. Focusing prospective treatment options around disrupting the Btk pathway may prove to be ideal pursuits for future clinical research in COPD.

Acknowledgments: We wish to thank William Sorensen for advice on statistical methods. This work was supported by Flight Attendant Medical Research Institute (FAMRI ID# 113016_CIA) awarded to Anna K. Kurdowska.

Author Contributions: Authors responsible for concepts and design were Anna K. Kurdowska and Jon M. Florence. Jon M. Florence, Anna K. Kurdowska and Agnieszka Krupa contributed to data collection. Anna K. Kurdowska, Jon M. Florence, Agnieszka Krupa, Laela M. Booshehri and Adrian L. Gajewski were responsible for the analysis and interpretation of data. Anna K. Kurdowska and Jon M. Florence drafted the manuscript.

Abbreviations

$ApoE^{-/-}$	apolipoprotein E-deficient
Btk	Bruton's tyrosine kinase
Btk Inh.	Bruton's tyrosine kinase inhibitor PCI-32765 (Ibrutinib)
COPD	Chronic obstructive pulmonary disease
Ly6G	Monoclonal antibody (clone 1A8) against Lymphocyte Antigen 6 Complex Locus G, a specific marker of mouse neutrophils
MECA-32	Monoclonal antibody (clone MECA-32) against mouse pan-endothelial cell antigen, a specific marker of mouse endothelial cells
MMPs	matrix metalloproteinases
MMP-9	matrix metalloproteinase-9
PSR	picro-sirius red
SHS	second hand smoke
WD	Western Diet

References

1. Birru, R.L.; Di, Y.P. Pathogenic mechanism of second hand smoke induced inflammation and COPD. *Front. Physiol.* **2012**, *3*, 348. [CrossRef] [PubMed]
2. Pappas, K.; Papaioannou, A.I.; Kostikas, K.; Tzanakis, N. The role of macrophages in obstructive airways disease: Chronic obstructive pulmonary disease and asthma. *Cytokine* **2013**, *64*, 613–625. [CrossRef] [PubMed]
3. Vlahos, R.; Bozinovski, S. Recent advances in pre-clinical mouse models of COPD. *Clin. Sci.* **2014**, *126*, 253–265. [CrossRef] [PubMed]
4. Lo Sasso, G.; Schlage, W.K.; Boué, S.; Veljkovic, E.; Peitsch, M.C.; Hoeng, J. The $ApoE^{-/-}$ mouse model: A suitable model to study cardiovascular and respiratory diseases in the context of cigarette smoke exposure and harm reduction. *J. Transl. Med.* **2016**, *14*, 146. [CrossRef] [PubMed]

5. Arunachalam, G.; Sundar, I.K.; Hwang, J.; Yao, H.; Rahman, I. Emphysema is associated with increased inflammation in lungs of atherosclerosis-prone mice by cigarette smoke: Implications in comorbidities of COPD. *J. Inflamm.* **2010**, *7*, 34. [CrossRef] [PubMed]
6. Titz, B.; Boué, S.; Phillips, B.; Talikka, M.; Vihervaara, T.; Schneider, T.; Nury, C.; Elamin, A.; Guedj, E.; Peck, M.J.; et al. Effects of Cigarette Smoke, Cessation, and Switching to Two Heat-Not-Burn Tobacco Products on Lung Lipid Metabolism in C57BL/6 and ApoE$^{-/-}$ Mice—An Integrative Systems Toxicology Analysis. *Toxicol. Sci.* **2016**, *149*, 441–457. [CrossRef] [PubMed]
7. Naura, A.S.; Hans, C.P.; Zerfaoui, M.; Errami, Y.; Ju, J.; Kim, H.; Matrougui, K.; Kim, J.G.; Boulares, A.H. High-fat diet induces lung remodeling in ApoE-deficient mice: An association with an increase in circulatory and lung inflammatory factors. *Lab. Investig.* **2009**, *89*, 1243–1251. [CrossRef] [PubMed]
8. Beckett, E.L.; Stevens, R.L.; Jarnicki, A.G.; Kim, R.Y.; Hanish, I.; Hansbro, N.G.; Deane, A.; Keely, S.; Horvat, J.C.; Yang, M.; et al. A new short-term mouse model of chronic obstructive pulmonary disease identifies a role for mast cell tryptase in pathogenesis. *J. Allergy Clin. Immunol.* **2013**, *131*, 752–762. [CrossRef] [PubMed]
9. Jobse, B.N.; McCurry, C.A.; Morissette, M.C.; Rhem, R.G.; Stampfli, M.R.; Labiris, N.R. Impact of inflammation, emphysema, and smoking cessation on V/Q in mouse models of lung obstruction. *Respir. Res.* **2014**, *15*, 42. [CrossRef] [PubMed]
10. Boue, S.; de Leon, H.; Schlage, W.K.; Peck, M.J.; Weiler, H.; Berges, A.; Vuillaume, G.; Martin, F.; Friedrichs, B.; Lebrun, S.; et al. Cigarette smoke induces molecular responses in respiratory tissues of ApoE$^{-/-}$ mice that are progressively deactivated upon cessation. *Toxicology* **2013**, *314*, 112–124. [CrossRef] [PubMed]
11. Krupa, A.; Fudala, R.; Florence, J.M.; Tucker, T.; Allen, T.C.; Standiford, T.J.; Luchowski, R.; Fol, M.; Rahman, M.; Gryczynski, Z.; et al. Bruton's tyrosine kinase mediates cross-talk between FcγRIIa and TLR4 signaling cascades in human neutrophils. *Am. J. Respir. Cell Mol. Biol.* **2013**, *48*, 240–249. [CrossRef] [PubMed]
12. Krupa, A.; Fol, M.; Rahman, M.; Stokes, K.Y.; Florence, J.M.; Leskov, I.L.; Khoretonenko, M.V.; Matthay, M.A.; Liu, K.D.; Calfee, C.S.; et al. Silencing Bruton's tyrosine kinase in alveolar neutrophils protects mice from LPS/immune complex induced acute lung injury. *Am. J. Physiol.-Lung Cell. Mol. Physiol.* **2014**, *307*, L435–L448. [CrossRef] [PubMed]
13. Jefferies, C.A.; Doyle, S.; Brunner, C.; Dunne, A.; Brint, E.; Wietek, C.; Walch, E.; Wirth, T.; O'Neill, L.A. Bruton's tyrosine kinase is a Toll/interleukin-1 receptor domain-binding protein that participates in nuclear factor κB activation by Toll-like receptor 4. *J. Biol. Chem.* **2003**, *278*, 26258–26264. [CrossRef] [PubMed]
14. Churg, A.; Zhou, S.; Wright, J.L. Series "matrix metalloproteinases in lung health and disease": Matrix metalloproteinases in COPD. *Eur. Respir. J.* **2012**, *39*, 197–209. [CrossRef] [PubMed]
15. Phillips, B.; Veljkovic, E.; Boue, S.; Schlage, W.K.; Vuillaume, G.; Martin, F.; Titz, B.; Leroy, P.; Buettner, A.; Elamin, A.; et al. An 8-Month Systems Toxicology Inhalation/Cessation Study in ApoE$^{-/-}$ Mice to Investigate Cardiovascular and Respiratory Exposure Effects of a Candidate Modified Risk Tobacco Product, THS 2.2, Compared With Conventional Cigarettes. *Toxicol. Sci.* **2016**, *149*, 411–432. [CrossRef] [PubMed]
16. Florence, J.M.; Krupa, A.; Booshehri, L.M.; Allen, T.C.; Kurdowska, A.K. Metalloproteinase-9 contributes to endothelial dysfunction in atherosclerosis via protease activated receptor-1. *PLoS ONE* **2017**, *12*, e0171427. [CrossRef] [PubMed]
17. Podowski, M.; Calvi, C.; Metzger, S.; Misono, K.; Poonyagariyagorn, H.; Lopez-Mercado, A.; Ku, T.; Lauer, T.; McGrath-Morrow, S.; Berger, A.; et al. Angiotensin receptor blockade attenuates cigarette smoke-induced lung injury and rescues lung architecture in mice. *J. Clin. Investig.* **2012**, *122*, 229–240. [CrossRef] [PubMed]
18. Simon, D.M.; Tsai, L.W.; Ingenito, E.P.; Starcher, B.C.; Mariani, T.J. PPARgamma deficiency results in reduced lung elastic recoil and abnormalities in airspace distribution. *Respir. Res.* **2010**, *11*, 69. [CrossRef] [PubMed]
19. Lucey, E.C.; Goldstein, R.H.; Stone, P.J.; Snider, G.L. Remodeling of alveolar walls after elastase treatment of hamsters. Results of elastin and collagen mRNA in situ hybridization. *Am. J. Respir. Crit. Care Med.* **1998**, *158*, 555–564. [CrossRef] [PubMed]
20. Oliveira, M.V.; Abreu, S.C.; Padilha, G.A.; Rocha, N.N.; Maia, L.A.; Takiya, C.M.; Xisto, D.G.; Suki, B.; Silva, P.L.; Rocco, P.R.M. Characterization of a Mouse Model of Emphysema Induced by Multiple Instillations of Low-Dose Elastase. *Front. Physiol.* **2016**, *7*, 457. [CrossRef] [PubMed]

21. Knudsen, L.; Weibel, E.; Gundersen, H.J.G.; Weinstein, F.V.; Ochs, M. Assessment of air space size characteristics by intercept (chord) measurement: An accurate and efficient stereological approach. *J. Appl. Physiol.* **2010**, *108*, 412–421. [CrossRef] [PubMed]
22. Wright, J.L.; Postma, D.S.; Kerstjens, H.A.M.; Timens, W.; Whittaker, P.; Churg, A. Airway remodeling in the smoke exposed guinea pig model. *Inhal. Toxicol.* **2007**, *19*, 915–923. [CrossRef] [PubMed]
23. Brajer, B.; Batura-Gabryel, H.; Nowicka, A.; Kuznar-Kaminska, B.; Szczepanik, A. Concentration of matrix metalloproteinase-9 in serum of patients with chronic obstructive pulmonary disease and a degree of airway obstruction and disease progression. *J. Physiol. Pharmacol.* **2008**, *59*, 145–152. [PubMed]
24. McAllister, D.A.; Maclay, J.D.; Mills, N.L.; Mair, G.; Miller, J.; Anderson, D.; Newby, D.E.; Murchison, J.T.; Macnee, W. Arterial Stiffness Is Independently Associated with Emphysema Severity in Patients with Chronic Obstructive Pulmonary Disease. *Am. J. Respir. Crit. Care Med.* **2007**, *176*, 1208–1214. [CrossRef] [PubMed]
25. Strulovici-Barel, Y.; Staudt, M.R.; Krause, A.; Gordon, C.; Tilley, A.E.; Harvey, B.G.; Kaner, R.J.; Hollmann, C.; Mezey, J.G.; Bitter, H.; et al. Persistence of circulating endothelial microparticles in COPD despite smoking cessation. *Thorax* **2016**, *71*, 1137–1144. [CrossRef] [PubMed]
26. Santos, S.; Peinado, V.I.; Ramírez, J.; Melgosa, T.; Roca, J.; Rodriguez-Roisin, R.; Barbera, J.A. Characterization of pulmonary vascular remodelling in smokers and patients with mild COPD. *Eur. Respir. J.* **2002**, *19*, 632–638. [CrossRef] [PubMed]
27. Can, U.; Yerlikaya, F.H.; Yosunkaya, S. Role of oxidative stress and serum lipid levels in stable chronic obstructive pulmonary disease. *J. Chin. Med. Assoc.* **2015**, *78*, 702–708. [CrossRef] [PubMed]
28. Austin, V.; Crack, P.J.; Bozinovski, S.; Miller, A.A.; Ross Vlahos, R. COPD and stroke: Are systemic inflammation and oxidative stress the missing links? *Clin. Sci.* **2016**, *130*, 1039–1050. [CrossRef] [PubMed]
29. Ouyang, Q.; Huang, Z.; Lin, H.; Ni, J.; Lu, H.; Chen, X.; Wang, Z.; Lin, L. Apolipoprotein E deficiency and high-fat diet cooperate to trigger lipidosis and inflammation in the lung via the Toll-like receptor 4 pathway. *Mol. Med. Rep.* **2015**, *12*, 2589–2597. [CrossRef] [PubMed]
30. Khedoe, P.P.; Rensen, P.C.; Berbée, J.F.; Hiemstra, P.S. Murine models of cardiovascular comorbidity in chronic obstructive pulmonary disease. *Am. J. Physiol.-Lung Cell. Mol. Physiol.* **2016**, *310*, L1011–L1027. [CrossRef] [PubMed]
31. Meijer, M.; Rijkers, G.T.; Van Overveld, F.J. Neutrophils and emerging targets for treatment in chronic obstructive pulmonary disease. *Expert Rev. Clin. Immunol.* **2013**, *9*, 1055–1068. [CrossRef] [PubMed]
32. Merkel, O.M.; Rubinstein, I.; Kissel, T. siRNA delivery to the lung: What's new? *Adv. Drug Deliv. Rev.* **2014**, *75*, 112–128. [CrossRef] [PubMed]
33. Barnes, P.J. Alveolar macrophages as orchestrators of COPD. *COPD* **2004**, *1*, 59–70. [CrossRef] [PubMed]

6

Fungi in Bronchiectasis: A Concise Review

Luis Máiz [1], Rosa Nieto [1], Rafael Cantón [2], Elia Gómez G. de la Pedrosa [2] and Miguel Ángel Martinez-García [3,*]

1 Servicio de Neumología, Unidad de Bronquiectasias y Fibrosis Quística, Hospital Universitario Ramón y Cajal, 28034 Madrid, Spain; luis.maiz@salud.madrid.org (L.M.); rosanr23@hotmail.com (R.N.)

2 Servicio de Microbiología, Hospital Universitario Ramón y Cajal and Instituto Ramón y Cajal de Investigación Sanitaria (IRYCIS), 28034 Madrid, Spain; rafael.canton@salud.madrid.org (R.C.); elia.gomez@gmail.com (E.G.G.d.l.P.)

3 Servicio de Neumología, Hospital Universitario y Politécnico la Fe, 46016 Valencia, Spain

* Correspondence: mianmartinezgarcia@gmail.com

Abstract: Although the spectrum of fungal pathology has been studied extensively in immunosuppressed patients, little is known about the epidemiology, risk factors, and management of fungal infections in chronic pulmonary diseases like bronchiectasis. In bronchiectasis patients, deteriorated mucociliary clearance—generally due to prior colonization by bacterial pathogens—and thick mucosity propitiate, the persistence of fungal spores in the respiratory tract. The most prevalent fungi in these patients are *Candida albicans* and *Aspergillus fumigatus;* these are almost always isolated with bacterial pathogens like *Haemophillus influenzae* and *Pseudomonas aeruginosa*, making very difficult to define their clinical significance. Analysis of the mycobiome enables us to detect a greater diversity of microorganisms than with conventional cultures. The results have shown a reduced fungal diversity in most chronic respiratory diseases, and that this finding correlates with poorer lung function. Increased knowledge of both the mycobiome and the complex interactions between the fungal, viral, and bacterial microbiota, including mycobacteria, will further our understanding of the mycobiome's relationship with the pathogeny of bronchiectasis and the development of innovative therapies to combat it.

Keywords: bronchiectasis; fungi; yeast; filamentous fungi; *Candida albicans*; *Aspergillus*; allergic bronchopulmonary aspergillosis; mycobiome

---

1. Introduction

Bronchiectasis is defined as chronic inflammatory bronchial disease with irreversible dilation of the bronchial lumen, and it can occur for a number of reasons. Clinically speaking, it usually presents itself with chronic cough and expectoration, and also with recurrent infectious exacerbations. It is mostly accompanied by chronic bacterial infection, as well as isolated yeast and filamentous fungi or molds whose pathogenic role has not yet been clarified [1,2].

The airways are constantly exposed to environmental fungi. The ones that are most commonly isolated in bronchiectasis patients are *Candida albicans* and *Aspergillus* spp. Of these, the various species of *Aspergillus* spp. have the greatest pathogenic potential [3]. The inhalation of fungal spores and conidias has little effect on healthy subjects as their immune mechanisms will function correctly. In chronic pulmonary diseases, such as bronchiectasis, however, fungal growth is enhanced by deteriorated mucociliary clearance, thick mucosity, and the fungis' capacity to evade the host's immune mechanisms [3]. Although there are no published data about the real prevalence of co-colonization of fungi and bacteria, in most cases, fungi are isolated with pathogens, such as *Haemophillus influenzae* or *Pseudomonas aeruginosa*, making difficult to determine their pathogenic significance. However, they are associated with a persistent inflammatory response in the airways that can be measured accurately, particularly in those patients with more marked respiratory deterioration.

Microbiological diagnostic techniques for fungal infection have developed enormously in recent years. Although the traditional diagnostic methods (microscopic tests, biochemical analysis, and cultures in selective media) are still used, in many instances they have been superseded by new molecular techniques, such as metagenomic analysis, as well as by the application of mass spectrometry (Matrix-Assisted Laser Desorption/Ionization Time-of-Flight—MALDI TOF) technique [4]. These breakthroughs have made it possible to identify new fungal pathogens, although more studies are needed to determine their clinical significance.

Anatomical modifications, as found in bronchiectasis and immunological alterations, as found in immunosuppressive states, can give rise to a wide range of respiratory fungal diseases, from simple colonizations to invasive aspergillosis or allergic bronchopulmonary aspergillosis (ABPA) [5]. These phenomena are difficult to diagnose in bronchiectasis patients, as their symptoms and radiological presentation are not easily distinguishable from those of the underlying disease. Furthermore, we are still lacking in uniform diagnostic criteria for some of these fungal diseases [6].

2. Pathogeny of Bronchiectasis

Bronchiectasis arises as a result of a vicious circle that is produced by bacterial infection and inflammation [7]. The damage to the mucociliary system impedes the elimination of secretions and propitiates the growth of microorganisms, such as bacteria, mycobacteria, and fungi in the airways. Infection and inflammation cause structural bronchial damage and perpetuate this pathogenically vicious circle. An imbalance between pro-inflammatory and anti-inflammatory products and an incomplete resolution of the infection and inflammation, despite treatment and the immune response, could play an important role in the progression of the disease [1]. The role of fungi in this process has yet to be defined.

3. Microbiology of Bronchiectasis

The airways of bronchiectasis patients tend to be colonized by potentially pathogenic microorganisms. The bacteria that are most commonly isolated in these patients are *H. influenzae*, *P. aeruginosa*, *Streptococcus pneumoniae*, *Staphylococcus aureus*, and *Moraxella catarrhalis* [8]. Other microorganisms are also often found, such as non-tuberculous mycobacteria (NTM) [9,10], yeasts, and filamentous fungi [11].

In the last ten years, the use of pyrosequencing methods to investigate all the genetic sequences of the microorganisms that are present in the respiratory secretions has revealed an extremely varied bacterial microbiota, which are comparable to that found in other chronic respiratory diseases [12].

4. Prevalence of Fungal Infection and Risk Factors

Healthy subjects quickly eliminate fungal conidias via the mucociliary system and then phagocytize them via cells in the immune system. In patients with chronic respiratory diseases, such as bronchiectasis, however, the deterioration of the mucociliary clearance system and thick mucosity allow for these pathogens to persist, and, furthermore, create colonization mechanisms [13,14]. The prevalence of fungal colonization in the airways varies according to the geographical area, the microbiological culturing, and identification methods used and the etiology of the bronchiectasis [15,16]. Any comparison of studies is also complicated by the differing definitions of colonization, infection, and persistence used therein [17,18].

C. albicans and *Aspergillus* spp. are the fungi that are most usually isolated in the respiratory secretions of patients with chronic respiratory disease, and they are also the ones that are most often cultured in patients with cystic fibrosis (CF) [19,20] and bronchiectasis [11,21,22]. *Aspergillus fumigatus* is isolated from respiratory secretions of patients with CF in between 9% and 57% of samples, and the rate is somewhat higher in the case of *C. albicans*.

5. Yeasts

The yeasts most often found in bronchiectasis belong to the *Candida* spp. genus, with *C. albicans* being the most common species. A recent analysis of the data derived from routine microbiological cultures in various Spanish hospitals showed that *C. albicans* was isolated in 45.2% of the patients that were studied [11]. Other fungal species were recovered from 5.2% of the patients.

It is also not uncommon to identify yeasts in these patients' respiratory samples. Yeasts such as *Trichosporon beigelli* and *Saccharomyces cerevisiae* form part of the normal microbiota of the upper respiratory tract, digestive system, and even foodstuffs, but their possible implication in the processes of colonization and infection is subject to debate. On the one hand, they could represent contamination derived from the collection of the respiratory sample, but on the other hand, these types of yeast have demonstrated a great immunogenic capacity, which could be linked to the impaired mucociliary clearance found in this group of patients [6].

Finally, the so-called black yeasts have recently been noted in patients with bronchiectasis and in CF. *Exophiala dermatitidis* is particularly prominent in this respect. In some cases in the literature it was the only fungus isolated in patients with a deteriorated respiratory function, and their clinical condition improved after the administration of antifungals and subsequent negative cultures [23].

Furthermore, as in the case of CF, chronic antibiotic treatment may be a major risk factor for respiratory fungal colonization and infection, although more studies are needed to corroborate this hypothesis. One study recently undertaken on bronchiectasis patients found that persistent *C. albicans* was most common in those patients who were receiving chronic antibiotic treatment [11].

6. Filamentous Fungi

The various species of the *Aspergillus* spp. genus are the most prevalent filamentous fungi found in bronchiectasis patients (24.2% in the aforementioned multi-centre study) [11]. *A. fumigatus* is the most common species, followed by *Aspergillus niger*, *Aspergillus terreus*, and *Aspegillus flavus*. However, there are huge variations in the prevalence of the fungi isolated in studies, for the reasons noted above. For example, the prevalence of *Aspergillus* spp. in bronchiectasis ranges from 7% to 24% [11,24].

A. fumigatus has been the main focus of almost all of the research into fungal diseases, as it is both the most prevalent and the most pathogenic. The other species of *Aspergillus* spp. tend to act more as colonizers than as pathogenic agents. The distribution of the species varies according to the geographical area, with a high prevalence of *A. niger* and *A. terreus* in Japan and of *A. flavus* in India and China [25].

Almost all of the research into the risk factors that are associated with the isolation of *Aspergillus* spp. and other fungi in the respiratory tract has been carried out on patients with CF [18], but even so, its role in this population has still not been totally clarified. It has been suggested that the incidence of *Aspergillus* spp. increases with age [26], with a greater severity of lung disease [26] and with chronic antibiotic treatment [21,27,28].

Although chronic antibiotic treatment may be one of the most significant risk factors for fungal respiratory infection, Máiz et al. did not find any such association with *Aspergillus* spp. Nevertheless, they did link its persistence to greater purulence in the sputum [11]. The lack of this association between *Aspergillus* spp. and antibiotic treatment could be due to the fact the culture of sputum samples may not be the most appropriate way to detect the presence of *Aspergillus* spp. in the lower respiratory tract [29–31], although the use of microbiological techniques that are not based on cultures from respiratory samples has been hotly debated in the case of bronchiectasis patients. The detection of the antigen of *Aspergillus* spp. or galactomannan in serum or bronchoalveolar lavage has been proposed as a microbiological criterion for probable invasive aspergillosis in immunocompetent patients with lung diseases, like Chronic obstructive pulmonary disease (COPD) and bronchiectasis, who also fulfil other clinical criteria, such as pulmonary deterioration, frequent exacerbations after antibiotic treatment, or high doses of steroids. These algorithms have only been applied to critical patients, however, further studies are required to validate the detection of galactomannan in immunocompetent patients who do not need to be admitted to an intensive care unit [32–34].

Other species of filamentous fungi that have been described in this group of patients include *Scedosporium apiospermum* and various species from the *Fusarium* and *Penicillium* geni. Filamentous fungi from the Mucorales family, such as *Rhizopus* spp. and *Mucor* spp., have also been found. Other species that have recently come to the fore include dematiaceous fungi, such as *Alternaria* spp. and *Bipolaris* spp, whose presence is associated with allergic stimuli of the bronchial airway [35].

Improvements in the methods used for the microbiological identification of filamentous fungi—including the recently introduced MALDI TOF technique—has made it possible to describe "new" species, such as *Geosmithia argillacea*, which is associated with the appearance of exacerbations in CF patients. Conventional identification techniques based on morphological characteristics usually define this as *Penicillium* spp.

Such descriptions of "new" species also extend to so-called cryptic species that are related to *A. fumigatus*: molecular biology techniques have revealed species associated with the Fumigati section, such as *A. ustus*, which would be defined as *A. fumigatus* by morphological identification, but nevertheless has a different profile of sensitivity to voriconazole [36]. Table 1 shows the species that are most frequently found in bronchiectasis patients.

Table 1. Species most frequently found in patients with bronchiectasis not associated with cystic fibrosis [6,11,21,23,37,38].

Yeasts	Filamentous Fungi
Candida albicans	*Aspergllus fumigatus*
Candida glabrata	*Aspergillus niger*
Candida parapsilosis	*Aspergullus terreus*
Saccharomyces cerevisiae	*Scedosporium apiospermum*
Trichosporon beigellii	*Penicillium* spp.
Exophiala dermatitidis	*Fusarium* spp.

7. Pathogenic Mechanisms

Apart from the case of *P. aeruginosa* [39], little is known about the pathogenic role that is played by other bacteria in bronchiectasis, but the role of fungi is even less documented. Most of the studies on the pathogeny of fungi in respiratory diseases have focused on CF and COPD, and the European Academy of Allergy and Clinical Immunology recently drew attention to our lack of knowledge about the connections between fungal infection, the microbiome, and bronchiectasis [40]. So far, any microbiome studies that could cast new light on this matter have placed a particular emphasis on CF [37] and bacterial ecology [41].

The alterations in ciliary clearance and the bronchial tree destruction that occur during the bronchiectasis process, along with the chronic inflammation that is associated with the colonization of the mucosa by various bacterial and viral microorganisms, favour pathogenic colonization by fungi. Moreover, the reduced ciliary clearance in the bronchial tree is particularly relevant in this respect. Whilst healthy people can eliminate most fungal spores or conidias via ciliary clearance—with the remainder being phagocytized by innate immune mechanisms—bronchiectasis patients are unable to eliminate the majority of spores, as the fungal presence is too big for their impaired mucociliary clearance. This means that fungi are retained in the mucosity of their respiratory tree and that, in the case of filamentous fungi, they can invade tissue (colonization-infection processes), cause tissue damage, and provide a stimulus to the humoral immune response [6].

There are three factors that can explain the contribution of fungi to the emergence of bronchiectasis: antigens and fungal proteases; genetic susceptibility; and, interactions that may arise with other microorganisms, such as mycobacteria.

Both yeasts, and, more particularly, molds have elements in their cellular wall (elastase, collagenase, trypsin, MUC5AC, chitin, β-glucan, gliotoxins) that can degrade the components of the tissue matrix [38,42–45]. Fungal proteases are produced once the fungus has invaded the mucosa and developed hyphas [46]. Animal models have shown that fungal proteases induce the production of cytokines and other pro-inflammatory mediators [47–49]. *Aspergillus* spp. spores are also capable of resisting phagocytic cells [50], neutrophils, and alveolar macrophages [51,52]. This hindrance to the elimination of conidias by the airway macrophages triggers a response in the fungal hyphae, the respiratory epithelial, dendritic and phagocytic cells, and the toll-like receptors [53]. Damage to this line of defence can favour exposure to fungal antigens, producing a Th1-type response in healthy people and a Th2-type response in ABPA patients [54]. Figure 1 presents a schematic summary of the pathogenic mechanisms of fungi in bronchiectasis.

There are various factors that are implicated in the genetic susceptibility to suffer from fungal diseases. For example, in the case of Allergic bronchopulmonary aspergillosis (ABPA), which is unleashed by a Th2 response, an association has been demonstrated with dysfunctions of the cystic fibrosis transmembrane conductance regulator [55], while variations in the prevalence of polymorphisms may explain the differences in the prevalence of ABPA from one geographical area to another.

Apart from fungal proteases and the susceptibility of the host, a third factor in the pathogeny of fungal bronchiectasis is a possible interaction with other microorganisms, such as mycobacteria. It has been demonstrated that Nontuberculous mycobacteria (NTM) can propitiate sensitization to *Aspergillus* and play a major role in the appearance of ABPA in a susceptible host [56].

CF patients have also presented an association between ABPA and isolations of *Aspergillus* and NTM in respiratory samples [57,58]. However, this apparent association could be spurious due to the deterioration of the lung function and the presence of common risk factors for their isolation (e.g., antimicrobial treatment).

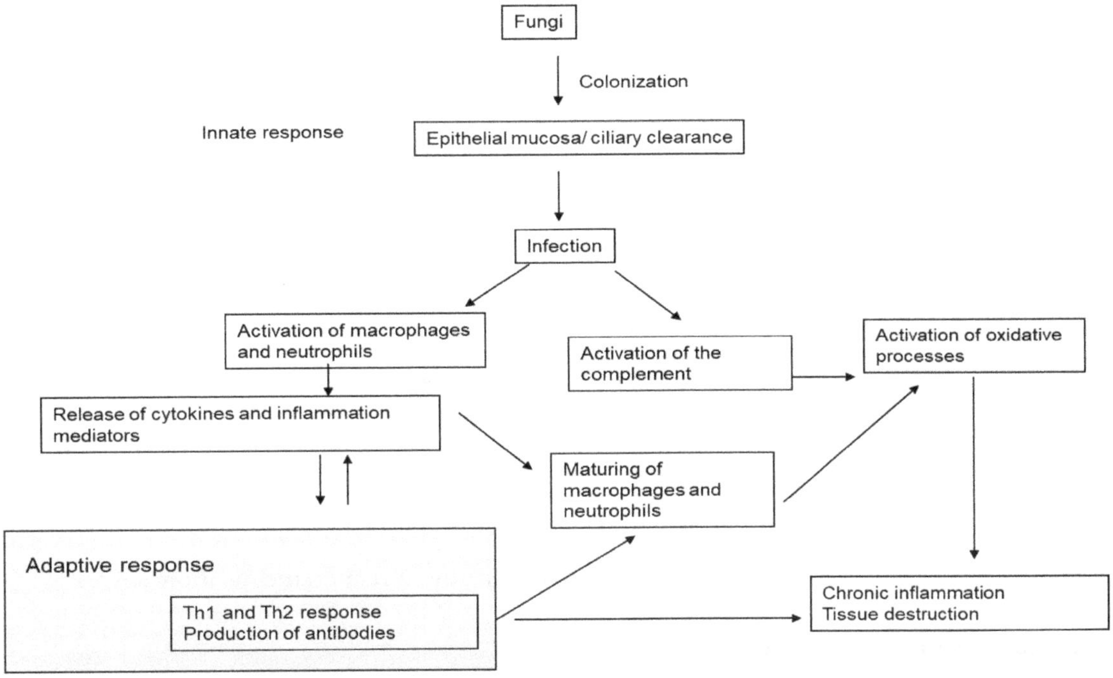

Figure 1. Pathogenic mechanisms of fungi in bronchiectasis.

8. Clinical Significance and Association with Other Microorganisms

The clinical significance of fungal growth in the cultures of respiratory samples that were taken from bronchiectasis patients has not been clearly established because, on the one hand, few studies have examined its epidemiology, and, on the other, the criteria usually applied to the definition of chronic colonization are adapted from definitions of chronic colonization by other microorganisms, such as *P. aeruginosa* [6]. The issue of clinical significance is complicated still further by the fact that fungi are not usually isolated on their own. More than one fungal species may be found (the most common being *A. fumigatus* and *C. albicans*) and they are often accompanied by other types of microorganisms, such as bacteria.

Apart from the aforementioned association with NTM [59], the model of the relationship with chronic bronchial infection described in the literature is very similar to that of CF patients, since there is a relationship between the appearance of filamentous fungi (especially *A. fumigatus*) and chronic bronchial infection by *P. aeruginosa*. No fungi are isolated, however, in the cultures of patients with chronic colonization by *H. influenzae* [11]. Finally, the possible role of respiratory viruses in bronchial inflammatory processes needs to be mentioned, as these could favour colonization by other types of microorganisms, including bacteria and fungi.

9. Clinical Spectrum of *Aspergillus*

Various species of *Aspergillus* can colonize the airways without any pathogenic consequences, but they are also capable of causing several types of disease: bronchitis due to *Aspergillus* spp., aspergilloma, chronic necrotizing aspergillosis, invasive aspergillosis, and asthmatic reactions (bronchial asthma, extrinsic allergic alveolitis, and ABPA) (Figure 2). *Aspergillus* spp. can create several different clinical pictures at the same time in a single patient, and these can evolve over time in accordance with the progression of the underlying pathology and the patient's immunity. All of this makes it even more difficult to diagnose and treat fungal disease in bronchiectasis patients. Of all the clinical pictures that are produced by fungi, the one most often associated with bronchiectasis is allergic bronchopulmonary mycosis.

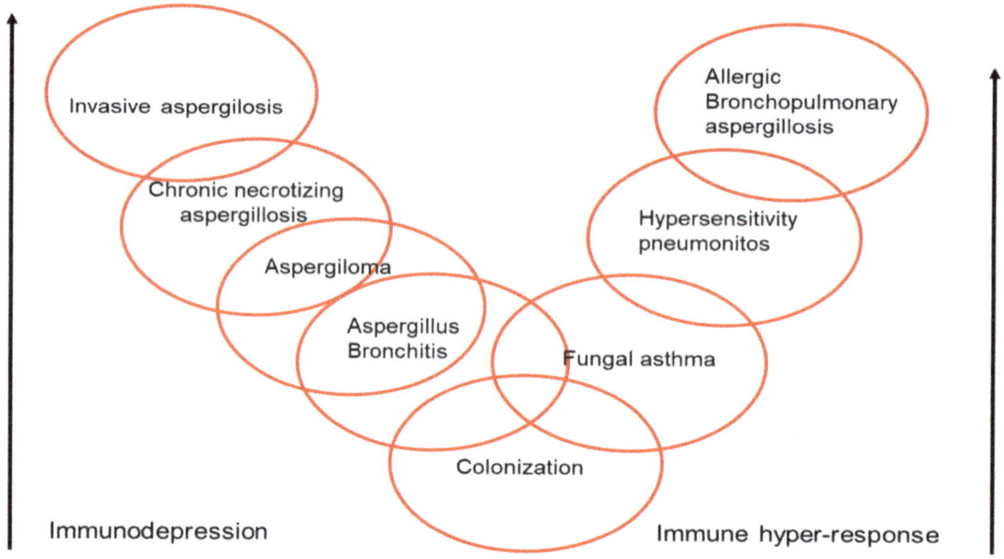

Figure 2. Pathogenic potential of *Aspergillus* spp. (arrow direction means more severity).

10. Allergic Bronchopulmonary Mycosis

Allergic bronchopulmonary mycosis is responsible for persistent asthmatic symptoms, pulmonary eosinophilia, radiological infiltrates, and proximal bronchiectasis. There are many fungi that are capable of triggering it [60,61], but *A. fumigatus* is behind more than 90% of cases, giving rise to what is known as ABPA. The manifestations of this group of diseases are affected both by the virulence of the fungus in question and by the patient's atopic immunological response. The prevalence of ABPA in idiopathic bronchiectasis is 10% [62]. *A. terreus* has been implicated in approximately 10% of patients with ABPA in Japan [63,64], but this species is not very pathogenic and is rarely associated with other types of fungal disease in bronchiectasis. *A. nidulans* has also been described as a cause of ABPA in bronchiectasis patients [65].

ABPA rarely causes bronchiectasis [66]. Both the European [2] and Spanish guidelines [1] for bronchiectasis recommend ruling out ABPA in all of the patients diagnosed with bronchiectasis, by screening by means of a total IgE serum test and specific IgE and IgG tests for *A. fumigatus*, or alternatively a prick test for *A. fumigatus* [2]. These recommendations are often ignored, however, as evidenced by a review recently undertaken in the United Kingdom [67].

It is difficult to diagnose ABPA in a bronchiectasis patient as both diseases share many clinical and radiological characteristics. An attempt to unify the diagnostic criteria for ABPA has recently been made in a review carried out by a working group from the International Society for Human and Animal Mycology [55].

ABPA intensifies the deterioration in the lung function and increases the number of exacerbations in both CF and bronchiectasis [68,69], but it is still not known whether the presence of *A. fumigatus* and the triggering of ABPA are a cause or consequence of pulmonary deterioration. The mechanisms by which sensitization to *A. fumigatus* gives rise to ABPA, and by which ABPA in its turn triggers bronchiectasis, have not been clearly established, but it has been speculated that they could be the result of remodelling of the airways subsequent to the inflammation that is caused by continuous exposure to *A. fumigatus* [38].

Although ABPA is associated, in both CF and bronchiectasis, with a greater prevalence of airway infection by other pathogenic microorganisms, such as NTM [56,57], it is not known whether this association is due to defects in the cystic fibrosis transmembrane conductance regulator that could occur in patients with bronchiectasis, or whether this explanation is only applicable to CF patients [70].

11. Mycobiome

The recent application of mass sequencing techniques with high-performance platforms and amplification of total DNA in the respiratory secretions of patients with chronic bronchopulmonary disease has made it possible to detect a wider range of microorganisms than was the case with conventional cultures [71]. Apart from classic bacteria like *P. aeruginosa*, *H. influenzae*, *S. pneumoniae*, and *S. aureus*, bacteria that grow exclusively in anaerobiosis have been found, along with molds and yeast; these are known collectively as the mycobiome [72]. Differences have been observed between the yeast identified in healthy individuals and those detected in patients with bronchiectasis or asthma [73], suggesting that they could have a different significance in different contexts.

Most of the research undertaken on the microbiome in respiratory disease has involved small sample sizes, as well as sputum samples (rather than bronchoaspiration), and as a result, its clinical importance is still unclear. The main focus has been on the bacterial microbiome in CF, asthma, and COPD [74–77], with only a few studies of bronchiectasis [12]. In the case of CF, fungi are detected more often during exacerbations, and, in many cases, after antimicrobial treatment, although one follow-up study of six patients who gave a series of respiratory samples and had their complete microbiome analyzed presented a relative stability of the various fungal species found, including *Candida* spp. [73].

Studies of the microbiome have demonstrated that resistance increases and bacterial diversity decreases after antibiotic treatment, although this effect disappears a few weeks after the completion of treatment, with a subsequent recovery of the previous microbial composition [77].

Apart from the infections that are already known to be caused by fungi, the lung mycobiome can have inflammatory effects that can cause or aggravate chronic respiratory disease. Like bacteria, fungi also contain pathogen-associated molecular patterns (PAMP), which are recognizable by pattern recognition receptors that activate immune cells (macrophages, B and T cells), thereby triggering inflammation. Given that fungi are omnipresent in the environment, the respiratory system's continuous exposure to them and their capacity to trigger an inflammatory process means that the mycobiome may contribute to lung damage, which makes it important to analyze it to establish its real pathogenic role [78]. Most studies have found that, as in the case of bacteria, a reduction in fungal diversity in respiratory diseases correlates with a poorer lung function (along the same lines as a reduction in bacterial diversity). This reduced diversity could be caused by the excessive growth of one fungal species or by the elimination of other species. Figure 3 shows the evolution of the mycobiome in patients with chronic respiratory disease [72].

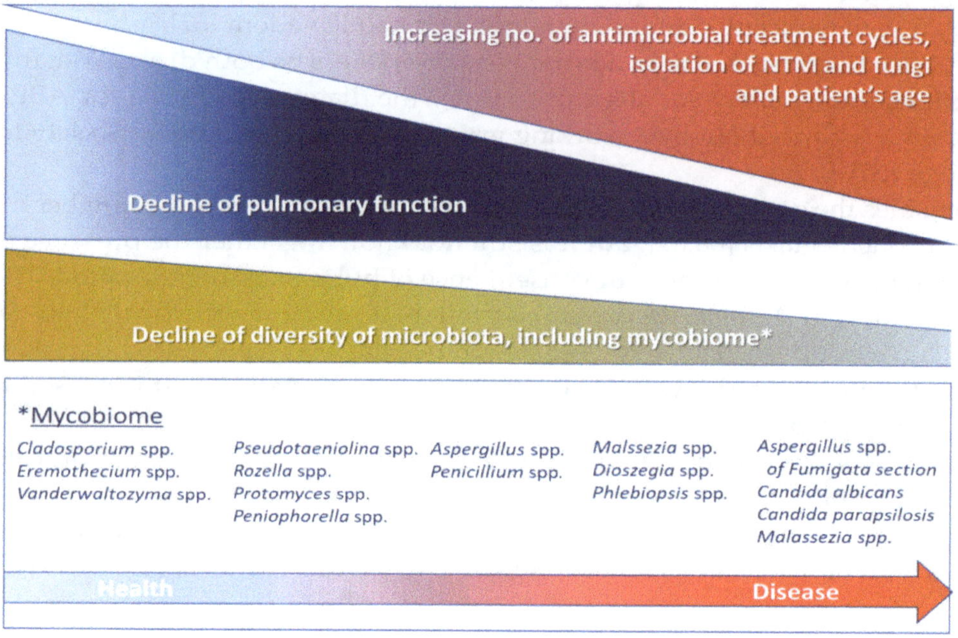

Figure 3. Evolution of the mycobiome in patients with chronic respiratory disease. Information has been obtained from reference [72].

There are several justifications for research into the lung mycobiome in patients with bronchiectasis. Firstly, the respiratory tract constitutes the main point of entry for fungal spores; secondly, it has been demonstrated that bronchiectasis is a risk factor for fungal disease; and, thirdly, fungi can exacerbate the respiratory deterioration of such patients. Increased knowledge of the complex interactions between the fungal, viral and bacterial microbiota would probably propitiate the development and implementation of innovative therapies. Improvements in sequencing techniques and their interpretation (as well as a reduction in their cost) could be useful in furthering our understanding of the microbiome in both healthy and sick people. Furthermore, research into the relationship between the digestive and respiratory microbiota could also provide insight into the pathogenesis of bronchiectasis.

12. Future Research

There are still many tasks pending with respect to fungi and bronchiectasis, such as, for example, establishing their prevalence and the best method for detecting them; assessing the pathogenic significance of individual species; verifying whether fungi are a cause or consequence of bronchiectasis; defining the risk factors for fungal infection and the importance of sensitization to fungi; and, evaluating tests to diagnose invasive aspergillosis in bronchiectasis patients and to detect interactions between the mycobiome and the host.

In a document recently published by the EMBARC Clinical Research Collaboration, Aliberti set out the following research priorities [79]:

1. Studies on bronchiectasis patients in a stable phase and in exacerbations, to evaluate how they are affected by fungi.

2. Studies on the microbiome (including bacteria and potentially pathogenic fungi) with detailed data on phenotypical studies.
3. Studies on the prevalence of fungi.
4. Studies on fungi (both alone and in joint infection with other pathogens) in bronchiectasis patients in a stable phase and in exacerbations, and on the impact of fungi on the severity and evolution of the disease in these patients.
5. Studies to evaluate whether chronic antibiotics are a predisposing risk factor for fungal respiratory diseases.

13. Conclusions

The growth of fungi in the conventional microbiological cultures of respiratory samples from bronchiectasis patients has been linked to the triggering of inflammatory response in the bronchi. The species that are most commonly found belong to the genera *Aspergillus* spp. and *Candida* spp.

Although we do not know the risk factors for fungal colonization and infection in bronchiectasis, chronic antibiotic treatment is one of the most important risk factors. The clinical significance of the growth of fungi in cultures of respiratory samples taken from bronchiectasis patients has still not been clearly defined. Further studies that would make it possible to standardize and evaluate both the microbiological criteria for defining chronic colonization and the methods used for culturing and identifying fungi would provide us with more precise knowledge of the genera and species involved, and of the role that fungi play in the clinical evolution of bronchiectasis patients.

Author Contributions: Drafting of the manuscript and critical revision of the manuscript: all authors.

References

1. Martínez-García, M.A.; Máiz, L.; Olveira, C.; Girón, R.M.; de la Rosa, D.; Blanco, M.; Cantón, R.; Vendrell, M.; Polverino, E.; de Gracia, J.; et al. Normativa sobre la valoración y el diagnóstico de las bronquiectasias en el adulto. *Arch. Bronconeumol.* **2017**. [CrossRef] [PubMed]
2. Polverino, E.; Goeminne, P.C.; McDonnell, M.J.; Aliberti, S.; Marshall, S.E.; Loebinger, M.R.; Murris, M.; Cantón, R.; Torres, A.; Dimakou, K.; et al. European Respiratory Society guidelines for the management of adult bronchiectasis. *Eur. Respir. J.* **2017**, *50*, 1700629. [CrossRef] [PubMed]
3. Chotirmall, S.H.; Al-Alawi, M.; Mirkovic, B.; Lavelle, G.; Logan, P.M.; Greene, C.M.; McElvaney, N.G. *Aspergillus*-associated airway disease, inflammation, and the innate immune response. *Biomed. Res. Int.* **2013**, *2013*, 723129. [CrossRef] [PubMed]
4. Ibáñez-Martínez, E.; Ruiz-Gaitán, A.; Pemán-García, J. Update on the diagnosis of invasive fungal infection. *Rev. Esp. Quimioter.* **2017**, *30* (Suppl. S1), 16–21. [PubMed]
5. Kosmidis, C.; Denning, D.W. The clinical spectrum of pulmonary aspergillosis. *Thorax* **2015**, *70*, 270–277. [CrossRef] [PubMed]
6. Moss, R.B. Fungi in cystic fibrosis and non-cystic fibrosis bronchiectasis. *Semin. Respir. Crit. Care Med.* **2015**, *36*, 207–216. [CrossRef] [PubMed]
7. Cole, P.J. Inflammation: A two-edged sword—The model of bronchiectasis. *Eur. J. Respir. Dis. Suppl.* **1986**, *147*, 6–15. [PubMed]
8. McDonnell, M.J.; Jary, H.R.; Perry, A.; MacFarlane, J.G.; Hester, K.L.; Small, T.; Molyneux, C.; Perry, J.D.; Walton, K.E.; De Soyza, A. Non cystic fibrosis bronchiectasis: A longitudinal retrospective observational cohort study of *Pseudomonas* persistence and resistance. *Respir. Med.* **2015**, *109*, 716–726. [CrossRef] [PubMed]
9. Wickremasinghe, M.; Ozerovitch, L.J.; Davies, G.; Wodehouse, T.; Chadwick, M.V.; Abdallah, S.; Shah, P.; Wilson, R. Non-tuberculous mycobacteria in patients with bronchiectasis. *Thorax* **2005**, *60*, 1045–1051. [CrossRef] [PubMed]
10. Máiz, L.; Girón, R.; Olveira, C.; Vendrell, M.; Nieto, R.; Martínez-García, M.A. Prevalence and factors associated with nontuberculous mycobacteria in non-cystic fibrosis bronchiectasis: A multicenter observational study. *BMC Infect. Dis.* **2016**, *16*, 437. [CrossRef] [PubMed]

11. Máiz, L.; Girón, R.; Olveira, C.; Vendrell, M.; Nieto, R.; Martínez-García, M.A. Prevalence and factors associated with isolation of *Aspergillus* and *Candida* from sputum in patients with non-cystic fibrosis bronchiectasis. *Respiration* **2015**, *89*, 396–403. [CrossRef] [PubMed]
12. Rogers, G.B.; van der Gast, C.J.; Cuthbertson, L.; Thomson, S.K.; Bruce, K.D.; Martin, M.L.; Serisier, D.J. Clinical measures of disease in adult non-CF bronchiectasis correlate with airway microbiota composition. *Thorax* **2013**, *68*, 731–737. [CrossRef] [PubMed]
13. Liu, J.C.; Modha, D.E.; Gaillard, E.A. What is the clinical significance of filamentous fungi positive sputum cultures in patients with cystic fibrosis? *J. Cyst. Fibros.* **2013**, *12*, 187–193. [CrossRef] [PubMed]
14. King, P.T.; Holdsworth, S.R.; Freezer, N.J.; Villanueva, E.; Holmes, P.W. Microbiologic follow-up study in adult bronchiectasis. *Respir. Med.* **2007**, *101*, 1633–1638. [CrossRef] [PubMed]
15. Máiz, L.; Cuevas, M.; Lamas, A.; Sousa, A.; Quirce, S.; Suárez, L. *Aspergillus fumigatus* and *Candida albicans* in cystic fibrosis: Clinical significance and specific immune response involving serum immunoglobulins G, A, and M. *Arch. Bronconeumol.* **2008**, *44*, 146–151. [CrossRef] [PubMed]
16. Pashley, C.H. Fungal culture and sensitisation in asthma, cystic fibrosis and chronic obstructive pulmonary disorder: What does it tell us? *Mycopathologia* **2014**, *178*, 457–463. [CrossRef] [PubMed]
17. Amin, R.; Dupuis, A.; Aaron, S.D.; Ratjen, F. The effect of chronic infection with *Aspergillus fumigatus* on lung function and hospitalization in patients with cystic fibrosis. *Chest* **2010**, *137*, 171–176. [CrossRef] [PubMed]
18. Sudfeld, C.R.; Dasenbrook, E.C.; Merz, W.G.; Carroll, K.C.; Boyle, M.P. Prevalence and risk factors for recovery of filamentous fungi in individuals with cystic fibrosis. *J. Cyst. Fibros.* **2010**, *9*, 110–116. [CrossRef] [PubMed]
19. Chotirmall, S.H.; O'Donoghue, E.; Bennett, K.; Gunaratnam, C.; O'Neill, S.J.; McElvaney, N.G. Sputum *Candida albicans* presages FEV_1 decline and hospital-treated exacerbations in cystic fibrosis. *Chest* **2010**, *138*, 1186–1195. [CrossRef] [PubMed]
20. Burns, J.L.; Van Dalfsen, J.M.; Shawar, R.M.; Otto, K.L.; Garber, R.L.; Quan, J.M.; Montgomery, A.B.; Albers, G.M.; Ramsey, B.W.; Smith, A.L. Effect of chronic intermittent administration of inhaled tobramycin on respiratory microbial flora in patients with cystic fibrosis. *J. Infect. Dis.* **1999**, *179*, 1190–1196. [CrossRef] [PubMed]
21. Angrill, J.; Agustí, C.; de Celis, R.; Rañó, A.; Gonzalez, J.; Solé, T.; Xaubet, A.; Rodriguez-Roisin, R.; Torres, A. Bacterial colonisation in patients with bronchiectasis: Microbiological pattern and risk factors. *Thorax* **2002**, *57*, 15–19. [CrossRef] [PubMed]
22. Nicotra, M.B.; Rivera, M.; Dale, A.M.; Shepherd, R.; Carter, R. Clinical, pathophysiologic, and microbiologic characterization of bronchiectasis in an aging cohort. *Chest* **1995**, *108*, 955–961. [CrossRef] [PubMed]
23. Mukaino, T.; Koga, T.; Oshita, Y.; Narita, Y.; Obata, S.; Aizawa, H. *Exophiala dermatitidis* infection in non-cystic fibrosis bronchiectasis. *Respir. Med.* **2006**, *100*, 2069–2071. [CrossRef] [PubMed]
24. Mortensen, K.L.; Johansen, H.K.; Fuursted, K.; Knudsen, J.D.; Gahrn-Hansen, B.; Jensen, R.H.; Howard, S.J.; Arendrup, M.C. A prospective survey of *Aspergillus* spp. in respiratory tract samples: Prevalence, clinical impact and antifungal susceptibility. *Eur. J. Clin. Microbiol. Infect. Dis.* **2011**, *30*, 1355–1363. [CrossRef] [PubMed]
25. Ishiguro, T.; Takayanagi, N.; Kagiyama, N.; Shimizu, Y.; Yanagisawa, T.; Sugita, Y. Clinical characteristics of biopsy-proven allergic bronchopulmonary mycosis: Variety in causative fungi and laboratory findings. *Intern. Med.* **2014**, *53*, 1407–1411. [CrossRef] [PubMed]
26. Milla, C.E.; Wielinski, C.L.; Regelmann, W.E. Clinical significance of the recovery of *Aspergillus* species from the respiratory secretions of cystic fibrosis patients. *Pediatr. Pulmonol.* **1996**, *21*, 6–10. [CrossRef]
27. Jubin, V.; Ranque, S.; Stremler Le Bel, N.; Sarles, J.; Dubus, J.C. Risk factors for *Aspergillus* colonization and allergic bronchopulmonary aspergillosis in children with cystic fibrosis. *Pediatr. Pulmonol.* **2010**, *45*, 764–771. [CrossRef] [PubMed]
28. Bargon, J.; Dauletbaev, N.; Köhler, B.; Wolf, M.; Posselt, H.G.; Wagner, T.O. Prophylactic antibiotic therapy is associated with an increased prevalence of *Aspergillus* colonization in adult cystic fibrosis patients. *Respir. Med.* **1999**, *93*, 835–838. [CrossRef]
29. El-Dahr, J.M.; Fink, R.; Selden, R.; Arruda, L.K.; Platts-Mills, T.A.; Heymann, P.W. Development of immune responses to *Aspergillus* at an early age in children with cystic fibrosis. *Am. J. Respir. Crit. Care Med.* **1994**, *150*, 1513–1518. [CrossRef] [PubMed]

30. Baxter, C.G.; Moore, C.B.; Jones, A.M.; Webb, A.K.; Denning, D.W. IgE-mediated immune responses and airway detection of *Aspergillus* and *Candida* in adult cystic fibrosis. *Chest* **2013**, *143*, 1351–1357. [CrossRef] [PubMed]
31. Nagano, Y.; Elborn, J.S.; Millar, B.C.; Walker, J.M.; Goldsmith, C.E.; Rendall, J.; Moore, J.E. Comparison of techniques to examine the diversity of fungi in adult patients with cystic fibrosis. *Med. Mycol.* **2010**, *48*, 166.e1–176.e1. [CrossRef] [PubMed]
32. Chabi, M.L.; Goracci, A.; Roche, N.; Paugam, A.; Lupo, A.; Revel, M.P. Pulmonary aspergillosis. *Diagn. Interv. Imaging* **2015**, *96*, 435–442. [CrossRef] [PubMed]
33. Ohn, M.; Robinson, P.; Selvadurai, H.; Fitzgerald, D.A. Question 11: How should Allergic Bronchopulmonary Aspergillosis [ABPA] be managed in Cystic Fibrosis? *Paediatr. Respir. Rev.* **2017**, *24*, 35–38. [CrossRef] [PubMed]
34. Huang, L.; He, H.; Jin, J.; Zhan, Q. Is Bulpa criteria suitable for the diagnosis of probable invasive pulmonary Aspergillosis in critically ill patients with chronic obstructive pulmonary disease? A comparative study with EORTC/ MSG and ICU criteria. *BMC Infect. Dis.* **2017**, *17*, 209. [CrossRef] [PubMed]
35. Knutsen, A.P.; Bush, R.K.; Demain, J.G.; Denning, D.W.; Dixit, A.; Fairs, A.; Greenberger, P.A.; Kariuki, B.; Kita, H.; Kurup, V.P.; et al. Fungi and allergic lower respiratory tract diseases. *J. Allergy Clin. Immunol.* **2012**, *129*, 280–291. [CrossRef] [PubMed]
36. Sabino, R.; Ferreira, J.A.; Moss, R.B.; Valente, J.; Veríssimo, C.; Carolino, E.; Clemons, K.V.; Everson, C.; Banaei, N.; Penner, J.; et al. Molecular epidemiology of *Aspergillus* collected from cystic fibrosis patients. *J. Cyst. Fibros.* **2015**, *14*, 474–481. [CrossRef] [PubMed]
37. Delhaes, L.; Monchy, S.; Fréalle, E.; Hubans, C.; Salleron, J.; Leroy, S.; Prevotat, A.; Wallet, F.; Wallaert, B.; Dei-Cas, E.; et al. The airway microbiota in cystic fibrosis: A complex fungal and bacterial community–implications for therapeutic management. *PLoS ONE* **2012**, *7*, e36313. [CrossRef] [PubMed]
38. Chotirmall, S.H.; Martin-Gomez, M.T. *Aspergillus* species in bronchiectasis: Challenges in the cystic fibrosis and non-cystic fibrosis airways. *Mycopathologia* **2017**. [CrossRef] [PubMed]
39. Finch, S.; McDonnell, M.J.; Abo-Leyah, H.; Aliberti, S.; Chalmers, J.D. A comprehensive analysis of the impact of *Pseudomonas aeruginosa* colonization on prognosis in adult bronchiectasis. *Ann. Am. Thorac. Soc.* **2015**, *12*, 1602–1611. [CrossRef] [PubMed]
40. Denning, D.W.; Pashley, C.; Hartl, D.; Wardlaw, A.; Godet, C.; Del Giacco, S.; Delhaes, L.; Sergejeva, S. Fungal allergy in asthma-state of the art and research needs. *Clin. Transl. Allergy* **2014**, *4*, 14. [CrossRef] [PubMed]
41. Rogers, G.B.; Zain, N.M.; Bruce, K.D.; Burr, L.D.; Chen, A.C.; Rivett, D.W.; McGuckin, M.A.; Serisier, D.J. A novel microbiota stratification system predicts future exacerbations in bronchiectasis. *Ann. Am. Thorac. Soc.* **2014**, *11*, 496–503. [CrossRef] [PubMed]
42. Lamy, B.; Moutaouakil, M.; Latge, J.P.; Davies, J. Secretion of a potential virulence factor, a fungal ribonucleotoxin, during human aspergillosis infections. *Mol. Microbiol.* **1991**, *5*, 1811–1815. [CrossRef] [PubMed]
43. Harvey, C.; Longbottom, J.L. Characterization of a second major antigen Ag 13 (antigen C) of *Aspergillus* fumigatus and investigation of its immunological reactivity. *Clin. Exp. Immunol.* **1987**, *70*, 247–254. [PubMed]
44. Frosco, M.; Chase, T., Jr.; Macmillan, J.D. Purification and properties of the elastase from *Aspergillus fumigatus*. *Infect. Immun.* **1992**, *60*, 728–734. [PubMed]
45. Chotirmall, S.H.; Mirkovic, B.; Lavelle, G.M.; McElvaney, N.G. Immunoevasive *Aspergillus* virulence factors. *Mycopathologia* **2014**, *178*, 363–370. [CrossRef] [PubMed]
46. Oosthuizen, J.L.; Gomez, P.; Ruan, J.; Hackett, T.L.; Moore, M.M.; Knight, D.A.; Tebbutt, S.J. Dual organism transcriptomics of airway epithelial cells interacting with conidia of Aspergillus fumigatus. *PLoS ONE* **2011**, *6*, e20527. [CrossRef] [PubMed]
47. Porter, P.C.; Yang, T.; Luong, A.; Delclos, G.L.; Abramson, S.L.; Kheradmand, F.; Corry, D.B. Proteinases as molecular adjuvants in allergic airway disease. *Biochim. Biophys. Acta* **2011**, *1810*, 1059–1065. [CrossRef] [PubMed]
48. Porter, P.; Polikepahad, S.; Qian, Y.; Knight, J.M.; Lu, W.; Tai, W.M.; Roberts, L.; Ongeri, V.; Yang, T.; Seryshev, A.; et al. Respiratory tract allergic disease and atopy: Experimental evidence for a fungal infectious etiology. *Med. Mycol.* **2011**, *49* (Suppl. 1), S158–S163. [CrossRef] [PubMed]

49. Amvar, S.; Warn, P.; Farnell, E.; Bromley, M.; Fraczek, M.; Bowyer, P.; Herrick, S. *Aspergillus fumigatus* proteases, Asp f 5 and Asp f 13, are essential for airway inflammation and remodelling in a murine inhalation model. *Clin. Exp. Allergy* **2015**, *45*, 982–993. [CrossRef] [PubMed]
50. Levitz, S.M.; Diamond, R.D. Mechanisms of resistance of *Aspergillus fumigatus* conidia to killing by neutrophils in vitro. *J. Infect. Dis.* **1985**, *152*, 33–42. [CrossRef] [PubMed]
51. Kurup, V.P. Interaction of *Aspergillus fumigatus* spores and pulmonary alveolar macrophages of rabbits. *Immunobiology* **1984**, *166*, 53–61. [CrossRef]
52. Levitz, S.M.; Selsted, M.E.; Ganz, T.; Lehrer, R.I.; Diamond, R.D. In vitro killing of spores and hyphae of *Aspergillus fumigatus* and *Rhizopus oryzae* by rabbit neutrophil cationic peptides and bronchoalveolar macrophages. *J. Infect. Dis.* **1986**, *154*, 483–489. [CrossRef] [PubMed]
53. Underhill, D.M.; Iliev, I.D. The mycobiota: Interactions between commensal fungi and the host immune system. *Nat. Rev. Immunol.* **2014**, *14*, 405–416. [CrossRef] [PubMed]
54. Becker, K.L.; Gresnigt, M.S.; Smeekens, S.P.; Jacobs, C.W.; Magis-Escurra, C.; Jaegerm, M.; Wang, X.; Lubbers, R.; Oosting, M.; Joosten, L.A.; et al. Pattern recognition pathways leading to a Th2 cytokine bias in allergic bronchopulmonary aspergillosis patients. *Clin. Exp. Allergy* **2015**, *45*, 423–437. [CrossRef] [PubMed]
55. Agarwal, R.; Chakrabarti, A.; Shah, A.; Gupta, D.; Meis, J.F.; Guleria, R.; Moss, R.; Denning, D.W. ABPA complicating asthma ISHAM working group. Allergic bronchopulmonary aspergillosis: Review of literature and proposal of new diagnostic and classification criteria. *Clin. Exp. Allergy* **2013**, *43*, 850–873. [CrossRef] [PubMed]
56. Kunst, H.; Wickremasinghe, M.; Wells, A.; Wilson, R. Nontuberculous mycobacterial disease and *Aspergillus*-related lung disease in bronchiectasis. *Eur. Respir. J.* **2006**, *28*, 352–357. [CrossRef] [PubMed]
57. Levy, I.; Grisaru-Soen, G.; Lerner-Geva, L.; Kerem, E.; Blau, H.; Bentur, L.; Aviram, M.; Rivlin, J.; Picard, E.; Lavy, A.; et al. Multicenter cross-sectional study of nontuberculous mycobacterial infections among cystic fibrosis patients, Israel. *Emerg. Infect. Dis.* **2008**, *14*, 378–384. [CrossRef] [PubMed]
58. Mussaffi, H.; Rivlin, J.; Shalit, I.; Ephros, M.; Blau, H. Nontuberculous mycobacteria in cystic fibrosis associated with allergic bronchopulmonary aspergillosis and steroid therapy. *Eur. Respir. J.* **2005**, *25*, 324–328. [CrossRef] [PubMed]
59. Moore, E.H. Atypical mycobacterial infection in the lung: CT appearance. *Radiology* **1993**, *187*, 777–782. [CrossRef] [PubMed]
60. Chowdhary, A.; Agarwal, K.; Kathuria, S.; Gaur, S.N.; Randhawa, H.S.; Meis, J.F. Allergic bronchopulmonary mycosis due to fungi other than Aspergillus: A global overview. *Crit. Rev. Microbiol.* **2014**, *40*, 30–48. [CrossRef] [PubMed]
61. Vincken, W.; Schandevul, W.; Roels, P. Allergic bronchopulmonary aspergillosis caused by *Aspergillus terreus*. *Am. Rev. Respir. Dis.* **1983**, *127*, 388–389. [PubMed]
62. Bahous, J.; Malo, J.L.; Paquin, R.; Cartier, A.; Vyas, P.; Longbottom, J.L. Allergic bronchopulmonary aspergillosis and sensitization to *Aspergillus fumigatus* in chronic bronchiectasis in adults. *Clin. Allergy* **1985**, *15*, 571–579. [CrossRef] [PubMed]
63. Laham, M.N.; Allen, R.C.; Greene, J.C. Allergic bronchopulmonary aspergillosis (ABPA) caused by *Aspergillus terreus*: Specific lymphocyte sensitization and antigen-directed serum opsonic activity. *Ann. Allergy* **1981**, *46*, 74–80. [PubMed]
64. Nakahara, Y.; Katoh, O.; Yamada, H.; Sumida, I.; Hanada, M. Allergic bronchopulmonary aspergillosis caused by *Aspergillus terreus* presenting lobar collapse. *Intern. Med.* **1992**, *31*, 140–142. [CrossRef] [PubMed]
65. Tillie-Leblond, I.; Tonnel, A.B. Allergic bronchopulmonary aspergillosis. *Allergy* **2005**, *60*, 1004–1013. [CrossRef] [PubMed]
66. Olveira, C.; Padilla, A.; Martínez-García, M.Á.; de la Rosa, D.; Girón, R.M.; Vendrell, M.; Máiz, L.; Borderías, L.; Polverino, E.; Martínez-Moragón, E.; et al. Etiology of bronchiectasis in a cohort of 2047 patients. An analysis of the Spanish Historical Bronchiectasis Registry. *Arch. Bronconeumol.* **2017**, *53*, 366–374. [CrossRef] [PubMed]
67. Hill, A.T.; Routh, C.; Welham, S. National BTS bronchiectasis audit 2012: Is the quality standard being adhered to in adult secondary care? *Thorax* **2014**, *69*, 292–294. [CrossRef] [PubMed]
68. Kraemer, R.; Deloséa, N.; Ballinari, P.; Gallati, S.; Crameri, R. Effect of allergic bronchopulmonary aspergillosis on lung function in children with cystic fibrosis. *Am. J. Respir. Crit. Care Med.* **2006**, *174*, 1211–1220. [CrossRef] [PubMed]

69. Greenberger, P.A.; Miller, T.P.; Roberts, M.; Smith, L.L. Allergic bronchopulmonary aspergillosis in patients with and without evidence of bronchiectasis. *Ann. Allergy* **1993**, *70*, 333–338. [PubMed]

70. Viviani, L.; Harrison, M.J.; Zolin, A.; Haworth, C.S.; Floto, R.A. Epidemiology of nontuberculous mycobacteria (NTM) amongst individuals with cystic fibrosis (CF). *J. Cyst. Fibros.* **2016**, *15*, 619–623. [CrossRef] [PubMed]

71. Dickson, R.P.; Huffnagle, G.B. The Lung Microbiome: New principles for respiratory bacteriology in health and disease. *PLoS Pathog.* **2015**, *11*, e1004923. [CrossRef] [PubMed]

72. Nguyen, L.D.; Viscogliosi, E.; Delhaes, L. The lung mycobiome: An emerging field of the human respiratory microbiome. *Front. Microbiol.* **2015**, *6*, 89. [CrossRef] [PubMed]

73. Willger, S.D.; Grim, S.L.; Dolben, E.L.; Shipunova, A.; Hampton, T.H.; Morrison, H.G.; Filkins, L.M.; O'Toole, G.A.; Moulton, L.A.; Ashare, A.; et al. Characterization and quantification of the fungal microbiome in serial samples from individuals with cystic fibrosis. *Microbiome* **2014**, *2*, 40. [CrossRef] [PubMed]

74. Kramer, R.; Sauer-Heilborn, A.; Welte, T.; Jauregui, R.; Brettar, I.; Guzman, C.A.; Höfle, M.G. High individuality of respiratory bacterial communities in a large cohort of adult cystic fibrosis patients under continuous antibiotic treatment. *PLoS ONE* **2015**, *10*, e0117436. [CrossRef] [PubMed]

75. De Dios Caballero, J.; Vida, R.; Cobo, M.; Máiz, L.; Suárez, L.; Galeano, J.; Baquero, F.; Cantón, R.; Del Campo, R. Individual patterns of complexity in cystic fibrosis lung microbiota, including predator bacteria, over a 1-Year Period. *MBio* **2017**, *8*, e00959-17. [CrossRef] [PubMed]

76. Del Campo, R.; Garriga, M.; Pérez-Aragón, A.; Guallarte, P.; Lamas, A.; Máiz, L.; Bayón, C.; Roy, G.; Cantón, R.; Zamora, J.; et al. Improvement of digestive health and reduction in proteobacterial populations in the gut microbiota of cystic fibrosis patients using a *Lactobacillus reuteri* probiotic preparation: A double blind prospective study. *J. Cyst. Fibros.* **2014**, *13*, 716–722. [CrossRef] [PubMed]

77. Tunney, M.M.; Einarsson, G.G.; Wei, L.; Drain, M.; Klem, E.R.; Cardwell, C.; Ennis, M.; Boucher, R.C.; Wolfgang, M.C.; Elborn, J.S. Lung microbiota and bacterial abundance in patients with bronchiectasis when clinically stable and during exacerbation. *Am. J. Respir. Crit. Care Med.* **2013**, *187*, 1118–1126. [CrossRef] [PubMed]

78. Tipton, L.; Ghedin, E.; Morris, A. The lung mycobiome in the next-generation sequencing era. *Virulence* **2017**, *8*, 334–341. [CrossRef] [PubMed]

79. Aliberti, S.; Masefield, S.; Polverino, E.; De Soyza, A.; Loebinger, M.R.; Menendez, R.; Ringshausen, F.C.; Vendrell, M.; Powell, P.; Chalmers, J.D.; et al. Research priorities in bronchiectasis: A consensus statement from the EMBARC Clinical Research Collaboration. *Eur. Respir. J.* **2016**, *48*, 632–647. [CrossRef] [PubMed]

7

Targeting the Bacterial Cytoskeleton of the *Burkholderia cepacia* Complex for Antimicrobial Development

Sonya C. Carnell [1], John D. Perry [2], Lee Borthwick [1], Daniela Vollmer [3], Jacob Biboy [3], Marcella Facchini [4], Alessandra Bragonzi [4], Alba Silipo [5], Annette C. Vergunst [6], Waldemar Vollmer [3], Anjam C. M. Khan [3] and Anthony De Soyza [1,*]

1 Institute of Cellular Medicine, Newcastle University, Newcastle NE2 4HH, UK; sonya.carnell@ncl.ac.uk (S.C.C.); lee.borthwick@ncl.ac.uk (L.B.)
2 Department of Microbiology, The Freeman Hospital, Newcastle NE7 7DN, UK; john.perry@nuth.nhs.uk
3 Centre for Bacterial Cell Biology, Institute for Cell and Molecular Biosciences, Newcastle University, Newcastle NE2 4HH, UK; daniela.vollmer@ncl.ac.uk (D.V.); Jacob.Biboy@newcastle.ac.uk (J.B.); waldemar.vollmer@newcastle.ac.uk (W.V.); anjam.khan@newcastle.ac.uk (A.C.M.K.)
4 Infections & Cystic Fibrosis Unit, San Raffaele Scientific Institute, 20132 Milan, Italy; facchini.marcella@hsr.it (M.F.); bragonzi.alessandra@hsr.it (A.B.)
5 Department of Chemical Sciences, University of Naples Federico II, Via Cintia 4, 80026 Napoli, Italy; silipo@unina.it
6 VBMI, INSERM, Univ. Montpellier, 30908 Nimes, France; annette.vergunst@univ-montp1.fr
* Correspondence: anthony.de-soyza@ncl.ac.uk

Abstract: *Burkholderia cepacia* complex (BCC) bacteria are a group of opportunistic pathogens that cause severe lung infections in cystic fibrosis (CF). Treatment of BCC infections is difficult, due to the inherent and acquired multidrug resistance of BCC. There is a pressing need to find new bacterial targets for antimicrobials. Here, we demonstrate that the novel compound Q22, which is related to the bacterial cytoskeleton destabilising compound A22, can reduce the growth rate and inhibit growth of BCC bacteria. We further analysed the phenotypic effects of Q22 treatment on BCC virulence traits, to assess its feasibility as an antimicrobial. BCC bacteria were grown in the presence of Q22 with a broad phenotypic analysis, including resistance to H_2O_2-induced oxidative stress, changes in the inflammatory potential of cell surface components, and in-vivo drug toxicity studies. The influence of the Q22 treatment on inflammatory potential was measured by monitoring the cytokine responses of BCC whole cell lysates, purified lipopolysaccharide, and purified peptidoglycan extracted from bacterial cultures grown in the presence or absence of Q22 in differentiated THP-1 cells. BCC bacteria grown in the presence of Q22 displayed varying levels of resistance to H_2O_2-induced oxidative stress, with some strains showing increased resistance after treatment. There was strain-to-strain variation in the pro-inflammatory ability of bacterial lysates to elicit TNFα and IL-1β from human myeloid cells. Despite minimal toxicity previously shown in vitro with primary CF cell lines, in-vivo studies demonstrated Q22 toxicity in both zebrafish and mouse infection models. In summary, destabilisation of the bacterial cytoskeleton in BCC, using compounds such as Q22, led to increased virulence-related traits in vitro. These changes appear to vary depending on strain and BCC species. Future development of antimicrobials targeting the BCC bacterial cytoskeleton may be hampered if such effects translate into the in-vivo environment of the CF infection.

Keywords: antimicrobial; cytoskeleton; Burkholderia

1. Introduction

The *Burkholderia cepacia* complex (BCC) constitutes a group of over 20 closely related opportunistic respiratory pathogen species associated with life-threatening infections in cystic fibrosis (CF) and other immunocompromised patients. Of these species, *B. cenocepacia* and *B. multivorans* are the most prevalent causes of infections in CF patients, and some strains have proved to be highly transmissible between CF patients. BCC infections may remain established for many months, or even years, with clinical outcomes highly variable and unpredictable; in some cases, they can lead to a severe and often fatal complication known as "cepacia syndrome". Cepacia syndrome is characterised by a rapid clinical decline, with high fevers and bacteraemia, progressing to severe pneumonia and death; its existence has led to BCC bacteria emerging as important respiratory pathogens within the CF community. Their intrinsic and acquired resistance to most clinically relevant antimicrobials makes BCC infections notoriously difficult to eradicate or manage. Understandably, due to concerns over this multidrug resistance in BCC and other respiratory pathogens, such as *Pseudomonas aeruginosa*, the development of new and novel antimicrobials is urgently required.

The majority of clinically available antibiotics generally target synthetic pathways, such as DNA synthesis, protein synthesis, and RNA synthesis (reviewed in [1]), suggesting that there is a need to identify new bacterial therapeutic targets that have an important cellular function or role. A number of groups have revealed the presence of the bacterial cytoskeleton, and its potential as an antimicrobial target has been recognized [2]. One cytoskeletal protein of particular interest is the widely conserved actin homolog, MreB. This plays a role in a number of cellular functions, including maintaining cell shape in rod-like bacteria. More recently the role of MreB has been found to be associated with cell-surface-located virulence factors, further emphasizing the suitability of this protein as an antimicrobial target. In the case of *P. aeruginosa*, MreB is required for motility and cell surface localisation of the type IV pilus, a cell surface adhesin important for adhesion to mammalian cells during infection and biofilm formation [3]. Additionally, Bulmer and colleagues have demonstrated the MreB-associated cytoskeletal protein MreC is required for expression of *Salmonella* Typhimurium type three secretion system-1 (T3SS-1) and flagella complexes, both important pathogenicity factors required for colonisation and invasion of the intestine in vivo [4].

To date, few inhibitors of MreB have been identified. *S*-(3,4-dichlorobenzyl) isothiourea hydrochloride (A22) is a small molecule inhibitor of MreB, originally identified as an inhibitor of replication in *E. coli* [5]. A22 has an antimicrobial effect on a range of Gram-negative bacteria; however, very little is known about the effects of A22 on virulence factor expression. Studies of *Shigella flexneri* have shown that exposure to sub-MIC levels of A22 can reduce its ability to invade CHO-K1 cells in vitro [6]. A further inhibitor of MreB, CBR-4830, was identified via a whole-cell antibacterial screen for growth inhibitors of efflux-compromised *P. aeruginosa* strains [7]. CBR-4830 is a novel indole MreB inhibitor chemically distinct from A22.

Recently, we assessed the antimicrobial activity of a panel of A22-related isothiourea hydrochloride derivatives against multi-drug resistant clinical isolates of *P. aeruginosa* and BCC [8]. Here, we extend the use of the lead candidate from this panel, *S*-(4-chlorobenzyl) isothiourea hydrochloride, named Q22, a putative MreB inhibitor (also described as C2 by Nicholson et al.), and study the effects of this compound on virulence-related traits of BCC bacteria [8]. We show that sub-lethal treatment of BCC with Q22 altered virulence phenotypes, including increased resistance to oxidative stress and pro-inflammatory potential, suggesting caution should be taken when targeting the bacterial cytoskeleton of BCC for antimicrobial development.

2. Results

2.1. *Q22 Treatment Alters Cell Morphology, Reduces Growth Rate, and Inhibits Growth of B. cenocepacia Species*

Having recently established the antimicrobial activity of both A22 and Q22 against a panel of BCC strains [8], we wanted to further analyse the effect of Q22 on growth and morphology of a panel of BCC bacteria (Table 1). Initially we used *B. cenocepacia* J2315 as a test organism to determine appropriate growth permissive levels of Q22 (Figure 1A). *B. cenocepacia* J2315 is a clinical ET-12 epidemic strain isolated from a CF patient [9]. Q22-treated *B. cenocepacia* J2315 cultures showed a reduction in growth rate in a concentration-dependent manner (Figure 1A; 0 µg/mL vs. 40 µg/mL Q22; $p \leq 0.05$)). Based on these results, 30 µg/mL Q22 was selected as an appropriate, sub-lethal, growth-permissive concentration for subsequent experiments. Upon exposure to 30 µg/mL Q22, all BCC strains tested, including those listed in Table 1, demonstrated a reduction in growth rate (as previously [8]). The degree of growth rate reduction varied between strains, and a lesser reduction was observed upon exposure to Q22 when compared to A22. Changes in cell morphology from rod to cocci forms were confirmed by scanning electron microscopy, supporting disruption of the MreB-based cytoskeleton (Figure 1B).

Table 1. Bacterial strains used in this study.

Species	Description	Source
B. cenocepacia LMG16656 (J2315)	Clinical isolate, CF patient, ET-12 epidemic strain	BCCM
B. cenocepacia LMG18829	Clinical isolate, CF patient, epidemic strain	BCCM
B. multivorans LMG13010	Clinical isolate, CF patient	BCCM
B. vietnamiensis LMG16232	Clinical isolate, CF patient	BCCM

BCCM, Belgian Coordinated Collection of Micro-organisms.

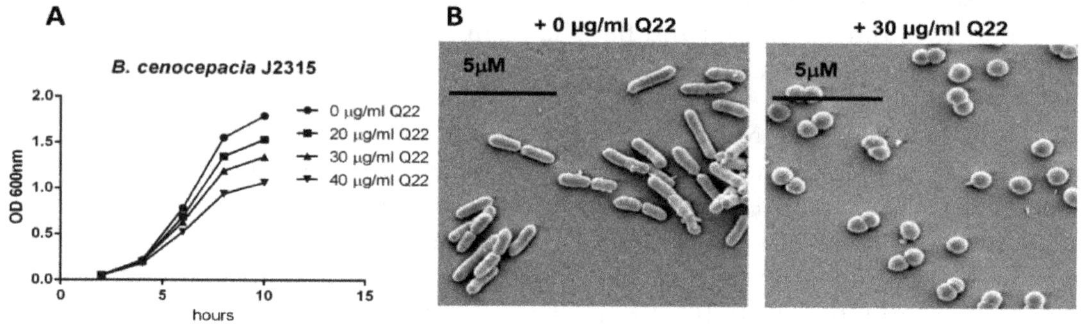

Figure 1. Growth and morphological changes induced by Q22 treatment. (**A**) Growth of *B. cenocepacia* J2315 in the absence or presence of increasing concentrations of Q22 (0, 20, 30, 40 µg/mL); (**B**) scanning electron microscope images of *B. cenocepacia* J2315, untreated and after treatment with 30 µg/mL Q22 at 6 h timepoint.

2.2. *Q22 Treatment Alters Ability of B. cenocepacia to Resist H_2O_2-Induced Oxidative Stress*

BCC bacteria are exposed to reactive oxygen species (ROS) during colonisation and infection of the CF lung, and have a number of strategies to combat this form of stress [10,11]. We evaluated the susceptibility of Q22-treated and untreated BCC cultures to H_2O_2 (Figure 2). The reduction in viability upon H_2O_2 exposure varied between BCC strains when grown without drug treatment, with *B. cenocepacia* strains LMG18829 and J2315 showing the greatest resistance at 20 mM H_2O_2 (Figure 2B,C).

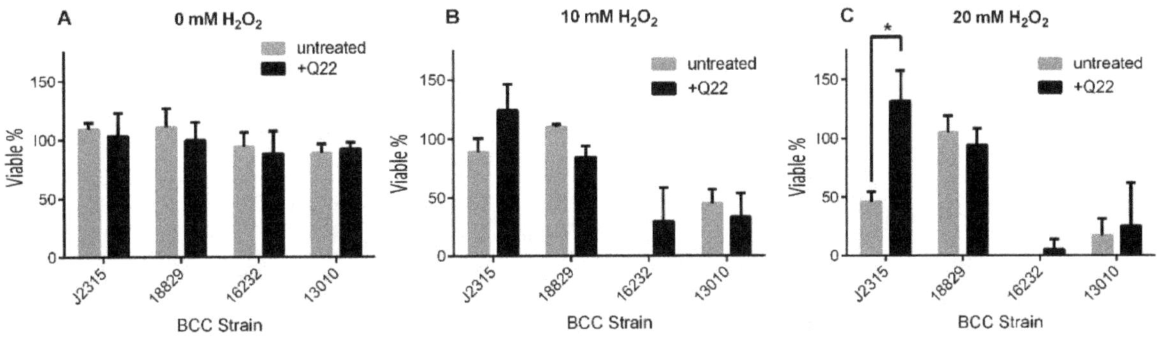

Figure 2. Survival of *B. cepacia* complex (BCC) strains exposed to H_2O_2 in vitro. Late-stationary-phase cells were treated with varying concentrations of H_2O_2, 0 mM (**A**), 10 mM (**B**), and 20 mM (**C**), as described under Section 4. Samples were plated in triplicate for colony counts, and percentage survival (expressed as % viability) was calculated relative to colony counts of untreated bacteria. * $p < 0.05$. Isolates included *B. cenocepacia* LMG16656 (J2315), *B. cenocepacia* LMG18829, *B. multivorans* LMG13010, and *B. vietnamiensis* LMG16232 (see Table 1).

When compared to untreated controls, we observed an increase in H_2O_2 resistance for strain J2315 that was statistically significant (Figure 2C, $p < 0.05$).

2.3. *Q22 Treatment Does Not Alter Lipopolysaccharide Profile of B. cenocepacia Strains*

We analysed the crude LPS profiles of WCLs prepared from BCC cultures exposed to Q22, to determine if this compound alters LPS composition when compared to untreated WCLs. WCLs were prepared from BCC strains grown in the presence and absence of 30 μg/mL Q22. Of the four strains tested, no significant differences in the LPS electrophoretic profile were observed. J2315 showed no difference in profile at all. To further assess if there were any changes in LPS structure, LPS was isolated from Q22-treated and untreated cultures of *B. cenocepacia* LMG18829, and lipid A extracted and analysed further by MALDI-TOF mass spectrometry (Table 2). Both LPS and lipid A showed a mixture of differently-acylated species, both carrying Ara4N residues on the polar heads. Interestingly, the Q22-treated LMG18829 strain also carried an unsubstituted tetra-acylated lipid A species, absent in the untreated strain (Table 2). However, no other significant differences in LPS structure were observed.

Table 2. Structural analysis of *B. cenocepacia* LMG18829 lipid A.

	***B. cenocepacia* LMG18829 Untreated**		***B. cenocepacia* LMG18829 + 30 μg/mL Q22**	
Lipid A Species	**Intensity (%)**	**Mass**	**Intensity (%)**	**Mass**
tetra-acylated lipid A			58.8	1444.9
tetra-acylated lipid A + Ara4N	100	1576.4	100	1576.1
tetra-acylated lipid A + 2 Ara4N	87.8	1707.5	60	1707.0
penta-acylated lipid A + Ara4N	48.7	1800.9	38.2	1801.0
penta-acylated lipid A + 2 Ara4N	39	1934.0	29	1932.2

Negative ion MALDI-TOF spectrum analysis of lipid A isolated from *B. cenocepacia* LMG18829, grown in the presence and absence of 30 μg/mL Q22.

2.4. *Q22 Treatment Alters Proinflammatory Potential of BCC Strains*

BCC LPS has potent endotoxic activity and can elicit high levels of pro-inflammatory cytokines [12,13]. To determine if chemical disruption of the bacterial cytoskeleton using compound Q22 alters the endotoxic potential of the bacteria, we stimulated differentiated THP-1 cells with WCLs, known to be rich in LPS, prepared from cultures exposed to Q22. Pro-inflammatory cytokine responses characteristic of those encountered within the host during BCC infection (TNFα and IL-1β) were measured. Data demonstrated a variable strain-dependent increase in cytokine induction when cells were stimulated with lysates obtained from bacteria exposed to Q22, compared to those obtained from untreated bacteria. This significant strain-specific increase was noted for both TNFα (Figure 3A; $p < 0.01$) and IL-1β (Figure 3B; $p < 0.05$) responses for Q22-treated *B. cenocepacia* strain J2315, as well as for TNFα (Figure 3A; $p < 0.01$) for Q22-treated *B. cenocepacia* strain LMG18829.

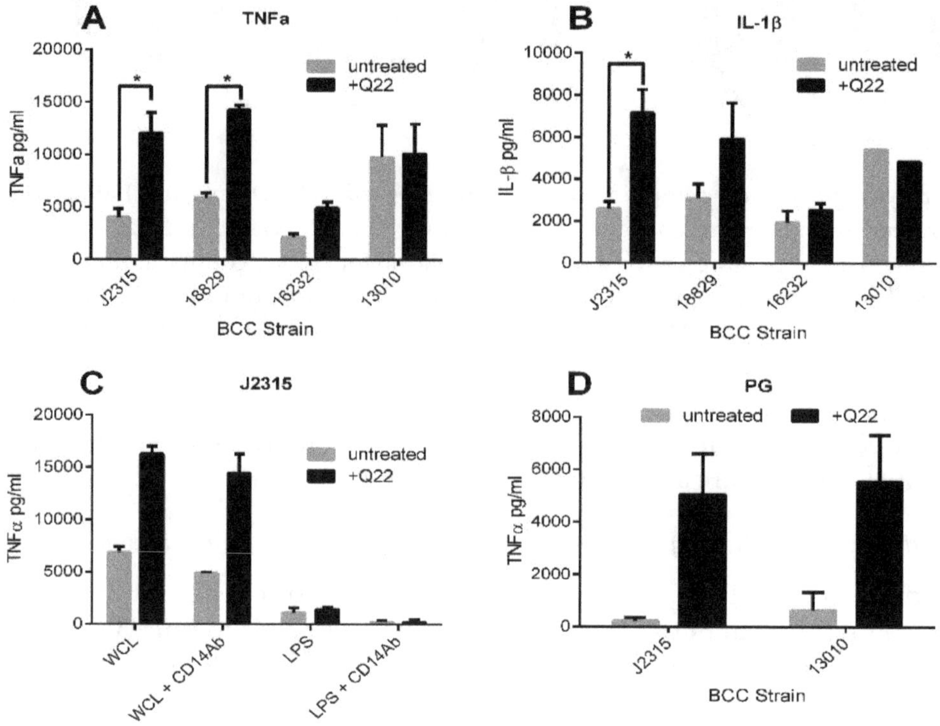

Figure 3. Cytokine responses of THP-1 cells, stimulated with Q22-treated and untreated preparations. Cytokine responses at 6 h post-stimulation with whole cell lysates of BCC strains *B. cenocepacia* J2315, *B. cenocepacia* LMG18829, *B. multivorans* LMG13010, and *B. vietnamiensis* LMG16232. (**A**) TNFα; (**B**) IL-1β. TNFα responses at 6 h post stimulation with whole cell lysates, purified lipopolysaccharide (LPS) (**C**), or purified peptidoglycan (PG) (**D**) from BCC strain *B. cenocepacia* J2315. Comparison of profiles from cells stimulated with and without a CD14 antibody pre-incubation step (**C**). * $p < 0.05$.

To determine whether this strain-specific increase in pro-inflammatory response was LPS-dependent, we pre-incubated THP-1 cells with a CD14 antibody prior to stimulation, to block the TLR4-dependent stimulatory pathway used by LPS. The increased TNFα response observed with *B. cenocepacia* J2315 Q22-treated lysates was not abolished with the CD14 antibody treatment, suggesting the increased cytokine release was not LPS-driven (Figure 3C). This was further confirmed by observing the TNFα response of THP-1 cells, stimulated with purified LPS extracted from *B. cenocepacia* J2315 cultures grown in the presence and absence of Q22. Results demonstrated no significant difference in TNFα response, obtained by stimulation with *B. cenocepacia* J2315 LPS purified from treated and untreated cultures (Figure 3C). This is in agreement with our finding that the LPS profile of *B. cenocepacia* J2315 was not changed after Q22 treatment.

Peptidoglycan (PG) is a significant structural and immune-stimulatory component of the bacterial cell wall, and could plausibly be affected by cytoskeletal disruption. To determine if the observed increase in pro-inflammatory potential of the *B. cenocepacia* WCLs could be attributed to PG, we isolated PG from two different BCC species, *B. cenocepacia* J2315 and *B. multivorans* LMG13010, each grown in the presence and absence of 30 μg/mL Q22. The purified PG was subsequently used to stimulate THP-1 cells, and TNFα responses were measured. Both BCC strains tested showed an increase in TNFα production when the bacteria were exposed to 30 μg/mL Q22 prior to PG extraction, when compared to untreated controls; however, only the increase between the treated and untreated *B. cenocepacia* J2315 samples was statistically significant ($p < 0.05$) (Figure 3D).

2.5. Q22 Toxicity In-Vivo Studies in Zebrafish and Mouse Models

Preliminary experiments demonstrated negligible toxicity in THP-1 cells or CF primary bronchial epithelial cells (data not shown) [14].

Ultimately, the potential for in-vivo toxicity must be considered when developing a compound for antimicrobial use; therefore, we aimed to determine the effects of Q22 in vivo, utilising the zebrafish embryo BCC infection model established by Vergunst and colleagues [15], and the BCC mouse lung infection model optimised by Bragonzi and co-workers [16]. We aimed to extend the in vivo toxicity testing in these models prior to Q22 infection protection assessment.

Zebrafish embryos, 30 h post-fertilisation, were incubated in different concentrations of Q22 in embryo water. Whereas 100% of untreated control embryos and embryos incubated in 6.4 μg/mL Q22 survived during a five-day observation period, a dose-dependent killing was observed with higher doses of Q22 than were anticipated to be needed for antimicrobial effects (Figure 4; $p < 0.0001$). A concentration of 64 μg/mL was lethal for the embryos on day five, but embryos started to die on day three when incubated in embryo water with 640 μg/mL, a concentration that killed most of the embryos on day four of the treatment. These results clearly indicate the toxicity of the compound for zebrafish larvae, even at concentrations that are close to the appropriate bacterial, sub-lethal, growth-permissive concentration of 30 μg/mL.

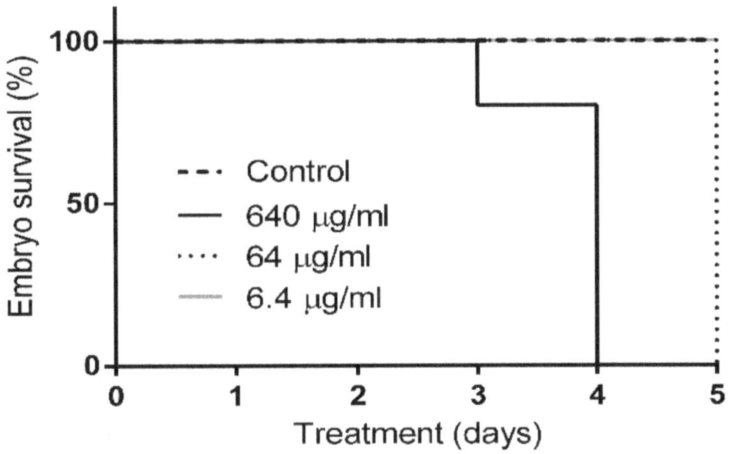

Figure 4. Toxicity of Q22 in the zebrafish embryo model. Zebrafish embryos were exposed to increasing concentrations of Q22 (6.4 μg/mL; 64 μg/mL; 640 μg/mL) at 30 high power field and monitored for survival for up to 120 h post-incubation. Data expressed as percentage survival.

Results of the preliminary toxicity study in mice demonstrated that mice exposed to higher doses of Q22 100 mg/kg (Group 1) and 50 mg/kg (Group 2) after IT administration of Q22 were moribund (could not right themselves after being placed in lateral recumbence), and thus were killed and the experiment terminated (Table 3). Those mice exposed to the lower dose, 25 mg/kg Q22 (Group 3), demonstrated reduced mobility when compared with control mice during the first two days of treatment, and lungs showed signs of inflammation and damage macroscopically after four days. All control mice were healthy after treatment (Group 4). Based on these results suggesting significant pulmonary toxicity, and in the interests of animal welfare, no further in-vivo experiments were performed.

Table 3. Toxicity of Q22 in the mouse model.

Group	Dose Q22 (mg/kg)	Results
1	100	Mice died immediately after intra-tracheal administration of Q22
2	50	Mice died immediately after intra-tracheal administration of Q22
3	25	Mice showed reduced mobility compared with controls during first 2 days after treatment. Lungs were inflamed and damaged after 4 days
4	0	Mice were healthy after treatment

Mice were injected IT with increasing concentrations of Q22 (25 mg/kg; 50 mg/kg; 100 mg/kg) and monitored for up to 4 days post administration.

3. Discussion

Although the emergence of drug-resistant bacteria is a pressing issue, there are few antimicrobials in development for the treatment of infections caused by these organisms [17]. We assessed the bacterial cytoskeleton as a potential novel antimicrobial target, using the highly antibiotic-resistant BCC as a model group of organisms. To target the bacterial cytoskeleton, we tested the A22-related compound *S*-(4-chlorobenzyl) isothiourea hydrochloride (named Q22 in this study) as a potential antimicrobial candidate, and measured phenotypic changes in the virulence traits of BCC. In addition to the expected changes in growth and morphology observed with other Gram-negative bacterial species [4,18,19], we also observed unexpected increases in resistance to H_2O_2-induced oxidative stress and the pro-inflammatory potential of Q22 treatment in selected strains. BCC strains are known to show a heterogeneity with other phenotypes, even across apparently clonal isolates [20]. Hence, the variation herein appears consistent with these prior data.

We are unable to provide a mechanistic explanation for this increased resistance to H_2O_2-induced stress in strain J2315. It is possible that the physiological changes in cell shape and structure may alter the release or access to oxidative stress-related enzymes, such as catalases, which may vary between strains. The concept of a drug treatment providing an opportunistic pathogen with the increased capacity to combat ROS is a concern. This is highly relevant, as protection against ROS, such as hydrogen peroxide, is important for the survival of BCC persister cells [21]. Persister cells are cells that have entered a dormant, multidrug-tolerant state, and are thought to play a role in the recalcitrance of biofilm-related infections in vivo.

Furthermore, in-vitro data generated during this study has suggested that Q22 treatment can increase the pro-inflammatory potential of certain BCC. As Q22 has been shown to depolymerise MreB in other Gram-negative organisms [22], it is possible that by depolymerising the bacterial cytoskeleton of BCC, Q22 may alter the structure of important bacterial pathogen-associated molecular patterns (PAMPs) located within the cell wall. Our data suggests that Q22 does not significantly affect the structure of the LPS component of the outer membrane, but may have an effect on the PG component. To confirm a role for PG in the changes in cytokine response of Q22-treated strains, we are currently investigating the structure of PG extracted from Q22-treated bacteria.

Recently, Q22 has been described as a breakdown product of an antibacterial compound, MAC13243, found to inhibit the bacterial lipoprotein targeting chaperone LolA, identified during a chemical genome screen [23]. Saturation transfer difference (STD) NMR analysis revealed that Q22 directly interacts with LolA in vitro. Therefore, we must consider that potential interactions of Q22 with LolA may contribute to the phenotypic changes seen here.

In conclusion, we have shown that sub-inhibitory concentrations of Q22 can alter and affect the phenotypic traits of certain BCC. Importantly, in contrast to earlier studies performed in vitro (unpublished data), our studies demonstrate that Q22 is highly toxic for zebrafish larvae and mice, which suggest that this compound is an unacceptable candidate for drug development for the treatment of human disease.

Furthermore, as destabilisation of the bacterial cytoskeleton using compounds such as Q22 can lead to unexpected increases of in-vitro, virulence-related traits, we believe future development of antimicrobials targeting the BCC bacterial cytoskeleton may be hampered if such effects translate into the in-vivo environment of CF infection, and consider that caution must be taken. Future studies that study a wider panel of isolates may help understand how widespread our observations are across the BCC. Further studies to help our understanding of the mechanistic basis of this increased virulence are imperative for developing alternative control strategies.

4. Materials and Methods

4.1. Ethics Statement

Mammalian studies were conducted according to protocols approved by the San Raffaele Scientific Institute (Milan, Italy) Institutional Animal Care and Use Committee (IACUC), and adhered strictly to the Italian Ministry of Health guidelines for the use and care of experimental animals. Zebrafish (Danio rerio) were kept and handled in compliance with the guidelines of the European Union for handling laboratory animals (http://ec.europa.eu/environment/chemicals/lab_animals/home_en.htm). Studies performed at VBMI are approved by the Direction Départementale de la Protection des Populations (DDPP) du Gard (ID 30-189-4). The experiments were terminated before the larvae reached the free feeding stage and did not classify as animal experiments according to the 2010/63/EU Directive. Approval date: 1 October 2014.

4.2. Bacterial Strains and Growth Conditions

The bacterial strains used in this study are included in the international BCC reference panel [20] and are described in Table 1. BCC strains were grown at 37 °C in Luria-Bertani (LB) broth, unless otherwise indicated. Q22, kindly provided by Prof. John Perry [8], was maintained in methanol at 1 mg/mL and stored at −20 °C. Bacterial stocks were maintained at −80 °C as 20% glycerol suspensions.

4.3. Q22 Treatment

Q22 treatment doses were based on sub-MIC concentrations, unless otherwise indicated [8]. To measure the effects of Q22 treatment on BCC cell morphology and growth, overnight bacterial cultures were subcultured 1:500 into fresh LB broth, in the absence or presence of Q22, and incubated at 37 °C with shaking. LB broth was supplemented with Q22 at the 0 h timepoint. Samples were removed at selected timepoints as indicated. BCC were additionally grown in the presence of corresponding volumes of methanol, as a diluent control. A viable count of bacteria in cultures grown in the presence and absence of Q22 was taken to confirm acceptable use of optical density as a measure of growth. Scanning electron microscope images of the resulting cells were taken.

4.4. Hydrogen Peroxide (H_2O_2) Protection Assay

The ability of BCC strains to survive H_2O_2 exposure was measured, as previously described [10]. Briefly, BCC cultures were grown and shaken at 37 °C in LB, supplemented with Q22, diluent control (methanol), or no supplementation until the late stationary phase. The optical density was determined and samples were standardised to a concentration of 1×10^8 cfu. Each strain was treated with varying H_2O_2 concentrations (0–20 mM) and incubated with shaking at 25 °C for 30 min. Control samples received distilled H_2O in place of the H_2O_2 treatment. Appropriate serial dilutions were plated in triplicate on LB agar plates. Colonies were counted after 48 h incubation, and percentage survival calculated by comparison with colony counts obtained from untreated samples.

4.5. Isolation of Bacterial Whole Cell Lysates (WCLs)

Whole cell lysates (WCLs) were prepared as described, with additional modifications [24]. Briefly, strains were grown overnight on Brain Heart Infusion (BHI) agar plates or in BHI broth to an optical density of ~1.8 at 600 nm. Broth grown bacteria were harvested by centrifugation and washed once with phosphate-buffered saline (PBS), to remove growth media and supplements prior to standardising to an optical density of 0.2 at 600 nm. Bacterial suspensions were disrupted by sonication with a Branson 150 sonifier (six cycles, 30 s on, 30 s off) and incubated with 200 µg/mL deoxyribonuclease II (Dnase II) (Sigma-Aldrich, Saint Louis, MO, USA) at 37 °C for 1 h. WCLs were treated with 2 mg/mL Proteinase K (Sigma-Aldrich) at 60 °C for 2 h, boiled for 20 min (inactivating Proteinase K), and stored at −80 °C until required.

4.6. Purification of Lipopolysaccharide (LPS)

Lipopolysaccharide (LPS) was extracted and purified using a modified version of the hot-water phenol method previously described [25]. Strains were grown to late log phase in nutrient broth containing 0.5% yeast extract at 37 °C. Bacteria were harvested by centrifugation at 1000× *g*, re-suspended in a minimal volume distilled water, and freeze-dried. Pellets were re-suspended in distilled water and sonicated on ice. The resulting sonicated suspension was subjected to Dnase II digestion (final concentration 200 µg/mL) at 37 °C for 2 h, followed by Proteinase K digestion (final concentration 1 mg/mL) at 60 °C for 2 h. After boiling for 20 min, an equal volume was mixed with hot phenol and incubated at 70 °C for 20 min with regular mixing. The suspension was cooled on ice and centrifuged at 800× *g*. The water-soluble phase was removed and dialysed against repeated changes of fresh distilled water for 72 h. Ultracentrifugation at 39,500× *g* for 6 h at 13 °C was undertaken, and the supernatant was discarded. The resulting pellet was dissolved in a minimal volume of ultrapure distilled water and freeze-dried. Protein and DNA contamination levels were assessed using a Pierce™ BCA Protein Assay (Thermo Scientific, Waltham, MA, USA) and UV spectrophotometry, respectively, to ensure an LPS purity level of at least 95% was obtained. LPS samples were analysed by sodium dodecyl sulphate polyacrylamide gel electrophoresis (SDS-PAGE) and visualised using a Pierce™ Silver Stain kit (Thermo Scientific).

After removal of organic solvents under a vacuum, the lipooligosaccharide (LOS) fraction was precipitated from concentrated phenol solution with water; the precipitate was washed with aqueous 80% phenol, and then three times with cold acetone and then lyophilized. The LOS fractions were analyzed by SDS-PAGE on 16% gels, which were stained with silver nitrate

4.7. Isolation of Lipid A

Free lipid A was obtained by hydrolysis of LOS (with 10 mM sodium acetate buffer pH 4.4, (100 °C, 3 h). The solution was extracted three times with chloroform/methanol/H_2O (100:100:30 *v*/*v*/*v*) and centrifuged (4 °C, 5000× *g*, 15 min). The organic phase contained the lipid A, and the water phase contained the core oligosaccharide.

4.8. Matrix Assisted Laser Desorption/Ionization Time of Flight (MALDI-TOF) Mass Spectrometry

MALDI-TOF mass spectra of the intact LOS were recorded in the negative polarity on a Perseptive (Framingham, MA, USA) Voyager STR equipped with delayed extraction technology. Ions formed by a pulsed UV laser beam (nitrogen laser, λ = 337 nm) were accelerated by 24 kV.

LOS and lipid A sample preparation: R-type LOS MALDI preparation was performed as recently reported in detail [26]. MALDI preparation of lipid A was performed as described [27]. Briefly, samples were dissolved in chloroform/methanol (1:1 *v*/*v*), whereas matrix solution was prepared by dissolving 2,4,6-trihydroxyacetophenone (THAP) in methanol/0.1% trifluoroacetic acid/acetonitrile (7:2:1). A sample/matrix solution mixture (1:1 *v*/*v*) was deposited (1 µL) onto the MALDI plate and left to dry at room temperature.

4.9. Purification of Peptidoglycan (PG)

Sacculi were isolated from BCC as described [28], with the following modifications. BCC cells (800 mL) were grown to an optical density of 0.6 at 600 nm and harvested by centrifugation at 7500× *g* for 15 min at 4 °C. The cell pellet was re-suspended in 6 mL of ice-cold sterile dH_2O. The cell suspension was added dropwise to 6 mL boiling 8% sodium dodecyl sulphate (SDS) solution. The solution was boiled for a further 30 min, and the resulting cell suspension pelleted by centrifugation at 130,000× *g* for 60 min at 25 °C. The pellet was washed repeatedly with dH_2O until the supernatant was free of SDS, as determined by a published assay [29].

4.10. Cell Culture

THP-1 human monocytes [30] were kindly donated by Prof. John Taylor and were maintained at 37 °C with 5% CO_2 in RPMI-1640 medium (Sigma-Aldrich), supplemented with 10% foetal calf serum (Sigma-Aldrich), 1% penicillin/streptomycin (Sigma-Aldrich) and 1% L-glutamine (Sigma-Aldrich). To differentiate the monocytes into macrophage-like cells, 300 μL cells at a concentration of 0.5×10^6 cells/mL was transferred into 24-well tissue culture plates and incubated at 37 °C with 5% CO_2 for 24 h in the presence of 2.5 ng/mL phorbol myristate acetate (PMA) (Sigma-Aldrich). Prior to stimulation, the differentiated cells were washed with PBS.

4.11. Stimulation Assays and Cytokine Quantification

Differentiated THP-1 cell lines were stimulated for 6 h with either 12.5 μL/mL bacterial whole cell lysate, 100 ng/mL LPS, or 100 μg/mL PG as indicated. Culture supernatants were harvested and assayed for cytokine (TNFα and IL-1β) production using Human DuoSet® ELISA Kits (R&D Systems, Abingdon-On-Thames, UK). Where indicated, differentiated THP-1 cells were pre-incubated with CD14 antibody (Monosan, Uden, The Netherlands, Mon1108, final concentration 400 ng/mL) for 1 h prior to stimulation.

4.12. Zebrafish Model

To determine the toxicity of compound Q22 in vivo, zebrafish embryos staged 30–32 h post-fertilisation (hpf) were incubated with E3 embryo medium (5 mM NaCl, 0.17 mM KCl, 0.33 mM $CaCl_2$, 0.33 mM $MgSO_4$) containing increasing concentrations (0, 6.4 μg/mL, 64 μg/mL or 640 μg/mL) of Q22. A stock solution of 6.4 mg/mL was freshly prepared in E3. Embryos, individually plated in a 24-well plate (experiment 1: $n = 10$ per treatment), or in groups of 10–20 embryos in 6-well plates (experiment 2: $n = 40$ per treatment; experiment 3: $n = 50$ per treatment) were incubated at 29 °C. Embryos were observed for five days post-administration, and embryo death was determined by the absence of a heartbeat.

4.13. Mouse Model

To determine the toxicity of compound Q22 in mammals, 8–10 week old male C57BL/6NCr mice, 20–22 g, from Charles River Laboratories, were housed in filtered cages under specific pathogen-free conditions, and permitted unlimited access to food and water. Groups of two mice were inoculated via the intratracheal (IT) route with varying doses (100 mg/kg; 50 mg/kg; 25 mg/kg) of Q22 dissolved in 60 μL distilled dH_2O. Control animals were exposed to 60 μL dH_2O as a negative control. For IT injection, mice were anesthetized by an intraperitoneal injection of Avertin (2,2,2-tribromethanol, 97%) in 0.9% NaCl, administered at a volume of 0.015 mL/g body weight. Mice were placed in a supine position. The trachea was directly visualised by ventral midline, exposed and intubated with a sterile, flexible 22 g cannula attached to a 1 mL syringe. After compound administration, moribund mice (those that could not right themselves after being placed in lateral recumbence) were killed before termination of the experiments. Remaining groups of mice were monitored twice daily for the parameters: vocalisation, piloerection, attitude, locomotion, breathing, curiosity, nasal secretion, grooming, and dehydration. Mice that lost >25% of their body weight and had evidence of severe clinical disease, such as scruffy coat, inactivity, loss of appetite, poor locomotion, or painful posture, were sacrificed before the termination of the experiments with an overdose of carbon dioxide. Mice were sacrificed by increasing CO_2 administration, and lungs were harvested and observed for damage and inflammation.

4.14. Statistical Methods

Statistical analysis was performed using a paired t-test where appropriate. Differences with p values of <0.05 were considered statistically significant. For zebrafish survival studies, the data were plotted using Kaplan–Meier survival curves (Prism GraphPad software version 6.03), and statistical significance was determined with a log rank test.

Author Contributions: Conceived and designed the experiments: S.C.C., A.S., A.C.M.K., W.V. Performed the experiments: S.C.C., L.B., D.V., J.B., A.B., M.F., A.C.V., A.S. Analyzed the data: S.C.C., A.S. Contributed reagents/materials/analysis tools: J.D.P., A.B., A.C.V., A.S. Wrote the paper: S.C.C., A.D.S.

Acknowledgments: The authors are grateful to Tracey Davies of Newcastle University Electron Microscopy Research Services for technical assistance, David Bulmer for performance of Q22 preliminary growth tests, and David McGeeney of Newcastle University Industrial Statistics Research Unit for statistical advice. The authors acknowledge support from EU COST Action BM1003 and the Newcastle Upon Tyne Hospitals Special Trustees.

References

1. Chopra, I. Research and development of antibacterial agents. *Curr. Opin. Microbiol.* **1998**, *1*, 495–501. [CrossRef]
2. Vollmer, W. The prokaryotic cytoskeleton: A putative target for inhibitors and antibiotics? *Appl. Microbiol. Biotechnol.* **2006**, *73*, 37–47. [CrossRef] [PubMed]
3. Cowles, K.N.; Gitai, Z. Surface association and the MreB cytoskeleton regulate pilus production, localization and function in Pseudomonas aeruginosa. *Mol. Microbiol.* **2010**, *76*, 1411–1426. [CrossRef] [PubMed]
4. Bulmer, D.M.; Kharraz, L.; Grant, A.J.; Dean, P.; Morgan, F.J.; Karavolos, M.H.; Doble, A.C.; McGhie, E.J.; Koronakis, V.; Daniel, R.A.; et al. The bacterial cytoskeleton modulates motility, type 3 secretion, and colonization in Salmonella. *PLoS Pathog.* **2012**, *8*, e1002500. [CrossRef] [PubMed]
5. Iwai, N.; Nagai, K.; Wachi, M. Novel S-benzylisothiourea compound that induces spherical cells in Escherichia coli probably by acting on a rod-shape-determining protein(s) other than penicillin-binding protein 2. *Biosci. Biotechnol. Biochem.* **2002**, *66*, 2658–2662. [CrossRef] [PubMed]
6. Noguchi, N.; Yanagimoto, K.; Nakaminami, H.; Wakabayashi, M.; Iwai, N.; Wachi, M.; Sasatsu, M. Anti-infectious effect of S-benzylisothiourea compound A22, which inhibits the actin-like protein, MreB, in Shigella flexneri. *Biol. Pharm. Bull.* **2008**, *31*, 1327–1332. [CrossRef] [PubMed]
7. Robertson, G.T.; Doyle, T.B.; Du, Q.; Duncan, L.; Mdluli, K.E.; Lynch, A.S. A Novel indole compound that inhibits Pseudomonas aeruginosa growth by targeting MreB is a substrate for MexAB-OprM. *J. Bacteriol.* **2007**, *189*, 6870–6881. [CrossRef] [PubMed]
8. Nicholson, A.; Perry, J.D.; James, A.L.; Stanforth, S.P.; Carnell, S.; Wilkinson, K.; Khan, C.A.; De Soyza, A.; Gould, F.K. In vitro activity of S-(3,4-dichlorobenzyl)isothiourea hydrochloride and novel structurally related compounds against multidrug-resistant bacteria, including Pseudomonas aeruginosa and Burkholderia cepacia complex. *Int. J. Antimicrob. Agents* **2012**, *39*, 27–32. [CrossRef] [PubMed]
9. Govan, J.R.; Doherty, C.J.; Nelson, J.W.; Brown, P.H.; Greening, A.P.; Maddison, J.; Dodd, M.; Webb, A.K. Evidence for transmission of Pseudomonas cepacia by social contact in cystic fibrosis. *Lancet* **1993**, *342*, 15–19. [CrossRef]
10. Lefebre, M.; Valvano, M. In vitro resistance of Burkholderia cepacia complex isolates to reactive oxygen species in relation to catalase and superoxide dismutase production. *Microbiology* **2001**, *147*, 97–109. [CrossRef] [PubMed]

11. Bylund, J.; Burgess, L.A.; Cescutti, P.; Ernst, R.K.; Speert, D.P. Exopolysaccharides from Burkholderia cenocepacia inhibit neutrophil chemotaxis and scavenge reactive oxygen species. *J. Biol. Chem.* **2006**, *281*, 2526–2532. [CrossRef] [PubMed]
12. De Soyza, A.; Ellis, C.D.; Khan, C.M.; Corris, P.A.; Demarco de Hormaeche, R. Burkholderia cenocepacia lipopolysaccharide, lipid A, and proinflammatory activity. *Am. J. Respir. Crit. Care Med.* **2004**, *170*, 70–77. [CrossRef] [PubMed]
13. Silipo, A.; Molinaro, A.; Ierano, T.; De Soyza, A.; Sturiale, L.; Garozzo, D.; Aldridge, C.; Corris, P.A.; Khan, C.M.; Lanzetta, R.; et al. The complete structure and pro-inflammatory activity of the lipooligosaccharide of the highly epidemic and virulent gram-negative bacterium Burkholderia cenocepacia ET-12 (strain J2315). *Chemistry* **2007**, *13*, 3501–3511. [CrossRef] [PubMed]
14. Brodlie, M.; McKean, M.C.; Johnson, G.E.; Perry, J.D.; Nicholson, A.; Verdon, B.; Gray, M.A.; Dark, J.H.; Pearson, J.P.; Fisher, A.J.; et al. Primary bronchial epithelial cell culture from explanted cystic fibrosis lungs. *Exp. Lung Res.* **2010**, *36*, 101–110. [CrossRef] [PubMed]
15. Vergunst, A.C.; Meijer, A.H.; Renshaw, S.A.; O'Callaghan, D. Burkholderia cenocepacia creates an intramacrophage replication niche in zebrafish embryos, followed by bacterial dissemination and establishment of systemic infection. *Infect. Immun.* **2010**, *78*, 1495–1508. [CrossRef] [PubMed]
16. Pirone, L.; Bragonzi, A.; Farcomeni, A.; Paroni, M.; Auriche, C.; Conese, M.; Chiarini, L.; Dalmastri, C.; Bevivino, A.; Ascenzioni, F. Burkholderia cenocepacia strains isolated from cystic fibrosis patients are apparently more invasive and more virulent than rhizosphere strains. *Environ. Microbiol.* **2008**, *10*, 2773–2784. [CrossRef] [PubMed]
17. Health Do. UK Five Year Antimicrobial Resistance Strategy. 2013. Available online: https://wwwgovuk/government/uploads/system/uploads/attachment_data/file/244058/20130902_UK_5_year_AMR_strategypdf (accessed on 10 January 2016).
18. Iwai, N.; Fujii, T.; Nagura, H.; Wachi, M.; Kitazume, T. Structure-activity relationship study of the bacterial actin-like protein MreB inhibitors: Effects of substitution of benzyl group in S-benzylisothiourea. *Biosci. Biotechnol. Biochem.* **2007**, *71*, 246–248. [CrossRef] [PubMed]
19. Srivastava, P.; Demarre, G.; Karpova, T.S.; McNally, J.; Chattoraj, D.K. Changes in nucleoid morphology and origin localization upon inhibition or alteration of the actin homolog, MreB, of Vibrio cholerae. *J. Bacteriol.* **2007**, *189*, 7450–7463. [CrossRef] [PubMed]
20. Mahenthiralingam, E.; Coenye, T.; Chung, J.W.; Speert, D.P.; Govan, J.R.; Taylor, P.; Vandamme, P. Diagnostically and experimentally useful panel of strains from the Burkholderia cepacia complex. *J. Clin. Microbiol.* **2000**, *38*, 910–913. [PubMed]
21. Van Acker, H.; Sass, A.; Bazzini, S.; De Roy, K.; Udine, C.; Messiaen, T.; Riccardi, G.; Boon, N.; Nelis, H.J.; Mahenthiralingam, E.; et al. Biofilm-grown Burkholderia cepacia complex cells survive antibiotic treatment by avoiding production of reactive oxygen species. *PLoS ONE* **2013**, *8*, e58943. [CrossRef] [PubMed]
22. Takacs, C.N.; Poggio, S.; Charbon, G.; Pucheault, M.; Vollmer, W.; Jacobs-Wagner, C. MreB drives de novo rod morphogenesis in Caulobacter crescentus via remodeling of the cell wall. *J. Bacteriol.* **2010**, *192*, 1671–1684. [CrossRef] [PubMed]
23. Barker, C.A.; Allison, S.E.; Zlitni, S.; Nguyen, N.D.; Das, R.; Melacini, G.; Capretta, A.A.; Brown, E.D. Degradation of MAC13243 and studies of the interaction of resulting thiourea compounds with the lipoprotein targeting chaperone LolA. *Bioorg. Med. Chem. Lett.* **2013**, *23*, 2426–2431. [CrossRef] [PubMed]
24. Borthwick, L.A.; Sunny, S.S.; Oliphant, V.; Perry, J.; Brodlie, M.; Johnson, G.E.; Ward, C.; Gould, K.; Corris, P.A.; De Soyza, A.; et al. Pseudomonas aeruginosa accentuates epithelial-to-mesenchymal transition in the airway. *Eur. Respir. J.* **2011**, *37*, 1237–1247. [CrossRef] [PubMed]
25. Westphal, O.; Jann, K. Bacterial lipopolysaccharide extraction with phenol-water and further applications of the procedure. *Methods Carbohydr. Chem.* **1965**, *5*, 83–91.
26. Sturiale, L.; Garozzo, D.; Silipo, A.; Lanzetta, R.; Parrilli, M.; Molinaro, A. New conditions for matrix-assisted laser desorption/ionization mass spectrometry of native bacterial R-type lipopolysaccharides. *Rapid Commun. Mass Spectrom.* **2005**, *19*, 1829–1834. [CrossRef] [PubMed]
27. Silipo, A.; Sturiale, L.; Garozzo, D.; de Castro, C.; Lanzetta, R.; Parrilli, M.; Grant, W.D.; Molinaro, A. Structure elucidation of the highly heterogeneous lipid A from the lipopolysaccharide of the gram-negative extremophile bacterium Halomonas magadiensis strain 21 m1. *Eur. J. Org. Chem.* **2004**, 2263–2271. [CrossRef]

28. Bui, N.K.; Eberhardt, A.; Vollmer, D.; Kern, T.; Bougault, C.; Tomasz, A.; Simorre, J.P.; Vollmer, W. Isolation and analysis of cell wall components from Streptococcus pneumoniae. *Anal. Biochem.* **2012**, *421*, 657–666. [CrossRef] [PubMed]
29. Hayashi, K. A rapid determination of sodium dodecyl sulfate with methylene blue. *Anal. Biochem.* **1975**, *67*, 503–506. [CrossRef]
30. Tsuchiya, S.; Yamabe, M.; Yamaguchi, Y.; Kobayashi, Y.; Konno, T.; Tada, K. Establishment and characterization of a human acute monocytic leukemia cell line (THP-1). *Int. J. Cancer* **1980**, *26*, 171–176. [CrossRef] [PubMed]

8

Taste Receptors Mediate Sinonasal Immunity and Respiratory Disease

Jennifer E. Douglas [1,2] and Noam A. Cohen [2,3,4,*]

1 Perelman School of Medicine, University of Pennsylvania, Philadelphia, PA 19104, USA; Jennifer.Douglas@uphs.upenn.edu
2 Monell Chemical Senses Center, Philadelphia, PA 19104, USA
3 Department of Otorhinolaryngology–Head and Neck Surgery, University of Pennsylvania Health System, Philadelphia, PA 19104, USA
4 Philadelphia Veterans Affairs Medical Center Surgical Services, Philadelphia, PA 19104, USA
* Correspondence: Noam.Cohen@uphs.upenn.edu

Academic Editor: Francesco B. Blasi

Abstract: The bitter taste receptor T2R38 has been shown to play a role in the pathogenesis of chronic rhinosinusitis (CRS), where the receptor functions to enhance upper respiratory innate immunity through a triad of beneficial immune responses. Individuals with a functional version of T2R38 are tasters for the bitter compound phenylthiocarbamide (PTC) and exhibit an anti-microbial response in the upper airway to certain invading pathogens, while those individuals with a non-functional version of the receptor are PTC non-tasters and lack this beneficial response. The clinical ramifications are significant, with the non-taster genotype being an independent risk factor for CRS requiring surgery, poor quality-of-life (QOL) improvements post-operatively, and decreased rhinologic QOL in patients with cystic fibrosis. Furthermore, indirect evidence suggests that non-tasters also have a larger burden of biofilm formation. This new data may influence the clinical management of patients with infectious conditions affecting the upper respiratory tract and possibly at other mucosal sites throughout the body.

Keywords: taste receptors; chronic rhinosinusitis; mucociliary clearance; airway physiology; biofilm; innate immunity; upper respiratory infection

---

1. Introduction

The upper airway is constantly exposed to a number of pathogens, toxins, and other irritative particulates that are typically successfully defended against by the upper airway innate immune defenses. Recently, the bitter taste system, far from its site of original identification in taste buds, has been implicated in this defense pathway with implications for the pathogenesis of upper respiratory infectious/inflammatory diseases and biofilm formation. This review will present recent evidence for the role of the bitter taste receptor T2R38 in chronic rhinosinusitis (CRS) and put forth support for an expanded role for individual taste differences in the clinical management of patients with upper respiratory infections.

Bitter taste is one of five unique tastes in addition to salty, sour, sweet, and umami that humans are capable of perceiving. Receptors for each of these tastes are present in the oral cavity, where bitter taste receptors (T2Rs) specifically signal the ingestion of potentially toxic substances and mediate aversive behavior [1]. As G protein-coupled receptors (GPCRs), T2Rs feature seven transmembrane domains but are unique in having a short extracellular N-terminus, in contrast with other taste receptors (e.g., T1R sweet taste receptors) [2–4]. Recently, T2Rs have also been identified in extraoral sites including, but not limited to, the upper and lower respiratory tracts, skin, thyroid, gastrointestinal tract, and testes [1,5–10]. Within the airway, the bitter taste receptor T2R38 has specifically been identified on ciliated epithelial cells [11–13]. T2Rs in upper respiratory cells appear to utilize most of the canonical bitter taste signaling cascade including phospholipase C β2 and TRPM5 (transient receptor potential cation channel subfamily M member 5), but interestingly not gustducin, the G-protein classically associated with T2Rs in the tongue (Figure 1) [11,14]. In the airway, a ligand for the human T2R38 appears to be acyl-homoserine lactones (AHLs), quorum sensing molecules secreted by gram-negative organisms [1]. Additionally, the extraoral expression of T2Rs has been hypothesized to cause many of the poorly understood off target effects of many medications, which are often bitter in taste [15].

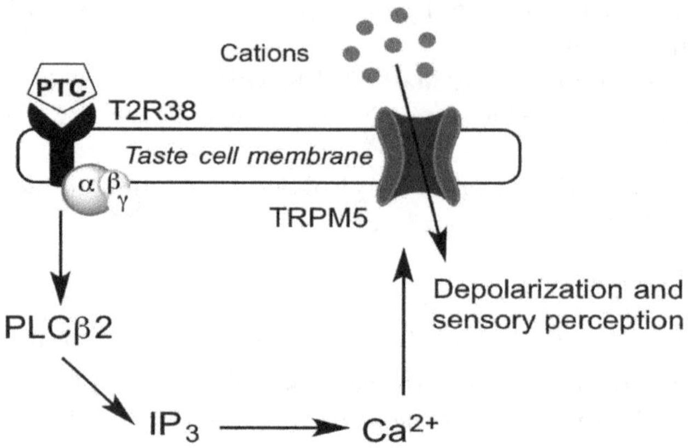

Figure 1. Intracellular taste receptor signaling. Binding of the bitter compound phenylthiocarbamide (PTC) to the T2R38 bitter taste receptor in sinonasal epithelial cells results in activation of an undetermined G-protein that then activates phosopholipase C isoform β2 (PLCβ2), resulting in increased inositol 1,4,5-trisphosphate (IP_3) [16]. IP_3 induces the release of calcium (Ca^{2+}) from the endoplasmic reticulum. Ca^{2+}-dependent activation of TRPM5 channels (transient receptor potential cation channel subfamily M member 5) depolarizes the membrane and results in bitterness perception [1,17,18].

The bitter taste receptor family includes approximately 25 different T2Rs, each of which is encoded by a corresponding bitter taste receptor gene (*TAS2Rs*) [19]. One of the most well-studied receptors among this group is the bitter taste receptor T2R38, which is encoded by the *TAS2R38* gene and was first characterized molecularly in 2005 [20]. It is specifically responsive to the bitter compounds phenylthiocarbamide (PTC), propylthiouracil (PROP), the plant compound goitrin (common in cruciferous vegetables), and other chemically similar substances [21]. Prior studies show that *TAS2R38* exists in two common haplotypes that are either functional and respond to its bitter agonists, or are non-functional and are not activated by its bitter agonists, based on three missense single nucleotide polymorphisms (SNPs) [20]. The specific coding logic is further detailed below. Many common bitter foods such as broccoli, Brussels sprouts, coffee, and beer contain compounds that agonize T2R38 and as such, genetic variability in *TAS2R38* influences dietary preferences through differences in psychophysical bitterness perception [22]. Further, the extraoral expression of T2R38 has been shown to influence upper respiratory immunity with clinically significant effects on CRS [14,23]. In the paragraphs below, we discuss the state of knowledge on the expression pattern of T2R38 in the upper respiratory epithelium, its role in the pathogenesis of CRS and other respiratory conditions, the emerging understanding of its influence on biofilm formation, and the implications for clinical treatment.

2. Genetic Variability of *TAS2R38*

As previously mentioned, the *TAS2R38* gene features two common haplotypes that confer significant phenotypic variability in bitterness sensitivity. There exist three SNPs within the gene that each produce an amino acid change (P49A, A262V, and V296I), resulting in two common haplotypes: a proline-alanine-valine (PAV) haplotype that is exquisitely sensitive to PTC due to successful signal transduction and intracellular calcium release (Figure 1), and an alanine-valine-isoleucine (AVI) haplotype that is relatively insensitive to PTC due to an absence of signal transduction. Thus, individuals can either be homozygous for the PAV allele (so-called "tasters" for their ability to taste PTC), homozygous for the AVI allele ("non-tasters" for their relative inability to taste PTC), or heterozygous (intermediate tasters with variable PTC sensitivity) [8]. Importantly, the AVI haplotype exists in a significant portion of the population, with frequency ranging from zero to 66.7% in various subgroups [24]. Of note, there are three less common *TAS2R38* haplotypes (AAI (alanine-alanine-isoleucine), PVI (proline-valine-isoleucine), and AAV (alanine-alanine-valine)), each of which show intermediate sensitivity to PTC; however, these sub-types make-up only 1%–5% of the Caucasian population and up to 20% of the African American population and will not be further discussed here [20,25].

3. Mechanisms of Upper Airway Immunity

There are two primary cell types within the upper airway epithelium, goblet cells and ciliated cells, which work synergistically to keep the mucosa clean. Goblet cells, which produce mucin, a proteinaceous substance that physically traps pathogens and other foreign particles within the airway surface liquid (ASL), and ciliated cells, which beat in a coordinated fashion to propel mucin out of the airway [26–29]. Together, these cells contribute to the crucial process of mucociliary clearance (MCC) that physically clears the area of trapped pathogens and particles (Figure 2).

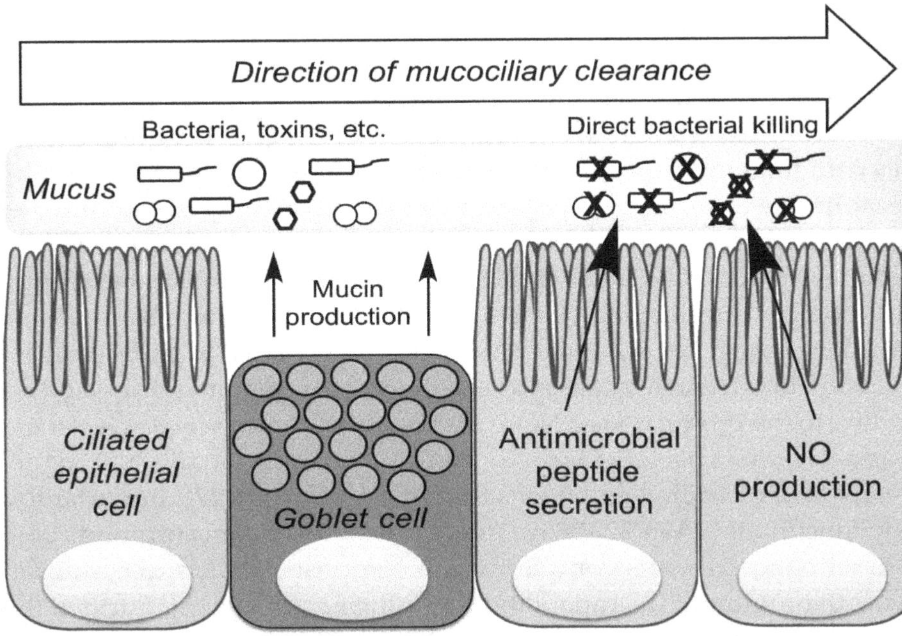

Figure 2. Mechanisms of upper airway innate immunity. Ciliated epithelial and goblet cells work in concert to rid the airway epithelium of foreign pathogens and other toxins through a process known as mucociliary clearance (MCC). Goblet cells secrete mucin that physically traps bacteria and other toxins while ciliated epithelial cells beat in a coordinated fashion to expel trapped pathogens from the airway. Ciliated cells also produce antimicrobial peptides and nitric oxide (NO), which both are directly bactericidal. NO also results in increased ciliary beat frequency, enhancing MCC.

Additionally, the epithelium produces a number of compounds that enhance the local immune response. Specifically, ciliated cells produce antimicrobial peptides (AMPs) as well as nitric oxide (NO) that work to inhibit pathogen colonization [30]. These peptides include defensins, lactoferrin, and cathelicidins. β-defensin 1 and 2, specifically, are effective against both gram-positive and gram-negative bacteria, with particular potency against gram-negative bacteria such as *Pseudomonas aeruginosa* and *Klebsiella pneumonia* [14]. Nitric oxide has parallel benefits: local increase in NO concentration enhances the process of MCC by increasing ciliary beat frequency (CBF), while also inducing direct DNA damage as a reactive oxygen species, leading to bacterial cell death [11].

Bacteria and other pathogens like fungi have naturally developed mechanisms to evade these immune responses and secrete compounds including pyocyanin and pyoverdin that paralyze cilia, or aflatoxin that slows cilia, thereby dismantling the crucial process of MCC [31,32]. Additionally, gram-negative microbes also secrete a class of compounds known as AHLs that communicate within a bacterial community to report microbial density, thereby coordinating virulence through biofilm formation, toxin secretion, and acquisition of antibiotic resistance [33,34]. Biofilms are a particularly challenging form of infection to treat as they represent a coalescence of single-cell, planktonic bacteria into a bacterial community with a glycocalyx scaffold that increases bacterial adherence, limits antibiotic penetration, and prevents phagocytosis by immune cells. Additionally, biofilms provide a chronic source of shedding bacteria, toxins, and antigens that stimulate the immune system and generate persistent localized inflammation. In patients with CRS, biofilms have been associated with persistent infections and poor treatment outcomes [35–37].

4. Taste Receptors and Upper Airway Immunity

As with the signaling pathway in taste buds, stimulation of taste receptors on airway cells with bitter agonists like denatonium benzoate (DB) induces an intracellular calcium release [14]. Additionally, early studies found that murine solitary chemosensory cells (SCCs) respond directly to AHLs, but the exact T2R responsible for this activation was undetermined [38]. Thus, early work demonstrated that non-ciliated murine nasal cells that express bitter taste signaling proteins are activated by gram-negative quorum-sensing molecules.

Our laboratory has utilized a culture technique known as the air-liquid interface culture (ALI) to facilitate a better understanding of these pathways in human upper airway immunity [39,40]. The technique recapitulates the natural polarization of the airway epithelium, enabling in vitro modeling of cell activation, signaling, and response to pathogen invasion [11,14].

Investigating human sinonasal epithelial cultures, our group demonstrated that the gram-negative AHLs *N*-butyryl-L-homoserine lactone (C4HSL) and *N*-3-oxo-dodecanoyl-L-homoserine lactone (C12HSL) activate T2R38, which in the human is exclusively expressed in ciliated cells, not SCCs [11,41]. Stimulation of T2R38 in human ciliated cell leads to intracellular calcium release and activation of nitric oxide synthase leading to the production of NO [11]. The NO diffuses across the cell membrane into the overlying mucus and has direct bactericidal activity. [42–45]. Additionally, NO triggers an increase in CBF, promoting removal of offending pathogens from the airway [46,47]. Importantly, NO production by activation of the functional (PAV) T2R38 occurs at physiologic concentrations of AHLs (1–10 μM), as evidenced by in vitro experiments comparing the response of ALIs to conditioned media from *P. aeruginosa* either with or without the capability of producing AHLs [11]. Further, this process occurs through a pathway consistent with what is known of intracellular taste receptor signal transduction, producing activation of phosopholipase C isoform β2 (PLCβ2) and the non-selective cation channel, TRPM5 [15,16,48]. This pathway occurs in a genotype-dependent manner akin to that in taste buds; T2R38-AVI individuals do not exhibit the crucial NO response to the gram-negative AHLs [14]. Thus, it follows that non-tasters might be at increased risk of gram-negative bacterial invasion and persistence, which may contribute to T2R specific alterations in the upper respiratory microbiome.

While AHLs in the human nose stimulate T2Rs on ciliated cells to activate NO production, AHLs in the mouse nose stimulate T2Rs on SCCs (discrete non-ciliated cells) to induce a cholinergic-mediated neurogenic inflammatory response [38,49,50]. While acetylcholine release has not been demonstrated following stimulation of human SCCs, in vitro studies have found that activation of T2Rs present on human SCCs by DB and other bitter tasting compounds such as absinthin, parthenolide, and amoraogentin results in a release of intracellular Ca^{2+}, which propagates to the surrounding epithelial cells via gap junctions and stimulates release of AMP stores [14] (Figure 3). Significantly, this immune activation does not occur with AHL stimulation of human SCCs. It is hypothesized that an as yet unidentified bacterial product/byproduct triggers T2Rs on human SCCs to activate this robust antimicrobial defense pathway.

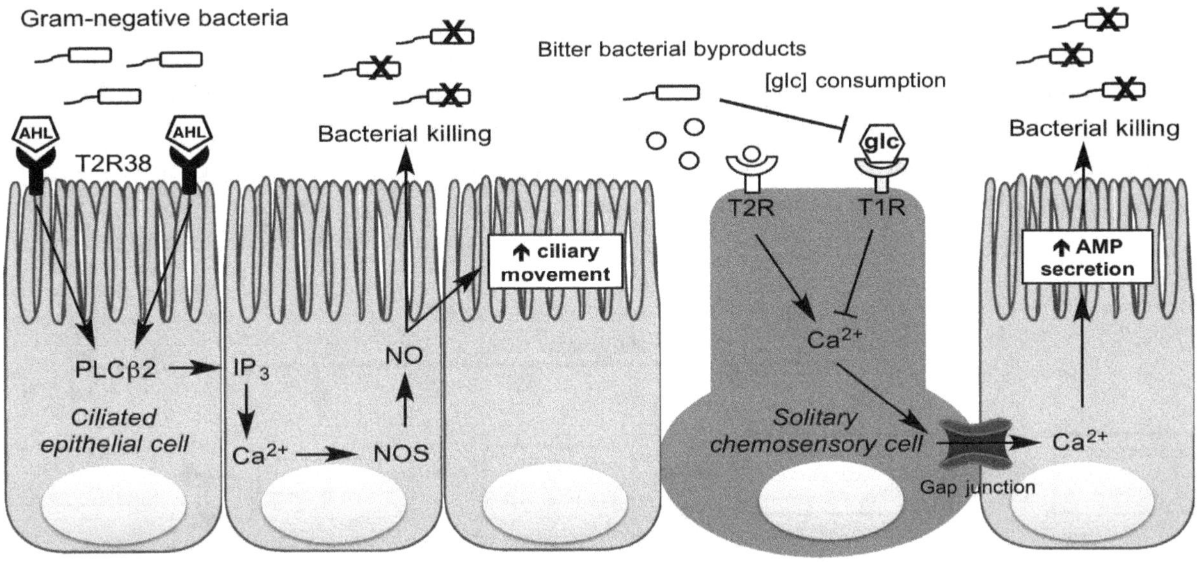

Figure 3. Taste receptor-dependent upper airway immunity. Ciliated epithelial cells express T2R38 while solitary chemosensory cells (SCCs) express both T2Rs and T1Rs. Gram-negative bacteria produce acyl-homoserine lactones (AHLs), which bind to and activate T2R38, producing an intracellular cascade activating PLCβ2 and production of IP_3. This increases nitric oxide (NO) production through the activation of nitric oxide synthase (NOS), which both directly kills bacteria and enhances ciliary beating. Additionally, presumed other bitter bacterial byproducts activate an as yet unknown T2R(s) on solitary chemosensory cells and, through typical taste receptor intracellular signaling including gustducin, yields increased Ca^{2+}. This Ca^{2+} diffuses into adjacent ciliated cells via gap junctions where it produces increased antimicrobial peptide (AMP) secretion, killing pathogens. Due to glucose (glc) consumption by bacteria, microbial colonization also decreases the T1R-mediated inhibition of SCC Ca^{2+} release, thereby contributing to enhanced antimicrobial peptide production.

Interestingly, T1R2+3 sweet taste receptors are also present on SCCs, where they are influenced in parallel by the presence of bacteria. Glucose is present in the airway due to a physiological "leak" across the epithelium [51]. Upon glucose binding the SCC sweet taste receptor, Ca^{2+} release is blocked, leading to decreased AMP release [14]. During microbial invasion, glucose concentration is decreased due to bacterial consumption. Thus, in the presence of local bacterial overgrowth/infection, the tonic sweet taste receptor brake on SCC activity is relieved, yielding local antimicrobial peptide secretion and reduction in the local microbes (Figure 3). Additionally, studies using sweet receptor antagonists such as lactisole demonstrate the specific inhibition in AMP release by the sweet receptor [14,52,53], while glucose transport inhibitors such as phloretin and phlorizin do not [14]. Clinically, this pathway has important implications, as individuals with diseases of glucose homeostasis such as diabetes mellitus have chronically elevated ASL glucose, and are known to suffer from a greater frequency of respiratory infections than patients without diabetes [54,55]. Diabetic patients with CRS also exhibit smaller improvements in QOL measures following sinus surgery [56].

5. Conditions of Defective Airway Immunity

Numerous diseases exist for which the pathways of airway immunity are important. We will discuss two of these conditions: CRS, which is a common syndrome effecting the upper airway and paranasal sinuses, and cystic fibrosis (CF), a disease affecting both the upper and lower airways. Patients suffering from CRS experience significant inflammation of the upper respiratory epithelium, with a resultant overproduction of mucin and a defect in MCC. Symptoms can include rhinorrhea, hyposmia, headaches, nasal obstruction, and facial pressure/pain. When these symptoms persist for three months or more and on a physical exam there are objective findings of nasal purulence or polyps, or paranasal sinus opacification on radiographic imaging, patients are given the diagnosis of CRS. The syndrome of CRS results in significant decrements in patient quality of life (QOL), as measured by the Sinonasal Outcome (SNOT-22) test, with individuals reporting lower QOL measures than patients with serious heart and lung diseases [57,58]. Treatment for CRS is initially medical, with courses of culture directed antibiotics, potent anti-inflammatories such as steroids, as well as topical irrigation with saline and/or steroid solutions. When symptoms persist despite medical therapy, patients are offered a surgical intervention known as functional endoscopic sinus surgery (FESS) to ventilate and drain the sinuses as well as optimize the exposure of the sinonasal epithelium to topical treatments (Figure 4).

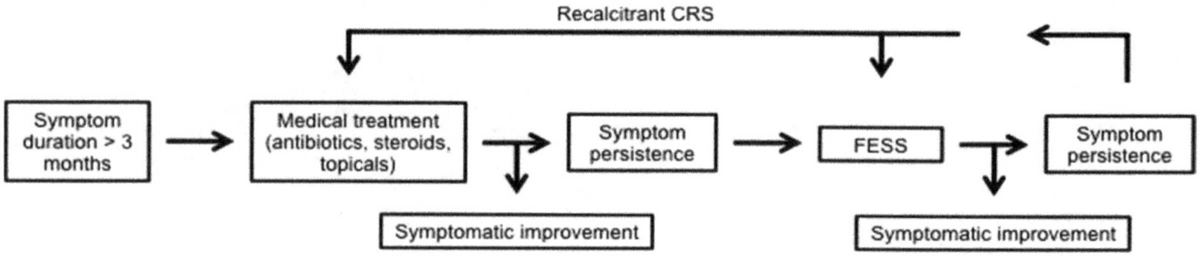

Figure 4. Treatment algorithm for chronic rhinosinusitis (CRS). CRS is diagnosed after symptoms, including headache, hyposmia, rhinorrhea, and nasal congestion persist for greater than three months. Treatment is initiated medically with oral antibiotics and steroids as well as topical steroids and nasal irrigation. Should symptoms persist, patients are offered surgical intervention with functional endoscopic sinus surgery (FESS). Continued symptoms of recalcitrant CRS are managed with repeated courses of culture-directed antibiotics, steroids, and topical treatment with revision sinus surgery when indicated.

While gram-positive bacteria such as *Streptococcus pneumoniae* are most frequently responsible for sinusitis and particularly acute sinusitis, recalcitrant CRS is more commonly linked with sinonasal biofilm formation and gram-negative bacteria such as *P. aeruginosa*, making antibiotic choice for coverage and penetration more complex [31]. The pathway mediated by bitter taste receptors in upper airway immunity directly influences these features characteristic of CRS.

Clinical studies first employed a retrospective analysis evaluating the frequency of *TAS2R38* genotypes within the non-polypoid CRS population undergoing FESS. Results found a disproportionate number of non-tasters (*TAS2R38*-AVI/AVI genotype) within the population, demonstrating that tasters (*TAS2R38*-PAV/PAV) are less likely to require surgical intervention for their CRS, likely due to enhanced upper airway immunity [59]. A follow-up prospective study confirmed that the non-taster genotype is an independent risk factor for CRS requiring surgical intervention [23]. More recently, a prospective study assessing post-operative improvement in SNOT-22 scores found that homozygous tasters experienced greater improvement in scores at one, three, and six months post-operatively as compared with heterozygotes and homozygous non-tasters [60]. Similar observations have recently been confirmed in a Canadian [61] and Polish cohort of patients [62]. However, an Italian cohort found no association between *TAS2R38* genotype and CRS either with or without polyps [63]. A significant limitation of this study is its small non-polyp population ($n = 17$), given that the genotype relationship has been previously shown to be exclusive to this CRS sub-group.

CF, in contrast, is an autosomal recessive genetic disorder caused by defective transcellular ion transport across the Cystic Fibrosis Transmembrane Conductance Regulator (CFTR), which is encoded by the *CFTR* gene. The disease is most commonly caused by the ΔF508 mutation but can be caused by one of almost 200 different mutations. [64,65]. While the preponderance of symptoms manifest in the lower airway epithelium, the disease affects all mucosal surfaces and nearly 50% of CF patients also suffer from CRS, with one-third of who require surgical management [66–69]. Because CF is characterized by a preponderance of *P. aeruginosa* colonization and biofilm formation, a link with bitter taste receptors has been hypothesized. A retrospective analysis identified that *TAS2R38* genotype correlates with both SNOT-22 scores and rhinologic-specific symptoms in CF patients [70]. Further, as the understanding of taste receptors in biofilm formation and gram-negative respiratory infections grows, an even more significant role for *TAS2R38* genotype in CF may be revealed.

6. Taste Influence on Biofilm

Biofilms not only influence CRS and CF, but also contribute significantly to treatment-resistant infections throughout the body [37,71]. Recently, a study sought to identify whether PTC sensitivity, as a proxy for *TAS2R38* genotype, is linked with biofilm formation based on the understanding of the role of T2R38 in upper airway immunity. Endoscopic nasal swabs were obtained from patients with CRS both with and without polyps, and analyzed using the Calgary biofilm detection assay. Results found an inverse linear relationship between biofilm formation and PTC sensitivity, indicating that patients with poor bitterness sensitivity (decreased T2R38 function) yielded more ex-vivo biofilm biomass [72]. While this correlation was true for the entire CRS cohort of patients, it was exclusively driven by those patients without polyps, likely due to different immunologic pathways driving polyp and non-polyp CRS [73]. Additionally, by using PTC taste sensitivity rather than *TAS2R38* genotype, this study is a proof of concept for the idea that a simple taste test can easily approximate genotype, simplifying the costly and time-consuming process of genotyping. However, further studies are necessary to definitively prove that bitterness sensitivity and expression of T2R38 in taste buds directly correlate with that in the nasal epithelium.

7. Conclusions

The understanding of the role of the bitter taste receptors in upper respiratory immunity continues to grow. What is clear is that bitter taste receptors, specifically T2R38, are expressed in the upper airway epithelium where they respond to bitter compounds produced by invading bacteria to potentiate the local innate immune response. Due to common individual genetic variation, non-taster individuals do not benefit from this taste receptor-dependent pathway of upper airway immunity and are at increased risk of gram-negative upper respiratory infections and non-polypoid CRS. Because of the role that biofilms play in the pathogenesis of recalcitrant respiratory disease, which has been directly correlated with *TAS2R38* genotype, it is likely that broader conclusions may be drawn about local immune responses at diverse sites throughout the body.

Going forward, taste receptors may be targeted for topical therapeutic intervention by using bitter compounds to directly activate the sinonasal bitter taste receptors. One could argue that a bitter taste panel may guide the ideal bitter compound(s) for individualized therapeutic intervention. This precision medicine could optimize individual treatment responsiveness, decreasing the use of oral steroids and antibiotics, limiting their contribution to the growing epidemic of antibiotic resistance [74]. Interestingly, this pathway has been largely tied to gram-negative bacteria. However, gram-positive bacteria are responsible for the large majority of CRS cases and the common pathogen *S. aureus* has been found to induce NO production in human upper airway epithelium, though through a process that is independent of T2R38 [75]. A better understanding of this process would have implications for the treatment of both acute and chronic sinusitis.

Additionally, future studies should aim to directly correlate the expression of T2R38 in the oral and nasal epithelium, as well as to assess the feasibility of instilling bitter compounds in nasal lavages or sprays to evaluate the benefit of taste receptor-targeted topical therapies. Because the T2R38 bitter taste receptor is one of only 25 different bitter taste receptors, it is necessary to understand how all bitter taste receptors, the so-called "bitterome", work in concert to influence upper airway innate defenses [76]. By contrast with the bitter taste system, the sweet taste system remains relatively poorly understood and presents an opportunity for significant advances in understanding. With this knowledge, it is likely that the principles first identified and characterized within the sinonasal epithelium will become applicable to many mucosal sites throughout the body, with implications for the use of extraoral taste receptors in the treatment of a diverse group of infectious processes.

Acknowledgments: Some of the research described here was supported by National Institutes of Health (NIH) R01DC013588 to Noam A. Cohen, National Institute on Deafness and Other Communication Disorders Administrative Research Supplement to Promote Emergence of Clinician-Scientists in Chemosensory Research to Jennifer E. Douglas, and NIH R21DC013886 to Noam A. Cohen and Danielle R. Reed. Reed and members of her lab, including Corrine J. Mansfield and Charles J. Arayata, have been instrumental in many of the genetic components of the research described here.

Abbreviations

CRS	Chronic rhinosinusitis
GPCRs	G protein-coupled receptors
AHLs	Acyl-homoserine lactones
PTC	Phenylthiocarbamide
QOL	Quality of life
PLCβ2	Phosopholipase C isoform β2
IP_3	Inositol 1,4,5-trisphosphate
Ca^{2+}	Calcium ions
TRPM5	Transient receptor potential cation channel subfamily M member 5
PROP	Propylthiouracil
SNPs	Single nucleotide polymorphisms
PAV	Proline-alanine-valine *TAS2R38* haplotype ("tasters")
AVI	Alanine-valine-isoleucine *TAS2R38* haplotype ("non-tasters")
ASL	Airway surface liquid
MCC	Mucociliary clearance
NO	Nitric oxide
AMPs	Antimicrobial peptides
CBF	Ciliary beat frequency
DB	Denatonium benzoate
SCCs	Solitary chemosensory cells
ALI	Air-liquid interface culture
C4HSL	*N*-butyryl-L-homoserine lactone
C12HSL	*N*-3-oxo-dodecanoyl-L-homoserine lactone
glc	Glucose
CF	Cystic fibrosis
SNOT-22	Sinonasal outcome test
FESS	Functional endoscopic sinus surgery

References

1. Kinnamon, S.C. Taste receptor signalling—From tongues to lungs. *Acta Physiol.* **2012**, *204*, 158–168. [CrossRef] [PubMed]
2. Chandrashekar, J.; Mueller, K.L.; Hoon, M.A.; Adler, E.; Feng, L.; Guo, W.; Zuker, C.S.; Ryba, N.J. T2Rs function as bitter taste receptors. *Cell* **2000**, *100*, 703–711. [CrossRef]
3. Adler, E.; Hoon, M.A.; Mueller, K.L.; Chandrashekar, J.; Ryba, N.J.; Zuker, C.S. A novel family of mammalian taste receptors. *Cell* **2000**, *100*, 693–702. [CrossRef]

4. Hoon, M.A.; Adler, E.; Lindemeier, J.; Battey, J.F.; Ryba, N.J.P.; Zuker, C.S. Putative mammalian taste receptors: A class of taste-specific gpcrs with distinct topographic selectivity. *Cell* **1999**, *96*, 541–551. [CrossRef]
5. Clark, A.A.; Liggett, S.B.; Munger, S.D. Extraoral bitter taste receptors as mediators of off-target drug effects. *FASEB J.* **2012**, *26*, 4827–4831. [CrossRef] [PubMed]
6. Laffitte, A.; Neiers, F.; Briand, L. Functional roles of the sweet taste receptor in oral and extraoral tissues. *Curr. Opin. Clin. Nutr. Metab. Care* **2014**, *17*, 379–385. [CrossRef] [PubMed]
7. Clark, A.A.; Dotson, C.D.; Elson, A.E.; Voigt, A.; Boehm, U.; Meyerhof, W.; Steinle, N.I.; Munger, S.D. Tas2r bitter taste receptors regulate thyroid function. *FASEB J.* **2015**, *29*, 164–172. [CrossRef] [PubMed]
8. Mueller, K.L.; Hoon, M.A.; Erlenbach, I.; Chandrashekar, J.; Zuker, C.S.; Ryba, N.J.P. The receptors and coding logic for bitter taste. *Nature* **2005**, *434*, 225–229. [CrossRef] [PubMed]
9. Wölfle, U.; Elsholz, F.A.; Kersten, A.; Haarhaus, B.; Müller, W.E.; Schempp, C.M. Expression and functional activity of the bitter taste receptors TAS2R1 and TAS2R38 in human keratinocytes. *Skin Pharmacol. Physiol.* **2015**, *28*, 137–146. [CrossRef] [PubMed]
10. Xu, J.; Cao, J.; Iguchi, N.; Riethmacher, D.; Huang, L. Functional characterization of bitter-taste receptors expressed in mammalian testis. *Mol. Hum. Reprod.* **2013**, *19*, 17–28. [CrossRef] [PubMed]
11. Lee, R.J.; Xiong, G.; Kofonow, J.M.; Chen, B.; Lysenko, A.; Jiang, P.; Abraham, V.; Doghramji, L.; Adappa, N.D.; Palmer, J.N.; et al. T2R38 taste receptor polymorphisms underlie susceptibility to upper respiratory infection. *J. Clin. Investig.* **2012**, *122*, 4145–4159. [CrossRef] [PubMed]
12. Shah, A.S.; Ben-Shahar, Y.; Moninger, T.O.; Kline, J.N.; Welsh, M.J. Motile cilia of human airway epithelia are chemosensory. *Science* **2009**, *325*, 1131–1134. [CrossRef] [PubMed]
13. Cohen, N.A. The genetics of the bitter taste receptor T2R38 in upper airway innate immunity and implications for chronic rhinosinusitis. *Laryngoscope* **2016**, *127*, 44–51. [CrossRef] [PubMed]
14. Lee, R.J.; Kofonow, J.M.; Rosen, P.L.; Siebert, A.P.; Chen, B.; Doghramji, L.; Xiong, G.; Adappa, N.D.; Palmer, J.N.; Kennedy, D.W.; et al. Bitter and sweet taste receptors regulate human upper respiratory innate immunity. *J. Clin. Investig.* **2014**, *124*, 1393–1405. [CrossRef] [PubMed]
15. Mennella, J.A.; Spector, A.C.; Reed, D.R.; Coldwell, S.E. The bad taste of medicines: Overview of basic research on bitter taste. *Clin. Ther.* **2013**, *35*, 1225–1246. [CrossRef] [PubMed]
16. Yamamoto, K.; Ishimaru, Y. Oral and extra-oral taste perception. *Semin. Cell Dev. Biol.* **2013**, *24*, 240–246. [CrossRef] [PubMed]
17. Taruno, A.; Vingtdeux, V.; Ohmoto, M.; Ma, Z.; Dvoryanchikov, G.; Li, A.; Adrien, L.; Zhao, H.; Leung, S.; Abernethy, M.; et al. CALHM1 ion channel mediates purinergic neurotransmission of sweet, bitter and umami tastes. *Nature* **2013**, *495*, 223–226. [CrossRef] [PubMed]
18. Lionakis, M.S.; Netea, M.G.; Holland, S.M. Mendelian genetics of human susceptibility to fungal infection. *Cold Spring Harb. Perspect. Med.* **2014**, *4*, a019638. [CrossRef] [PubMed]
19. Kuhn, C.; Bufe, B.; Batram, C.; Meyerhof, W. Oligomerization of TAS2R bitter taste receptors. *Chem. Sens.* **2010**, *35*, 395–406. [CrossRef] [PubMed]
20. Bufe, B.; Breslin, P.A.S.; Kuhn, C.; Reed, D.R.; Tharp, C.D.; Slack, J.P.; Kim, U.-K.; Drayna, D.; Meyerhof, W. The molecular basis of individual differences in phenylthiocarbamide and propylthiouracil bitterness perception. *Curr. Biol.* **2005**, *15*, 322–327. [CrossRef] [PubMed]
21. Meyerhof, W.; Batram, C.; Kuhn, C.; Brockhoff, A.; Chudoba, E.; Bufe, B.; Appendino, G.; Behrens, M. The molecular receptive ranges of human TAS2R bitter taste receptors. *Chem. Sens.* **2010**, *35*, 157–170. [CrossRef] [PubMed]
22. Lipchock, S.V.; Mennella, J.A.; Spielman, A.I.; Reed, D.R. Human bitter perception correlates with bitter receptor messenger rna expression in taste cells. *Am. J. Clin. Nutr.* **2013**, *98*, 1136–1143. [CrossRef] [PubMed]
23. Adappa, N.D.; Zhang, Z.; Palmer, J.N.; Kennedy, D.W.; Doghramji, L.; Lysenko, A.; Reed, D.R.; Scott, T.; Zhao, N.W.; Owens, D.; et al. The bitter taste receptor T2R38 is an independent risk factor for chronic rhinosinusitis requiring sinus surgery. *Int. Forum Allergy Rhinol.* **2014**, *4*, 3–7. [CrossRef] [PubMed]
24. Guo, S.W.; Reed, D.R. The genetics of phenylthiocarbamide perception. *Ann. Hum. Biol.* **2001**, *28*, 111–142. [PubMed]
25. Behrens, M.; Gunn, H.C.; Ramos, P.C.M.; Meyerhof, W.; Wooding, S.P. Genetic, functional, and phenotypic diversity in TAS2R38-mediated bitter taste perception. *Chem. Senses* **2013**, *38*, 475–484. [CrossRef] [PubMed]
26. Cohen, N.A. Sinonasal mucociliary clearance in health and disease. *Ann. Otol. Rhinol. Laryngol. Suppl.* **2006**, *115*, 20–26. [CrossRef]

27. Gudis, D.; Zhao, K.Q.; Cohen, N.A. Acquired cilia dysfunction in chronic rhinosinusitis. *Am. J. Rhinol. Allergy* **2012**, *26*, 1–6. [CrossRef] [PubMed]
28. Antunes, M.B.; Gudis, D.A.; Cohen, N.A. Epithelium, cilia, and mucus: Their importance in chronic rhinosinusitis. *Immunol. Allergy Clin. N. Am.* **2009**, *29*, 631–643. [CrossRef] [PubMed]
29. Eliezer, N.; Sade, J.; Silberberg, A.; Nevo, A.C. The role of mucus in transport by cilia. *Am. Rev. Respir. Dis.* **1970**, *102*, 48–52. [PubMed]
30. Knowles, M.R.; Boucher, R.C. Mucus clearance as a primary innate defense mechanism for mammalian airways. *J. Clin. Investig.* **2002**, *109*, 571–577. [CrossRef] [PubMed]
31. Jimenez, P.N.; Koch, G.; Thompson, J.A.; Xavier, K.B.; Cool, R.H.; Quax, W.J. The multiple signaling systems regulating virulence in *Pseudomonas aeruginosa*. *Microbiol. Mol. Biol. Rev.* **2012**, *76*, 46–65. [CrossRef] [PubMed]
32. Lee, R.J.; Workman, A.D.; Carey, R.M.; Chen, B.; Rosen, P.L.; Doghramji, L.; Adappa, N.D.; Palmer, J.N.; Kennedy, D.W.; Cohen, N.A. Fungal aflatoxins reduce respiratory mucosal ciliary function. *Sci. Rep.* **2016**, *6*, 33221. [CrossRef] [PubMed]
33. Eberhard, A.; Burlingame, A.L.; Eberhard, C.; Kenyon, G.L.; Nealson, K.H.; Oppenheimer, N.J. Structural identification of autoinducer of photobacterium fischeri luciferase. *Biochemistry* **1981**, *20*, 2444–2449. [CrossRef] [PubMed]
34. Mitchell, R.J.; Lee, S.K.; Kim, T.; Ghim, C.M. Microbial linguistics: Perspectives and applications of microbial cell-to-cell communication. *BMB Rep.* **2011**, *44*, 1–10. [CrossRef] [PubMed]
35. Costerton, J.W.; Stewart, P.S.; Greenberg, E.P. Bacterial biofilms: A common cause of persistent infections. *Science* **1999**, *284*, 1318–1322. [CrossRef] [PubMed]
36. Ferguson, B.J.; Stolz, D.B. Demonstration of biofilm in human bacterial chronic rhinosinusitis. *Am. J. Rhinol.* **2005**, *19*, 452–457. [PubMed]
37. Bendouah, Z.; Barbeau, J.; Hamad, W.A.; Desrosiers, M. Biofilm formation by *Staphylococcus aureus* and *Pseudomonas aeruginosa* is associated with an unfavorable evolution after surgery for chronic sinusitis and nasal polyposis. *Otolaryngol. Head Neck Surg.* **2006**, *134*, 991–996. [CrossRef] [PubMed]
38. Tizzano, M.; Gulbransen, B.D.; Vandenbeuch, A.; Clapp, T.R.; Herman, J.P.; Sibhatu, H.M.; Churchill, M.E.A.; Silver, W.L.; Kinnamon, S.C.; Finger, T.E. Nasal chemosensory cells use bitter taste signaling to detect irritants and bacterial signals. *Proc. Natl. Acad. Sci. USA* **2010**, *107*, 3210–3215. [CrossRef] [PubMed]
39. Ramanathan, M., Jr.; Lane, A.P. A comparison of experimental methods in molecular chronic rhinosinusitis research. *Am. J. Rhinol.* **2007**, *21*, 373–377. [CrossRef] [PubMed]
40. Dimova, S.; Brewster, M.E.; Noppe, M.; Jorissen, M.; Augustijns, P. The use of human nasal in vitro cell systems during drug discovery and development. *Toxicol. In Vitro* **2005**, *19*, 107–122. [CrossRef] [PubMed]
41. Lee, R.J.; Chen, B.; Redding, K.M.; Margolskee, R.F.; Cohen, N.A. Mouse nasal epithelial innate immune responses to *Pseudomonas aeruginosa* quorum-sensing molecules require taste signaling components. *Innate Immun.* **2013**, *20*, 606–617. [CrossRef] [PubMed]
42. Fang, F.C. Perspectives series: Host/pathogen interactions. Mechanisms of nitric oxide-related antimicrobial activity. *J. Clin. Investig.* **1997**, *99*, 2818–2825. [CrossRef] [PubMed]
43. Marcinkiewicz, J. Nitric oxide and antimicrobial activity of reactive oxygen intermediates. *Immunopharmacology* **1997**, *37*, 35–41. [CrossRef]
44. Jones, M.L.; Ganopolsky, J.G.; Labbé, A.; Wahl, C.; Prakash, S. Antimicrobial properties of nitric oxide and its application in antimicrobial formulations and medical devices. *Appl. Microbiol. Biotechnol.* **2010**, *88*, 401–407. [CrossRef] [PubMed]
45. Schairer, D.O.; Chouake, J.S.; Nosanchuk, J.D.; Friedman, A.J. The potential of nitric oxide releasing therapies as antimicrobial agents. *Virulence* **2012**, *3*, 271–279. [CrossRef] [PubMed]
46. Salathe, M. Regulation of mammalian ciliary beating. *Annu. Rev. Physiol.* **2007**, *69*, 401–422. [CrossRef] [PubMed]
47. Jain, B.; Rubinstein, I.; Robbins, R.A.; Leise, K.L.; Sisson, J.H. Modulation of airway epithelial cell ciliary beat frequency by nitric oxide. *Biochem. Biophys. Res. Commun.* **1993**, *191*, 83–88. [CrossRef] [PubMed]
48. Perez, C.A.; Margolskee, R.F.; Kinnamon, S.C.; Ogura, T. Making sense with trp channels: Store-operated calcium entry and the ion channel TRPM5 in taste receptor cells. *Cell Calcium* **2003**, *33*, 541–549. [CrossRef]
49. Tizzano, M.; Finger, T.E. Chemosensors in the nose: Guardians of the airways. *Physiology* **2013**, *28*, 51–60. [CrossRef] [PubMed]
50. Saunders, C.J.; Christensen, M.; Finger, T.E.; Tizzano, M. Cholinergic neurotransmission links solitary chemosensory cells to nasal inflammation. *Proc. Natl. Acad. Sci. USA* **2014**, *111*, 6075–6080. [CrossRef] [PubMed]

51. Kalsi, K.K.; Baker, E.H.; Fraser, O.; Chung, Y.L.; Mace, O.J.; Tarelli, E.; Philips, B.J.; Baines, D.L. Glucose homeostasis across human airway epithelial cell monolayers: Role of diffusion, transport and metabolism. *Pflug. Arch.* **2009**, *457*, 1061–1070. [CrossRef] [PubMed]
52. Jiang, P.; Cui, M.; Zhao, B.; Liu, Z.; Snyder, L.A.; Benard, L.M.; Osman, R.; Margolskee, R.F.; Max, M. Lactisole interacts with the transmembrane domains of human T1R3 to inhibit sweet taste. *J. Biol. Chem.* **2005**, *280*, 15238–15246. [CrossRef] [PubMed]
53. Jiang, P.; Cui, M.; Zhao, B.; Snyder, L.A.; Benard, L.M.; Osman, R.; Max, M.; Margolskee, R.F. Identification of the cyclamate interaction site within the transmembrane domain of the human sweet taste receptor subunit T1R3. *J. Biol. Chem.* **2005**, *280*, 34296–34305. [CrossRef] [PubMed]
54. Garnett, J.P.; Baker, E.H.; Baines, D.L. Sweet talk: Insights into the nature and importance of glucose transport in lung epithelium. *Eur. Respir. J.* **2012**, *40*, 1269–1276. [CrossRef] [PubMed]
55. Koziel, H.; Koziel, M.J. Pulmonary complications of diabetes mellitus. Pneumonia. *Infect. Dis. Clin. N. Am.* **1995**, *9*, 65–96.
56. Zhang, Z.; Adappa, N.D.; Lautenbach, E.; Chiu, A.G.; Doghramji, L.; Howland, T.J.; Cohen, N.A.; Palmer, J.N. The effect of diabetes mellitus on chronic rhinosinusitis and sinus surgery outcome. *Int. Forum Allergy Rhinol.* **2014**, *4*, 315–320. [CrossRef] [PubMed]
57. Gliklich, R.E.; Metson, R. The health impact of chronic sinusitis in patients seeking otolaryngologic care. *Otolaryngol. Head Neck Surg.* **1995**, *113*, 104–109. [CrossRef]
58. Hopkins, C.; Gillett, S.; Slack, R.; Lund, V.J.; Browne, J.P. Psychometric validity of the 22-item sinonasal outcome test. *Clin. Otolaryngol.* **2009**, *34*, 447–454. [CrossRef] [PubMed]
59. Adappa, N.D.; Howland, T.J.; Palmer, J.N.; Kennedy, D.W.; Doghramji, L.; Lysenko, A.; Reed, D.R.; Lee, R.J.; Cohen, N.A. Genetics of the taste receptor T2R38 correlates with chronic rhinosinusitis necessitating surgical intervention. *Int. Forum Allergy Rhinol.* **2013**, *3*, 184–187. [CrossRef] [PubMed]
60. Adappa, N.D.; Farquhar, D.; Palmer, J.N.; Kennedy, D.W.; Doghramji, L.; Morris, S.A.; Owens, D.; Mansfield, C.; Lysenko, A.; Lee, R.J.; et al. TAS2R38 genotype predicts surgical outcome in nonpolypoid chronic rhinosinusitis. *Int. Forum Allergy Rhinol.* **2016**, *6*, 25–33. [CrossRef] [PubMed]
61. Mfuna Endam, L.; Filali-Mouhim, A.; Boisvert, P.; Boulet, L.P.; Bosse, Y.; Desrosiers, M. Genetic variations in taste receptors are associated with chronic rhinosinusitis: A replication study. *Int. Forum Allergy Rhinol.* **2014**, *4*, 200–206. [CrossRef] [PubMed]
62. Dżaman, K.; Zagor, M.; Sarnowska, E.; Krzeski, A.; Kantor, I. The correlation of TAS2R38 gene variants with higher risk for chronic rhinosinusitis in polish patients. *Otolaryngol. Pol.* **2016**, *70*, 13–18. [CrossRef] [PubMed]
63. Gallo, S.; Grossi, S.; Montrasio, G.; Binelli, G.; Cinquetti, R.; Simmen, D.; Castelnuovo, P.; Campomenosi, P. TAS2R38 taste receptor gene and chronic rhinosinusitis: New data from an Italian population. *BMC Med. Genet.* **2016**, *17*, 54. [CrossRef] [PubMed]
64. Ferril, G.R.; Nick, J.A.; Getz, A.E.; Barham, H.P.; Saavedra, M.T.; Taylor-Cousar, J.L.; Nichols, D.P.; Curran-Everett, D.; Kingdom, T.T.; Ramakrishnan, V.R. Comparison of radiographic and clinical characteristics of low-risk and high-risk cystic fibrosis genotypes. *Int. Forum Allergy Rhinol.* **2014**, *4*, 915–920. [CrossRef] [PubMed]
65. Johansen, H.K.; Nir, M.; Høiby, N.; Koch, C.; Schwartz, M. Severity of cystic fibrosis in patients homozygous and heterozygous for ΔF508 mutation. *Lancet* **1991**, *337*, 631–634. [CrossRef]
66. Jorissen, M.B.; de Boeck, K.; Cuppens, H. Genotype-phenotype correlations for the paranasal sinuses in cystic fibrosis. *Am. J. Respir. Crit. Care Med.* **1999**, *159*, 1412–1416. [CrossRef] [PubMed]
67. Ramsey, B.; Richardson, M.A. Impact of sinusitis in cystic fibrosis. *J. Allergy Clin. Immunol.* **1992**, *90*, 547–552. [CrossRef]
68. Marks, S.C.; Kissner, D.G. Management of sinusitis in adult cystic fibrosis. *Am. J. Rhinol.* **1997**, *11*, 11–14. [CrossRef] [PubMed]
69. Mainz, J.G.; Koitschev, A. Management of chronic rhinosinusitis in CF. *J. Cyst. Fibros.* **2009**, *8*, S10–S14. [CrossRef]
70. Adappa, N.D.; Workman, A.D.; Hadjiliadis, D.; Dorgan, D.J.; Frame, D.; Brooks, S.; Doghramji, L.; Palmer, J.N.; Mansfield, C.; Reed, D.R.; et al. T2R38 genotype is correlated with sinonasal quality of life in homozygous ΔF508 cystic fibrosis patients. *Int. Forum Allergy Rhinol.* **2016**, *6*, 356–361. [CrossRef] [PubMed]
71. Høiby, N.; Ciofu, O.; Bjarnsholt, T. *Pseudomonas aeruginosa* biofilms in cystic fibrosis. *Future Microbiol.* **2010**, *5*, 1663–1674. [CrossRef] [PubMed]

72. Adappa, N.D.; Truesdale, C.M.; Workman, A.D.; Doghramji, L.; Mansfield, C.; Kennedy, D.W.; Palmer, J.N.; Cowart, B.J.; Cohen, N.A. Correlation of T2R38 taste phenotype and in vitro biofilm formation from nonpolypoid chronic rhinosinusitis patients. *Int. Forum Allergy Rhinol.* **2016**, *6*, 783–791. [CrossRef] [PubMed]
73. Tyler, M.A.; Russell, C.B.; Smith, D.E.; Rottman, J.B.; Padro Dietz, C.J.; Hu, X.; Citardi, M.J.; Fakhri, S.; Assassi, S.; Luong, A. Large scale gene expression profiling reveals distinct type 2 inflammatory patterns in chronic rhinosinusitis subtypes. *J. Allergy Clin. Immunol.* **2016**. [CrossRef] [PubMed]
74. Genoway, K.A.; Philpott, C.M.; Javer, A.R. Pathogen yield and antimicrobial resistance patterns of chronic rhinosinusitis patients presenting to a tertiary rhinology centre. *J. Otolaryngol. Head Neck Surg.* **2011**, *40*, 232–237. [PubMed]
75. Carey, R.M.; Workman, A.D.; Chen, B.; Adappa, N.D.; Palmer, J.N.; Kennedy, D.W.; Lee, R.J.; Cohen, N.A. *Staphylococcus aureus* triggers nitric oxide production in human upper airway epithelium. *Int. Forum Allergy Rhinol.* **2015**, *5*, 808–813. [CrossRef] [PubMed]
76. Roudnitzky, N.; Behrens, M.; Engel, A.; Kohl, S.; Thalmann, S.; Hübner, S.; Lossow, K.; Wooding, S.P.; Meyerhof, W. Receptor polymorphism and genomic structure interact to shape bitter taste perception. *PLoS Genet.* **2015**, *11*, e1005530. [CrossRef] [PubMed]

9

Characterizing Non-Tuberculous Mycobacteria Infection in Bronchiectasis

Paola Faverio [1], Anna Stainer [1], Giulia Bonaiti [1], Stefano C. Zucchetti [1], Edoardo Simonetta [1], Giuseppe Lapadula [2], Almerico Marruchella [1], Andrea Gori [2], Francesco Blasi [3], Luigi Codecasa [4], Alberto Pesci [1], James D. Chalmers [5], Michael R. Loebinger [6] and Stefano Aliberti [3,*]

1 Dipartimento Cardio-Toraco-Vascolare, University of Milan Bicocca, Respiratory Unit, San Gerardo Hospital, ASST di Monza, Via Pergolesi 33, 20900 Monza, Italy; paola.faverio@gmail.com (P.F.); annetta.stainer@gmail.com (A.S.); giu28686@hotmail.it (G.B.); s.zucchetti2@campus.unimib.it (S.C.Z.); edo.simonetta@gmail.com (E.S.); almx@libero.it (A.M.); alberto.pesci@unimib.it (A.P.)
2 Department of Internal Medicine, Division of Infectious Diseases, San Gerardo Hospital, ASST di Monza, Via Pergolesi 33, 20900 Monza, Italy; giuseppe.lapadula@gmail.com (G.L.); andrea.gori@unimib.it (A.G.)
3 Department of Pathophysiology and Transplantation, University of Milan, Cardio-Thoracic Unit and Cystic Fibrosis Adult Center, Fondazione IRCCS Cà Granda Ospedale Maggiore Policlinico, Via Francesco Sforza 35, 20122 Milan, Italy; francesco.blasi@unimi.it
4 Villa Marelli Institute, Niguarda Ca' Granda Hospital, 20122 Milan, Italy; luigiruffo.codecasa@ospedaleniguarda.it
5 Scottish Centre for Respiratory Research, University of Dundee, Dundee DD1 9SY, UK; j.chalmers@dundee.ac.uk
6 Host Defence Unit, Royal Brompton and Harefield NHS Foundation Trust, London, UK Imperial College London, London SW3 6NP, UK; M.Loebinger@rbht.nhs.uk
* Correspondence: stefano.aliberti@unimi.it

Academic Editor: William Chi-shing Cho

Abstract: Chronic airway infection is a key aspect of the pathogenesis of bronchiectasis. A growing interest has been raised on non-tuberculous mycobacteria (NTM) infection. We aimed at describing the clinical characteristics, diagnostic process, therapeutic options and outcomes of bronchiectasis patients with pulmonary NTM (pNTM) disease. This was a prospective, observational study enrolling 261 adult bronchiectasis patients during the stable state at the San Gerardo Hospital, Monza, Italy, from 2012 to 2015. Three groups were identified: pNTM disease; chronic *P. aeruginosa* infection; chronic infection due to bacteria other than *P. aeruginosa*. NTM were isolated in 32 (12%) patients, and among them, a diagnosis of pNTM disease was reached in 23 cases. When compared to chronic *P. aeruginosa* infection, patients with pNTM were more likely to have cylindrical bronchiectasis and a "tree-in-bud" pattern, a history of weight loss, a lower disease severity and a lower number of pulmonary exacerbations. Among pNTM patients who started treatment, 68% showed a radiological improvement, and 37% achieved culture conversion without recurrence, while 21% showed NTM isolation recurrence. NTM isolation seems to be a frequent event in bronchiectasis patients, and few parameters might help to suspect NTM infection. Treatment indications and monitoring still remain an important area for future research.

Keywords: non-cystic fibrosis bronchiectasis; non-tuberculous mycobacteria; pulmonary infection

---

1. Introduction

Bronchiectasis represents a significant disease entity with increasing prevalence and substantial impact on patients' morbidity and mortality, as well as healthcare utilization [1]. Chronic airway infection plays a key role in the pathogenesis of the disease sustaining a vicious cycle of inflammation and structural damage [2]. *P. aeruginosa* defines a specific clinical phenotype of bronchiectasis, and its presence is clearly associated with worse patient outcomes [3–5]. The most frequently-isolated bacteria in sputum from bronchiectasis patients include *H. influenzae*, *P. aeruginosa*, *M. catarrhalis* and *S. aureus*. Among other pathogens, recent reports demonstrated an increasing role of non-tuberculous mycobacteria (NTM) with a frequency ranging from one to 18% in bronchiectasis patients [6,7].

Anatomic alteration of the bronchi along with airway clearance impairment seem to be the primum movens of chronic NTM infection, although some authors have also speculated about a possible role of NTM in directly causing bronchiectasis [8,9]. Treatment in pulmonary NTM (pNTM) remains extremely challenging in bronchiectasis. These patients usually meet per se two out of three criteria for pNTM disease recommended by the 2007 American Thoracic Society (ATS)/Infectious Diseases Society of America (IDSA), regardless of the presence of NTM, having both respiratory signs/symptoms and radiographic abnormalities (bronchiectasis) [8]. Thus, translating current evidence and recommendations for the general population with pNTM disease to a specific population of bronchiectasis patients might not be fully appropriate. In view of this scenario, specific evidence on NTM infection in bronchiectasis is needed to help physicians in identifying patients with pNTM disease and treating them appropriately [10].

The objective of this study was to describe the clinical, functional and radiological characteristics of bronchiectasis patients with pNTM infection, as well as the diagnostic process, therapeutic options and outcomes. We also aimed at comparing the characteristics of bronchiectasis patients with pNTM with those with a chronic infection due to *P. aeruginosa* or other bacteria.

2. Results

2.1. NTM Infection and pNTM Disease in Bronchiectasis

Among 261 bronchiectasis patients (median age: 69 years, 59% female) attending the clinic over the study period, 141 (median age: 69 years, 58% female) had a positive microbiology finding in the respiratory sample; see Figure 1. Among the entire study population, 136 (52%) patients underwent bronchoscopy; when considering only those with a positive respiratory sample, the percentage of patients who underwent bronchoscopy is as high as 61%. At least one NTM was isolated in 32 patients (23% among patients with an isolated pathogen and 12% among all bronchiectasis patients). The most common NTM were *Mycobacterium avium* complex (MAC) (24 patients, 17%), including 13 *M. avium* and 11 *M. intracellulare*, and *M. chelonae* (two patients, 1.4%); see Table 1. *M. gordonae* was isolated in four patients and was considered as a contaminant. Two NTM were isolated in one patient: *M. abscessus* spp. and subsequently *M. chelonae* (no treatment was initiated in this case). None of the NTM isolates were resistant to macrolides. NTM isolation was obtained from bronchoscopic specimens in 59% of the patients and from sputum samples in the remaining 41%. A co-infection with other bacteria was detected in 21 (66%) NTM patients, including *P. aeruginosa* (10 patients), *S. aureus* (eight methicillin-susceptible and one methicillin-resistant *S. aureus*), *H. influenzae* (six patients) and *M. catarrhalis* (two cases). A total of 22 (16%) patients had a nodular-bronchiectatic pattern for the high-resolution computed tomography (HRCT) scan, eight (5.7%) patients a cavitary pattern and two (1.4%) patients a bronchiectatic pattern. All patients, but four, had daily respiratory symptoms, either cough or sputum production.

Among the 32 patients with a NTM isolation, a diagnosis of pNTM disease according to the 2007 ATS/IDSA guidelines was reached in 23 (72%) cases: 18 subjects started antibiotic treatment; four patients refused any pharmacological treatment; while one patient had severe liver disease contraindicating antibiotic treatment. Among the nine patients in whom the ATS/IDSA diagnosis of pNTM disease was not reached, a lack of either the clinical (four cases) or microbiological criterion (five cases) was observed. All, but one, did not start a specific antibiotic treatment, but were monitored during follow-up. The only patient who started antibiotic treatment without reaching the ATS/IDSA criteria had a MAC isolation on sputum and a cavitary pattern on HRCT.

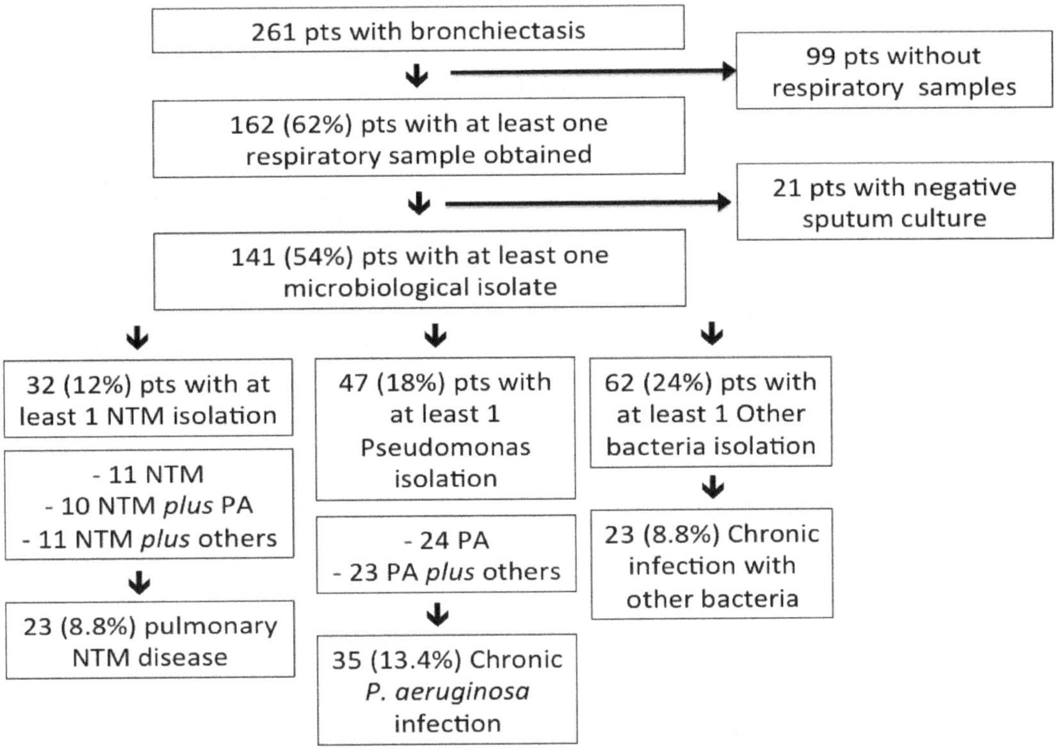

Figure 1. Division of the entire population according to microbiological isolations. PA = *P. aeruginosa*; NTM = non-tuberculous mycobacteria; pts = patients.

Table 1. Non-tuberculous mycobacteria isolated in the study population.

Non-Tuberculous Mycobacteria		
Mycobacterium avium complex		24
–	*M. avium*	13
–	*M. intracellulare*	11
M. gordonae	–	4
M. chelonae	–	2
M. kansasii	–	1
M. abscessus spp.	–	1
M. shimoidei	–	1

2.2. Characteristics of Bronchiectasis Patients with NTM

Among the entire study population, 23 (8.8%) patients belonged to the pNTM group, 35 (13.4%) to the *P. aeruginosa* group and 23 (8.8%) to the other bacteria group (including *H. influenzae* in 12 cases, *S. aureus* in four cases, *K. pneumoniae* in three cases, *M. catarrhalis* in two cases, *E. coli* and *S. pneumoniae* in one case). Four patients with both pNTM and *P. aeruginosa* were included in the pNTM group. Seven patients with concomitant chronic infection with other bacteria and either pNTM or *P. aeruginosa* were included in the pNTM or *P. aeruginosa* group, respectively; see Figure 1. Demographics, comorbidities, clinical, radiological, functional and laboratory data of the three study groups are reported in Table 2, and disease severity is summarized in Table 3.

Patients with pNTM were more likely to have cylindrical bronchiectasis and a "tree-in-bud" pattern, as well as a history of weight loss in comparison to patients with *P. aeruginosa*. Furthermore, patients with pNTM, including both those on active treatment and those in follow-up, showed a lower disease severity and a lower number of pulmonary exacerbations at one-year follow-up compared to patients with *P. aeruginosa*.

Table 2. Demographics, comorbidities, radiological characteristics, symptoms, pulmonary function and laboratory data according to the three study groups: pulmonary non-tuberculous mycobacteria disease (pNTM); chronic infection with *P. aeruginosa* (*Pseudomonas*) and chronic infection with bacteria other than *P. aeruginosa* (other bacteria).

Variables	pNTM (n = 23)	*Pseudomonas* (n = 31)	Other Bacteria (n = 16)	p-Value
Demographics	–	–	–	–
Male, n (%)	10 (44)	15 (48)	6 (38)	0.79
Age, median (IQR)	70 (62–76)	72 (66–76)	60 (51–71)	0.77
BMI, median (IQR)	20.6 (18.7–25.1)	22.6 (21.6–25.2)	21.4 (18.1–27.2)	0.15
BMI < 18.5, n (%)	3 (19)	4 (13)	4 (27)	0.68
Prior tuberculosis, n (%)	4 (22)	3 (10)	1 (6)	0.39
Either smoker or ex-smoker, n (%)	11 (65)	13 (42)	6 (38)	0.23
Comorbidities, n (%)	–	–	–	–
Chronic obstructive pulmonary disease	6 (35)	13 (42)	2 (13)	0.76
Asthma	1 (6)	3 (10)	4 (25)	1
Sinusitis	1 (6)	5 (16)	6 (38)	0.65
Cardiopathy	4 (25)	14 (45)	7 (44)	0.22
Arterial hypertension	6 (38)	17 (55)	6 (38)	0.36
Angina	0	2 (7)	1 (6)	0.54
Prior stroke	0	1 (3)	0	1
Vasculopathy	2 (13)	4 (13)	0	1
Atrial fibrillation	0	4 (13)	0	0.28
Valvulopathy	1 (6)	6 (19)	2 (13)	0.39
Congestive heart failure	0	2 (7)	0	0.54
Pulmonary hypertension	0	2 (7)	2 (13)	0.54
Diabetes	3 (18)	6 (19)	1 (6)	1
Liver disease	1 (6)	1 (3)	0	1
Cirrhosis	1 (6)	1 (3)	0	1
Chronic renal failure	0	2 (7)	0	0.54
Neurological disease	0	2 (7)	1 (6)	0.54
Rheumatological disease	0	5 (16)	1 (6)	0.15
Vasculitis	0	1 (3)	1 (6)	1
Gastroesophageal reflux disease	5 (31)	10 (32)	8 (50)	1
Immuno-deficit	0	1 (3)	4 (25)	1
Solid cancer	7 (39)	6 (19)	2 (13)	0.18
Haematological malignancy	0	2 (7)	1 (6)	0.54
Radiologic characteristics, n (%)	–	–	–	–
Cylindric	13 (87) *	16 (52) *	12 (75)	0.048
Cystic	2 (13)	11 (38)	3 (19)	0.16
Varicose	0	2 (7)	1 (6)	0.54
Tree-in-bud pattern	13 (57) *	7 (23) *	7 (44)	0.011
Symptoms, n (%)	–	–	–	–
Daily cough	9 (56)	22 (71)	8 (50)	0.35
Daily sputum	5 (31)	18 (58)	10 (63)	0.13
Haemoptysis	4 (25)	4 (13)	5 (31)	0.42
Dyspnoea	9 (56)	18 (58)	9 (56)	1
Recurrent pneumonias	1 (6)	0	5 (31)	0.34
Weight loss	6 (38) *	3 (10) *	3 (19)	0.045
Asthenia	7 (44)	16 (52)	7 (44)	0.76
PFTs	–	–	–	–
FEV_1 %, median (IQR)	85 (56–100)	61.5 (49–81)	82 (52–100)	0.074
Laboratories collected during stable phase		–	–	–
WBC × 10^3/mL, median (IQR)	6.4 (5.4–7.7)	7.4 (5.8–8.6)	7.13 (5.48–9.61)	0.19
CRP mg/mL, median (IQR)	0.57 (0.15–2.3)	0.5 (0.26–1.38)	0.97 (0.17–3.18)	0.76

* $p < 0.05$ (pNTM vs. *Pseudomonas*). BMI = body mass index, FEV_1 = forced expiratory volume in 1 s, WBC = white blood cells, CRP = C-reactive protein, PFT = pulmonary function test.

Table 3. Disease severity and outcomes according to the three study groups: pulmonary non-tuberculous mycobacteria disease (pNTM); chronic infection with *P. aeruginosa* (*Pseudomonas*) and chronic infection with bacteria other than *P. aeruginosa* (other bacteria).

Bronchiectasis Severity and Outcome	pNTM (n = 23)	*Pseudomonas* (n = 31)	Other Bacteria (n = 16)	p-Value
BSI, median (IQR)	7 (6–10) *	12 (9–15) *	6 (4–9)	0.004
One-year exacerbations, median (IQR)	0 (0–2) *	1 (0.75–3.25) *	0 (0–2)	0.043
One-year hospitalization (at least one/y), n (%)	2 (9)	5 (16)	0	0.94
One-year mortality, n (%)	1 (4.3)	1 (3.2)	0	0.76
Two-year mortality, n (%)	2 (8.7)	2 (6.5)	0	1
Three-year mortality, n (%)	4 (17.4)	4 (12.9)	0	0.9

* $p < 0.05$ (pNTM vs. *Pseudomonas*). BSI = bronchiectasis severity index.

In order to limit the confounding effect of multiple pathogens isolated from the same patient, a subset analysis of patients with only NTM isolates (11 cases) vs. patients with NTM and other pathogens co-infection (12 cases) was performed. No differences between groups were identified in regards to all of the items evaluated in Tables 2 and 3.

2.3. Treatment and Outcomes of Bronchiectasis Patients with pNTM

Therapeutic regimens for pNTM are summarized in Figure 2. The regimen schedule was chosen according to both the isolated pathogen and the radiologic pattern after multidisciplinary discussion between pulmonologists and infectious disease physicians: six patients were on a three-times a week schedule and 13 patients were on a daily regimen (patients infected by NTM other than MAC and with a cavitary pattern on the HRCT scan were included in the latter group). All regimens included standard antibiotic doses adjusted for either renal or liver function in the case of insufficiency. All medications were given orally with the exception of amikacin and streptomycin. Median (IQR) treatment duration was 18 (14–18) months. Nine patients experienced adverse events due to the antibiotic treatment, including gastric intolerance (five cases), liver toxicity (two cases), thrombocytopenia (one case) and visual toxicity (one case). A second line regimen was initiated in five patients (26%) because of the presence of adverse events during the first line regimen in four cases and because of treatment failure in one case; see Figure 2.

Among pNTM patients who started treatment, 13 (68%) showed a radiological improvement. Among them, seven also experienced culture conversion after treatment with no recurrence (treatment success). Median (IQR) duration of treatment for pNTM before culture conversion was 3 (2–4.5) months. Three (16%) patients were still on active first line treatment at the time of the present analysis. A total of four (21%) MAC patients had MAC isolation recurrence after treatment. One MAC patient had a new isolation of *M. gordonae* on one sputum sample after treatment that was considered contaminant. Median (IQR) duration of treatment for pNTM before culture conversion was 9 (5–16) months. Four (21%) patients died during NTM therapy due to causes not directly related to pNTM: two were not related to respiratory diseases, and two were caused by lung cancer. No differences were found between groups in regards to solid cancer rates. Among the four patients who refused or postponed treatment, none died. No statistically-significant differences were detected among groups in regards to all-cause mortality at one-, two- and three-year follow-up; see Table 3.

Four out of the five pNTM patients who did not receive treatment showed no radiological progression within the study period. They had a median (IQR) one-year exacerbations and hospitalizations rate of 2 (0.5–3) and 0 (0–1.5), respectively. Three cases had also other pathogens isolated on respiratory samples: *P. aeruginosa* (two cases), *M. catarrhalis* (one case), *H. influenzae* (one case) and methicillin-resistant *S. aureus* (one case).

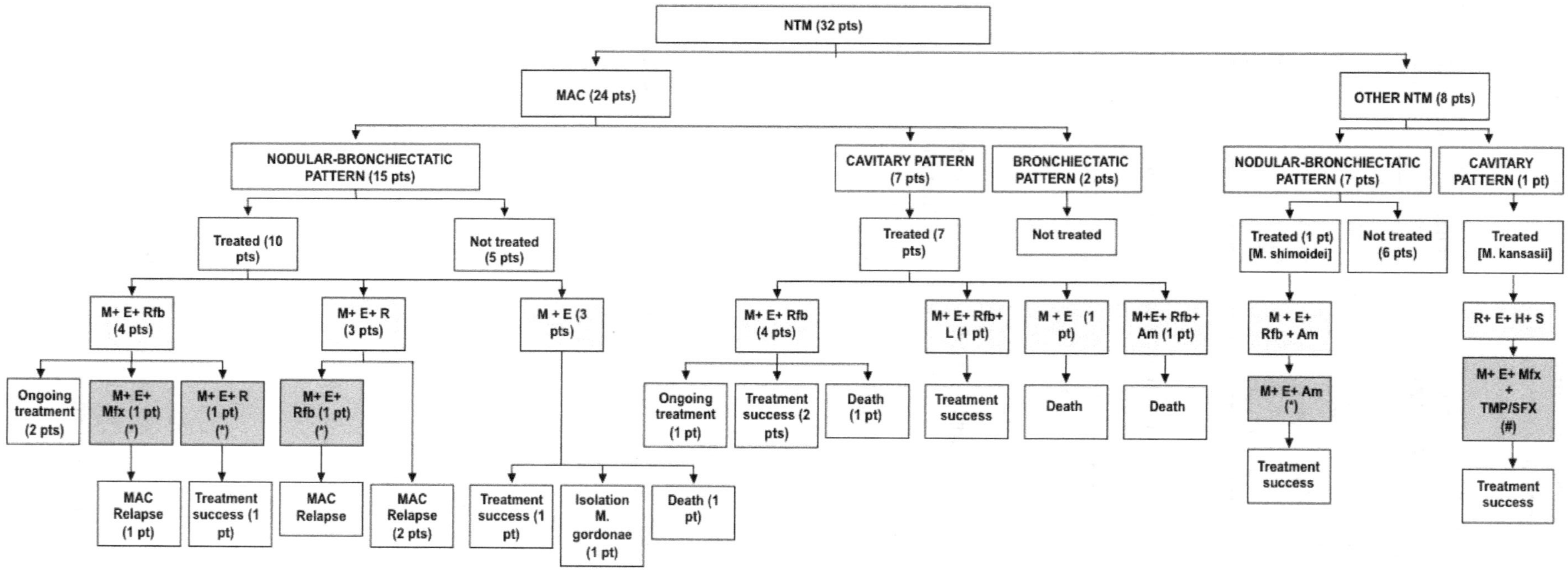

Am = amikacin; **E** = ethambutol, **H** = isoniazid, **L** = levofloxacin; **M** = macrolide (azithromycin or clarithromycin), **Mfx** = moxifloxacin; **R** = rifampicin; **Rfb** = rifabutin, **S** = streptomycin; **TMP-SMX** = trimethoprim sulfamethoxazole, **MAC** = Mycobacterium avium complex. **pts** = patients

(*) second line treatment started because of adverse events during the first-line regimen; (#) second line treatment started because of first-line regimen failure

First line treatment | Second line treatment

Figure 2. Therapeutic regimens and outcomes of adult bronchiectasis patients with pulmonary non-tuberculous mycobacteria disease according to the type of mycobacterium and the radiologic pattern.

Patients in the *Pseudomonas* and other bacteria groups also received long-term antibiotic therapy: patients in the *Pseudomonas* group received long-term macrolide therapy in five cases (16%) and long-term inhaled antibiotic therapy in four cases (13%) during the study period. Patients in the other bacteria group received long-term macrolide therapy in two cases (13%) and long-term inhaled antibiotic therapy in one case (6%) during the study period.

3. Discussion

This study shows that NTM are isolated in 12% of adult patients with bronchiectasis, while a specific diagnosis of pNTM disease requiring treatment is reached in 8.8% of them. When considering patients with at least one isolated pathogen, the prevalence of NTM is as high as 23%. MAC is the most frequent mycobacteria, while a co-infection with other bacteria is present in the majority of the patients (66%), including *P. aeruginosa* in almost one third of them. Patients with pNTM are more likely to have cylindrical bronchiectasis and a "tree-in-bud" pattern on HRCT, a history of weight loss, a lower disease severity and a lower number of pulmonary exacerbations compared to patients with chronic infection with *P. aeruginosa*. Among pNTM patients treated according to 2007 ATS/IDSA guidelines, only 37% achieved treatment success without recurrence, while 21% showed NTM isolation recurrence, and 21% died during treatment.

Our prevalence of 12% of NTM isolation and 8.8% of pNTM disease is in line with a recent meta-analysis reporting a 9.3% overall prevalence of NTM isolation in bronchiectasis patients worldwide and with other data coming from European cohorts and showing NTM isolations in 2%–10% of the subjects [7,11–14]. Notably, NTM isolation in our cohort was mainly obtained from bronchoscopic specimens. The high number of bronchoscopies we conducted according to our standard operating procedures might have increased the rate of NTM isolations and, consequently, of pNTM disease diagnosis (72% of cases with a NTM isolation). Differently from our study, Máiz et al. evaluated the prevalence of NTM isolation and pNTM disease in a cohort of 218 adult bronchiectasis patients in Spain considering only sputum samples [11]. The authors found a lower prevalence of both NTM isolation and pNTM disease (8.3% and 2.3%, respectively) compared to our cohort. These previous data suggest that the higher the number of bronchoscopies performed, the higher the probability of NTM isolation and, consequently, of pNTM disease diagnosis. In addition, the presence of a tree-in-bud pattern on HRCT scan and the inability to produce an adequate sputum sample were considered an indication to perform bronchial aspirate (BAS)/bronchoalveolar lavage (BAL) according to our standard operating procedures. This may also explain the high prevalence of pNTM disease diagnosis in our cohort. Our finding of MAC being the most frequent NTM in bronchiectasis also confirms previous data published by both Máiz and Mirsaeidi, who identified MAC in 50% and 80% of all NTM isolates, respectively [11,15]. Furthermore, our data show that in NTM patients, the most common co-infection is with *P. aeruginosa* (31%), and this is in line with previous experiences showing a prevalence ranging from 27% to −52% [14,16]. Finally, we also identified *S. aureus* and *H. influenzae* as other pathogens co-infecting bronchiectasis patients with NTM, as previously described [14].

Very scarce evidence supports experts' opinion in suggesting when to perform culture for mycobacteria in bronchiectasis patients [17]. According to our results, few clinical parameters might be helpful in discriminating between NTM vs. chronic *Pseudomonas* infection in bronchiectasis. Key findings that should be investigated and might lead physicians to consider a patient at higher risk for NTM infection include weight loss, a tree-in-bud pattern and cylindrical bronchiectasis at HRCT scan. Similarly to our results, Máiz and colleagues reported that a low body mass index was independently associated with NTM isolation [11]. Notably, Koh et al. identified the presence of bronchiolitis, lobular consolidations and cavities as radiological findings related to pNTM in 105 bronchiectasis patients [18].

Although two thirds of our patients had radiological improvement during treatment, only 37% achieved culture conversion without recurrence, while 21% showed NTM isolation recurrence. Similar results with a treatment success rate of 40%–60% and high rates of NTM isolation relapse or re-infection (up to 50% of patients who completed treatment) have also been found in larger MAC cohorts [19–21].

According to these results, it seems that, despite a successful antibiotic course, a large percentage of bronchiectasis patients develop NTM recurrence.

In this scenario, the vicious cycle connected with bronchiectasis leading to impaired airway clearance and chronic airways infection could be considered one of the main risk factors for pNTM disease recurrence, together with other host (e.g., immunodeficiency) and environmental risk factors. We might identify two possible repercussions on patients' management: from a diagnostic point of view, a higher relevance should be given to bronchiectasis severity, extension and radiological worsening during follow-up in the prognostic definition of the disease. This, along with clinical and microbiological criteria, could guide physicians in the decision making process whether to treat or not patients with pNTM disease. From a therapeutic point of view, physicians should keep in mind that a successful patient's management requires therapeutic strategies for both NTM infection and bronchiectasis. Airway clearance techniques, bronchodilators if indicated and exacerbations/infections prevention should be started as soon as possible and continued after a specific antibiotic course. A long-term macrolide regimen for frequent exacerbators is probably the only therapeutic strategy that comes into conflict with proven or suspected pNTM disease, since macrolide monotherapy is contraindicated in this latter case.

Other interesting observations can be pointed out in our cohort of bronchiectasis patients with pNTM disease. Given the prolonged antimicrobial course with a number of potential side effects (developed in 47% of our patients), a significant proportion of patients decides to postpone or refuse treatment even when suggested otherwise (17% in our cohort, none died); similar results with treatment discontinuation or refusal in 10%–30% of patients have also been described in other cohorts [20,21]. Furthermore, the morbidity and mortality related to patients' multiple comorbid conditions can often complicate short- and long-term outcomes [22], as described in our cohort where four patients died during pNTM treatment and one patient did not start antimicrobial therapy because of the severity of the comorbid conditions.

Although we present data from one of the largest cohorts of pNTM infection in adult bronchiectasis patients described so far in Europe, some limitations of our study should be acknowledged. On the one hand, the monocentric design limited our possibility to draw conclusions concerning the comparison of NTM patients with those with other chronic infections and impacts the generalizability of these and other results. Among four patients with pNTM disease who experienced recurrence after treatment of the same NTM species, we were not able to differentiate between true relapse vs. re-infection. On the other hand, the prospective nature of our study performed in a referral centre for bronchiectasis gave us the opportunity to work on a homogeneous cohort of patients with high quality data and with a complete clinical and microbiological history. Furthermore, a few possible confounders should be listed. Firstly, an important proportion of pNTM patients is on a prolonged antibiotic regimen with multiple drugs, including macrolides, which may have affected the exacerbation rate. Secondly, since all patients with a tree-in-bud pattern on HRCT scan without sputum production underwent bronchoscopy, the presence of tree-in-bud itself may self-select for NTM. Thirdly, some patients in the pNTM group had also other respiratory isolates, including *P. aeruginosa* (six cases) and other pathogens (six cases). One of the main limitations of the present study is the impossibility to perform statistical analysis on patients with only NTM infection and no other pathogen isolated due to the small sample size (11 patients had only NTM infection); therefore, in the NTM pulmonary disease group, four patients had both NTM pulmonary disease and *P. aeruginosa* chronic infection.

Future studies should focus on determining whether patients with NTM isolation and bronchiectasis may benefit from different diagnostic criteria to define pNTM disease. Finally, given the frequently unsatisfactory outcomes after treatment, further research is needed to evaluate whether patients with pNTM disease and bronchiectasis may require specific therapeutic regimens, schemes and durations of treatment.

In conclusion, the isolation of NTM seems to be a frequent event in bronchiectasis patients, especially among those with cylindrical bronchiectasis and a "tree-in-bud" pattern on HRCT, a history of weight loss, a low disease severity and a low number of pulmonary exacerbations. Treatment indication in this specific population, as well as monitoring patients' response still remain important areas for future research.

4. Materials and Methods

4.1. Study Design

This was a prospective, observational study of adult patients with bronchiectasis attending the outpatient clinic at the San Gerardo Hospital, Monza, Italy, from 2012–2015. Consecutive patients aged $\geq$18 years with a diagnosis of bronchiectasis on HRCT scan in a stable state were recruited. Patients with cystic fibrosis or traction bronchiectasis due to pulmonary fibrosis were excluded. The Institutional Review Board of the San Gerardo Hospital approved the study (ethical permission code: 234, 30 September 2013), and patients signed an informed consent.

4.2. Data Collection and Microbiological Analysis

At the time of clinical assessment, all patients underwent the same comprehensive diagnostic work-up as recommended by the 2010 British Thoracic Society (BTS) guidelines [17]. Demographics, comorbidities, disease severity, respiratory symptoms, microbiology, radiological, functional and laboratory findings in the stable state, long-term treatments and outcomes (including exacerbations, hospitalizations and mortality) during a three-year follow-up were recorded. HRCT imaging was performed using a 64-slice CT scanner. Sequential scanning was performed at maximal inspiration from the apex to the diaphragm using 1-mm contiguous slices (1-mm set), while patients were in the supine position. Images were reviewed by a consultant radiologist with 15-year experience of reporting HRCT and a consultant respiratory physician with a major interest in bronchiectasis in order to define nodular-bronchiectatic vs. cavitary vs. bronchiectatic patterns. They etiology of bronchiectasis was evaluated as previously described [23]. The severity of bronchiectasis was evaluated according to the bronchiectasis severity index (BSI) [24,25].

All bacteriology, including culture for both bacteria and mycobacteria, was performed on either spontaneous sputum (for patients with a productive cough) or BAS/BAL samples. BAS/BAL were collected in patients showing a HRCT appearance of a tree-in-bud pattern without productive cough. Murray–Washington criteria for sputum quality were used in all cases, with all samples having less than 10 squamous cells and more than 25 leukocytes per low-power microscope field.

4.3. Study Definitions and Outcomes

pNTM disease was defined according to the 2007 ATS/IDSA guidelines as the presence of both clinical (pulmonary symptoms and radiographic abnormalities) and microbiological criteria (NTM positive culture results from at least two separate sputum samples or one bronchoscopic specimen) [8]. Chronic infection was defined by the isolation of potentially-pathogenic bacteria in sputum culture on two or more occasions, at least 3 months apart over a 1-year period [26]. A bronchiectasis exacerbation was defined as a clinical diagnosis of exacerbation for which antibiotics were prescribed in the presence of at least one (and usually more than one) of the following symptoms: increasing cough, increasing sputum volume, worsening sputum purulence, worsening dyspnoea, increased fatigue/malaise, fever and haemoptysis [17].

Study outcomes included exacerbations, hospitalizations and all-cause mortality at one-year follow-up, as well as all-cause mortality at two- and three-year follow-up.

4.4. Study Groups

The study population was divided according to the presence of bacteria and NTM: (1) patients with pNTM disease; (2) those with chronic *P. aeruginosa* infection; and (3) those with chronic infection due to bacteria other than *P. aeruginosa*. Patients with both pNTM disease and chronic infection with either *P. aeruginosa* or other bacteria were included in the pNTM disease group, whereas patients with a chronic infection with both *P. aeruginosa* and other bacteria were included in the *P. aeruginosa* group.

4.5. Statistical Analysis

Data were analysed using SPSS 21.0 for MAC OS (SPSS Inc., Chicago, IL, USA). Characteristics of the population (including respiratory symptoms), radiological features, pulmonary function tests (PFTs) and microbiological isolation, as well as study outcomes were considered for statistical analysis. Continuous variables are expressed as median (interquartile range (IQR) 25th–75th percentile). The difference of median (IQR) was evaluated by the Wilcoxon–Mann–Whitney U two-sample test. Categorical data are expressed as frequencies and percentages and compared using the chi-square or Fisher exact test where appropriate. All tests were 2-tailed, and a p-value <0.05 was considered statistically significant.

Author Contributions: Study concept and design: Stefano Aliberti and Paola Faverio. Acquisition of data: Paola Faverio, Anna Stainer, Giulia Bonaiti, Stefano C. Zucchetti, Edoardo Simonetta, Stefano Aliberti, and Giuseppe Lapadula. Analysis and interpretation of data: Stefano Aliberti, Paola Faverio, Anna Stainer, Giulia Bonaiti, Luigi Codecasa, James D. Chalmers, and Michael R. Loebinger. Drafting of the manuscript: Stefano Aliberti, Paola Faverio, Anna Stainer, Giulia Bonaiti, Almerico Marruchella, Luigi Codecasa, James D. Chalmers, and Michael R. Loebinger. Critical revision of the manuscript for important intellectual content: all authors. Statistical analysis: Paola Faverio and Stefano Aliberti. Study supervision: Stefano Aliberti, Michael R. Loebinger, James D. Chalmers, Andrea Gori, Francesco Blasi, and Alberto Pesci. Read and approved the final manuscript: all authors.

Abbreviations

NTM	non-tuberculous mycobacteria
pNTM	pulmonary NTM
ATS	American Thoracic Society
IDSA	Infectious Diseases Society of America
MAC	*Mycobacterium avium* complex
HRCT	high-resolution computed tomography
BAS	bronchial aspirate
BAL	bronchoalveolar lavage
BTS	British Thoracic Society
BSI	bronchiectasis severity index

References

1. Poppelwell, L.; Chalmers, J.D. Defining severity in non-cystic fibrosis bronchiectasis. *Expert. Rev. Respir. Med.* **2014**, *8*, 249–262. [CrossRef] [PubMed]
2. Chalmers, J.D.; Aliberti, S.; Blasi, F. Management of bronchiectasis in adults. *Eur. Respir. J.* **2015**, *45*, 1446–1462. [CrossRef] [PubMed]
3. Aliberti, S.; Lonni, S.; Dore, S.; McDonnell, M.J.; Goeminne, P.C.; Dimakou, K.; Fardon, T.C.; Rutherford, R.; Pesci, A.; Restrepo, M.I.; et al. Clinical phenotypes in adult patients with bronchiectasis. *Eur. Respir. J.* **2016**, *47*, 1113–1122. [CrossRef] [PubMed]
4. McDonnell, M.J.; Jary, H.R.; Perry, A.; MacFarlane, J.G.; Hester, K.L.M.; Small, T.; Molyneux, C.; Perry, J.D.; Walton, K.E.; de Soyza, A. Non cystic fibrosis bronchiectasis: A longitudinal retrospective observational cohort study of Pseudomonas persistence and resistance. *Respir. Med.* **2015**, *109*, 716–726. [CrossRef] [PubMed]

5. Finch, S.; McDonnell, M.J.; Abo-Leyah, H.; Aliberti, S.; Chalmers, J.D. A comprehensive analysis of the impact of *Pseudomonas aeruginosa* colonization on prognosis in adult bronchiectasis. *Ann. Am. Thorac. Soc.* **2015**, *12*, 1602–1611. [PubMed]
6. Bonaiti, G.; Pesci, A.; Marruchella, A.; Lapadula, G.; Gori, A.; Aliberti, S. Nontuberculous mycobacteria in noncystic fibrosis bronchiectasis. *BioMed Res. Int.* **2015**, *2015*, 197950–197958. [CrossRef] [PubMed]
7. Chu, H.; Zhao, L.; Xiao, H.; Zhang, Z.; Zhang, J.; Gui, T.; Gong, S.; Xu, L.; Sun, X. Prevalence of nontuberculous mycobacteria in patients with bronchiectasis: A meta-analysis. *Arch. Med. Sci.* **2014**, *29*, 661–668. [CrossRef] [PubMed]
8. Griffith, D.E.; Aksamit, T.; Brown-Elliott, B.A.; Catanzaro, A.; Daley, C.; Gordin, F.; Holland, S.M.; Horsburgh, R.; Huitt, G.; Iademarco, M.F.; et al. An official ATS/IDSA statement: Diagnosis, treatment, and prevention of nontuberculous mycobacterial diseases. *Am. J. Respir. Crit. Care Med.* **2007**, *175*, 367–416. [CrossRef] [PubMed]
9. Okumura, M.; Iwai, K.; Ogata, H.; Mizutani, S.; Yoshimori, K.; Itoh, K.; Nakajima, Y.; Kudoh, S. Pulmonary Mycobacterium avium complex (MAC) disease showing middle lobe syndrome—Pathological findings of 2 cases suggesting different mode of development. *Kekkaku* **2002**, *77*, 615–620. [PubMed]
10. Aliberti, S.; Masefield, S.; Polverino, E.; de Soyza, A.; Loebinger, M.R.; Menendez, R.; Ringshausen, F.C.; Vendrell, M.; Powell, P.; Chalmers, J.D. Research priorities in bronchiectasis: A consensus statement from the EMBARC clinical research collaboration. *Eur. Respir. J.* **2016**, *48*, 632–647. [CrossRef] [PubMed]
11. Máiz, L.; Girón, R.; Olveira, C.; Vendrell, M.; Nieto, R.; Martínez-García, M.A. Prevalence and factors associated with nontuberculous mycobacteria in non-cystic fibrosis bronchiectasis: A multicenter observational study. *BMC Infect. Dis.* **2016**, *16*, 437–444. [CrossRef] [PubMed]
12. Martínez-Cerón, E.; Prados, C.; Gómez-Carrera, L.; Cabanillas, J.J.; López-López, G.; Álvarez-Sala, R. Non-tuberculous mycobacterial infection in patients with non-cystic fibrosis bronchiectasias. *Rev. Clín. Esp.* **2012**, *212*, 127–130. [CrossRef] [PubMed]
13. Fowler, S.J.; French, J.; Screaton, N.J.; Foweraker, J.; Condliffe, A.; Haworth, C.S.; Exley, A.R.; Bilton, D. Nontuberculous mycobacteria in bronchiectasis: Prevalence and patient characteristics. *Eur. Respir. J.* **2006**, *28*, 1204–1210. [CrossRef] [PubMed]
14. Wickremasinghe, M.; Ozerovitch, L.J.; Davies, G.; Wodehouse, T.; Chadwick, M.V.; Abdallah, S.; Shah, P.; Wilson, R. Non-tuberculous mycobacteria in patients with bronchiectasis. *Thorax* **2005**, *60*, 1045–1051. [CrossRef] [PubMed]
15. Mirsaeidi, M.; Hadid, W.; Ericsoussi, B.; Rodgers, D.; Sadikot, R.T. Non-tuberculous mycobacterial disease is common in patients with non-cystic fibrosis bronchiectasis. *Int. J. Infect. Dis.* **2013**, *17*, 1000–1004. [CrossRef] [PubMed]
16. Zoumot, Z.; Boutou, A.K.; Gill, S.S.; van Zeller, M.; Hansell, D.M.; Wells, A.U.; Wilson, R.; Loebinger, M.R. Mycobacterium avium complex infection in non-cystic fibrosis bronchiectasis. *Respirology* **2014**, *19*, 714–722. [CrossRef] [PubMed]
17. Pasteur, M.C.; Bilton, D.; Hill, A.T. British thoracic society bronchiectasis non-CF guideline group. British thoracic society guideline for non-CF bronchiectasis. *Thorax* **2010**, *65*, 1–58. [CrossRef] [PubMed]
18. Koh, W.J.; Lee, K.S.; Kwon, O.J.; Jeong, Y.J.; Kwak, S.H.; Kim, T.S. Bilateral bronchiectasis and bronchiolitis at thin-section CT: Diagnostic implications in nontuberculous mycobacterial pulmonary infection. *Radiology* **2005**, *235*, 282–288. [CrossRef] [PubMed]
19. Wallace, R.J.; Brown-Elliott, B.A.; McNulty, S.; Philley, J.V.; Killingley, J.; Wilson, R.W.; York, D.S.; Shepherd, S.; Griffith, D.E. Macrolide/Azalide therapy for nodular/bronchiectatic mycobacterium avium complex lung disease. *Chest* **2014**, *146*, 276–282. [CrossRef] [PubMed]
20. Field, S.K.; Fisher, D.; Cowie, R.L. Mycobacterium avium complex pulmonary disease in patients without HIV infection. *Chest* **2004**, *126*, 566–581. [CrossRef] [PubMed]
21. Xu, H.B.; Jiang, R.H.; Li, L. Treatment outcomes for Mycobacterium avium complex: A systematic review and meta-analysis. *Eur. J. Clin. Microbiol. Infect. Dis.* **2014**, *33*, 347–358. [CrossRef] [PubMed]
22. Park, I.K.; Olivier, K.N. Nontuberculous mycobacteria in cystic fibrosis and non-cystic fibrosis bronchiectasis. *Semin. Respir. Crit. Care Med.* **2015**, *36*, 217–224. [CrossRef] [PubMed]
23. Lonni, S.; Chalmers, J.D.; Goeminne, P.C.; McDonnell, M.J.; Dimakou, K.; de Soyza, A.; Polverino, E.; van de Kerkhove, C.; Rutherford, R.; Davison, J.; et al. Etiology of non-cystic fibrosis bronchiectasis in adults and its correlation to disease severity. *Ann. Am. Thorac. Soc.* **2015**, *12*, 1764–1770. [CrossRef] [PubMed]

24. Chalmers, J.D.; Goeminne, P.; Aliberti, S.; McDonnell, M.J.; Lonni, S.; Davidson, J.; Poppelwell, L.; Salih, W.; Pesci, A.; Dupont, L.J.; et al. The bronchiectasis severity index. An international derivation and validation study. *Am. J. Respir. Crit. Care Med.* **2014**, *189*, 576–585. [CrossRef] [PubMed]
25. McDonnell, M.J.; Aliberti, S.; Goeminne, P.C.; Dimakou, K.; Zucchetti, S.C.; Davidson, J.; Ward, C.; Laffey, J.G.; Finch, S.; Pesci, A.; et al. Multidimensional severity assessment in bronchiectasis: An analysis of seven European cohorts. *Thorax* **2016**. [CrossRef] [PubMed]
26. Pasteur, M.C.; Helliwell, S.M.; Houghton, S.J.; Webb, S.C.; Foweraker, J.E.; Coulden, R.A.; Flower, C.D.; Bilton, D.; Keogan, M.T. An investigation into causative factors in patients with bronchiectasis. *Am. J. Respir. Crit. Care Med.* **2000**, *162*, 1277–1284. [CrossRef] [PubMed]

10

Aspergillus fumigatus Detection and Risk Factors in Patients with COPD–Bronchiectasis Overlap

Stephanie Everaerts [1,2], Katrien Lagrou [3,4], Kristina Vermeersch [2], Lieven J. Dupont [1,2], Bart M. Vanaudenaerde [2] and Wim Janssens [1,2,*]

1. Department of Respiratory Diseases, University Hospitals Leuven, Herestraat 49, B-3000 Leuven, Belgium; stephanie.everaerts@kuleuven.be (S.E.); lieven.dupont@uzleuven.be (L.J.D.)
2. Department of Chronic Diseases, Metabolism & Aging, Laboratory of Respiratory Diseases, KU Leuven, Herestraat 49, B-3000 Leuven, Belgium; kristina.vermeersch@uzleuven.be (K.V.); bart.vanaudenaerde@kuleuven.be (B.M.V.)
3. Department of Laboratory Medicine, University Hospitals Leuven, Herestraat 49, B-3000 Leuven, Belgium; katrien.lagrou@uzleuven.be
4. Department of Microbiology and Immunology, KU Leuven, Herestraat 49, B-3000 Leuven, Belgium

* Correspondence: wim.janssens@uzleuven.be

Abstract: The role of *Aspergillus fumigatus* in the airways of chronic obstructive pulmonary disease (COPD) patients with bronchiectasis is currently unclear. We searched for a sensitive and noninvasive method for *A. fumigatus* detection in the sputum of COPD patients and addressed potential risk factors for its presence. Induced sputum samples of 18 COPD patients and 17 COPD patients with bronchiectasis were analyzed for the presence of *A. fumigatus* by culture, galactomannan detection, and PCR. Of the patients with COPD–bronchiectasis overlap, 23.5% had a positive culture for *A. fumigatus* versus 10.5% of COPD patients without bronchiectasis ($p = 0.39$). The median sputum galactomannan optical density index was significantly higher in patients with COPD and bronchiectasis compared with patients with COPD alone ($p = 0.026$) and ranged between the levels of healthy controls and *A. fumigatus*-colonized cystic fibrosis patients. Both the presence of bronchiectasis and the administration of systemic corticosteroids were associated with sputum galactomannan ($p = 0.0028$ and $p = 0.0044$, respectively) and showed significant interaction (p interaction = 0.022). PCR for *Aspergillus* was found to be a less sensitive method, but was critically dependent on the extraction technique. The higher sputum galactomannan levels suggest a more abundant presence of *A. fumigatus* in the airways of patients with COPD–bronchiectasis overlap compared with patients with COPD without bronchiectasis, particularly when systemic corticosteroids are administered.

Keywords: sputum galactomannan; *Aspergillus* PCR; *Aspergillus* colonization; corticosteroids

---

1. Introduction

Chronic obstructive pulmonary disease (COPD) is a highly prevalent disease, characterized by progressive airflow limitation, which is caused by an abnormal inflammatory response to chronic inhalation of irritants, mainly cigarette smoke [1]. Both small airways (obstructive bronchiolitis) and parenchyma (emphysema) are affected. Bronchiectasis is defined by the presence of irreversibly dilated and chronically inflamed bronchi. COPD and bronchiectasis have overlapping clinical features, but the diagnostic criteria are very different. Whereas an irreversible obstructive lung function is obligatory in COPD, bronchiectasis is diagnosed by structural airway abnormalities observed on computed tomography (CT) of the thorax. The combined presence of COPD and bronchiectasis in one patient is not rare. In cohorts of COPD patients, bronchiectasis has been described in 30–60% of patients [2–5], whereas bronchiectasis cohorts report COPD as the underlying cause in approximately

30% of patients [6,7].The recognition of an overlap is relevant, since these patients not only have a worse prognosis [2,7,8], but their diagnostic and therapeutic approach is also different.

The pathogenesis of bronchiectasis is generally explained by a vicious circle of inflammation, structural damage, impaired mucus clearance, bacterial colonization, and infection [9]. The underlying mechanism for the development of bronchiectasis in a subset of COPD patients remains largely unknown. *Aspergillus fumigatus* is a ubiquitous fungus, which is cleared from the airways by the innate immune system. A damaged airway epithelium, inherited or acquired defects of the innate immune system, and immunosuppressive drugs such as corticosteroids (CS) predispose to aspergillosis. *A. fumigatus* colonization and sensitization associate with bronchiectasis and unfavorable outcomes in asthma and cystic fibrosis (CF) [10–13]. In COPD, a history of exacerbations and the isolation of pathogenic bacteria in sputum were suggested as potential risk factors for *A. fumigatus* [14]. Although the clinical relevance is not clear, several retrospective studies showed that more than 20% of COPD patients with *A. fumigatus* detected in respiratory samples eventually developed aspergillosis [15,16]. If *A. fumigatus* plays a causal role in the development of bronchiectasis is still a matter of debate.

One major reason for our limited understanding is the lack of sensitive and noninvasive methods to detect *A. fumigatus* in the airways. Mycological culture is not sensitive nor standardized and has led to an underestimation of *A. fumigatus* in the airways [17]. Other methods focus mainly on invasive fungal disease and require invasive procedures, such as immunohistochemistry on airway biopsies or galactomannan detection on bronchoalveolar lavage fluid. Galactomannan is a polysaccharide cell wall component of *Aspergillus* species, which is not present in resting conidia but is secreted by the hyphae during fungal growth. The determination of galactomannan by enzyme immunoassay in serum and bronchoalveolar lavage fluid is validated for diagnosing an invasive *Aspergillus* disease, mainly in immunocompromised patients. Molecular-based techniques such as polymerase chain reaction (PCR) and next-generation sequencing are hampered by complex DNA extraction, high costs, and limited experience with sputum samples. To investigate the role of *A. fumigatus* in patients with COPD, we explored the feasibility of galactomannan detection and *A. fumigatus* PCR on sputum samples.

We assumed a more abundant presence of *A. fumigatus* in the sputum of patients with COPD-bronchiectasis overlap and addressed the role of CS as a potential risk factor.

2. Results

2.1. Study Group Characteristics

Thirty-six COPD patients were included, of which 17 had bronchiectasis, with a median modified Reiff score of 4. There were no significant differences between the two groups, apart from a significantly lower median value of pack-years ($p = 0.048$) in patients with bronchiectasis. The results are shown in Table 1.

Table 1. Characteristics of the study groups.

characteristic	COPD without Bronchiectasis	COPD with Bronchiectasis
Subjects, *n*	19	17
Hospitalized, %	42	65
Age, y	71 (60–75)	68 (63–79)
Male, %	84	88
BMI, kg/m^2	25 (20–30)	22 (19–27)
Pack-years *	48 (40–55)	40 (25–45)
FEV1, % pred	51 (39–58)	41 (37–52)
DLCO, % pred	47 (40–57)	44 (26–53)
GOLD		
I/II/III/IV, %	0/53/47/0	6/29/65/0
A/B/C/D, %	21/0/16/63	12/17/6/65
Eosinophils, %	1.4 (0.1–3.1)	2.3 (0.8–4.6)

Table 1. *Cont.*

Characteritic	COPD without Bronchiectasis	COPD with Bronchiectasis
Eosinophils, µL	200 (0–300)	200 (100–350)
Total IgE, kU/L	83 (16–592)	43 (33–298)
mMRC	2 (1–2)	2 (1.5–3.5)
CAT	14 (12–20)	19 (13–24)
SGRQ	41.9 (30.6–53.4)	54.9 (37.3–66.7)
≥2 exacerbations/y, %	79	71
ICS, %	89	82
Modified Reiff score	NA	4 (2.5–6.5)

Data are presented as *n*, % or median (interquartile range). COPD: chronic obstructive pulmonary disease, y: year, BMI: body mass index, FEV1: forced expiratory volume in 1 s, % pred: percentage predicted, DLCO: diffusion capacity of the lung for carbon monoxide, GOLD: Global initiative for chronic Obstructive Lung Disease stadia, mMRC: modified Medical Research Council breathlessness scale, CAT: COPD Assessment Test, SGRQ: Saint Georges Respiratory Questionnaire, ICS: inhaled corticosteroids. * p-value < 0.05. All other variables were not significantly different between the groups.

2.2. *A. fumigatus Antibodies*

Patients with COPD-bronchiectasis overlap had a median *A. fumigatus* IgG value of 35.4 mg/L versus 17.4 mg/L in COPD patients without bronchiectasis ($p = 0.14$). On the basis of both ImmunoCAP measurement and skin prick test, three patients without (15.7%) and five patients with bronchiectasis (29.4%) were sensitized to *A. fumigatus* ($p = 0.37$). The results are summarized in Table 2.

Table 2. *A. fumigatus*-related results.

Test	COPD without Bronchiectasis	COPD with Bronchiectasis	*p*-Value
Subjects, *n*	19	17	
***A. fumigatus* IgG, mg/L**	17.4 (13.4–37.3)	35.4 (25.5–51.6)	0.14
***A. fumigatus* sensitization, %**	15.7	29.4	0.37
***A. fumigatus* sputum culture, %**	10.5	23.5	0.39
Sputum galactomannan, ODI	0.7 (0.4–1.5)	3.7 (0.6–5.7)	**0.026**

Data are presented as *n*, median (interquartile range) or %. COPD: chronic obstructive pulmonary disease, *A. fumigatus*: *Aspergillus fumigatus*, ODI: optical density index. *p*-Value < 0.05 is captured in bold.

2.3. *Fungal Sputum Culture*

Four COPD patients with bronchiectasis (23.5%) had a positive *A. fumigatus* culture versus two COPD patients without bronchiectasis (10.5%) ($p = 0.39$). *Aspergillus nidulans* was found in samples of two COPD–bronchiectasis-overlap patients which were also positive for *A. fumigatus*. When only inocula of 10 µL were considered, three out of six positive cultures were negative. Of the non-inoculated control plates and of the healthy control samples, none grew *A. fumigatus*, but a positive *A. fumigatus* culture was confirmed in all samples of cystic fibrosis patients with previously known *A. fumigatus* colonization.

2.4. *Sputum Galactomannan*

The median sputum galactomannan ODI was significantly higher in patients with COPD-bronchiectasis overlap compared with patients with only COPD (3.7 versus 0.7, $p = 0.026$) (Table 2). The results of galactomannan measurements in Sputasol, sterile water, and three vials of amoxicillin clavulanate were 0.0, 0.1, and 0.0 respectively. Thirteen sputum samples were retested and had a median galactomannan inter-assay difference of 0.4, with a median coefficient of variation of 9.4% (Supplementary Materials Table S1). The majority of patients was using inhalation corticosteroids (ICS) (Table 1); we found no difference in sputum galactomannan between patients without ICS or with medium or high dose ICS (Figure 1). In contrast to ICS, both bronchiectasis and systemic CS were significantly associated with sputum galactomannan ODI ($p = 0.0028$ and $p = 0.0044$ respectively) in a two-way analysis of variance model. Furthermore, CS showed a stronger association with galactomannan in the patients with COPD–bronchiectasis overlap compared with COPD patients without bronchiectasis (p interaction = 0.022). The results are presented in Figure 2 and Table 3. As galactomannan detection on sputum has not been validated, we compared our results to negative and positive control samples and found them to be significantly different (p = 0.0012, Figure 3). Moreover, all but one subjects with a positive *A. fumigatus* culture had a sputum galactomannan ODI above 4 (Supplementary Materials Table S2).

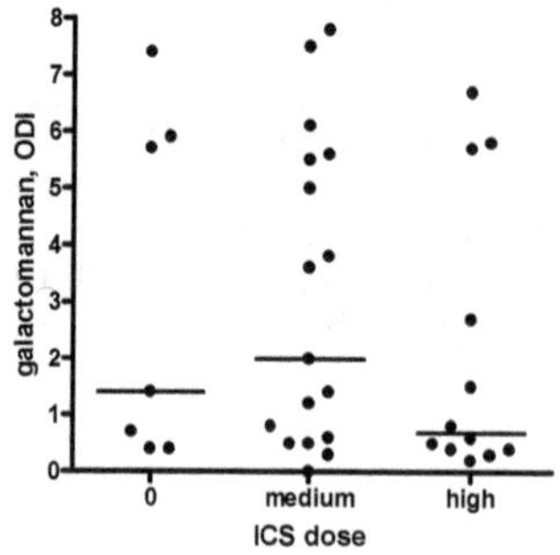

Figure 1. Inhaled corticosteroids and sputum galactomannan. Sputum galactomannan is presented as optical density index. Every dot represents one sample, and the horizontal lines reflect the median values. There was no significant difference in galactomannan values dependent on ICS dose. ODI: optical density index, ICS: inhaled corticosteroids.

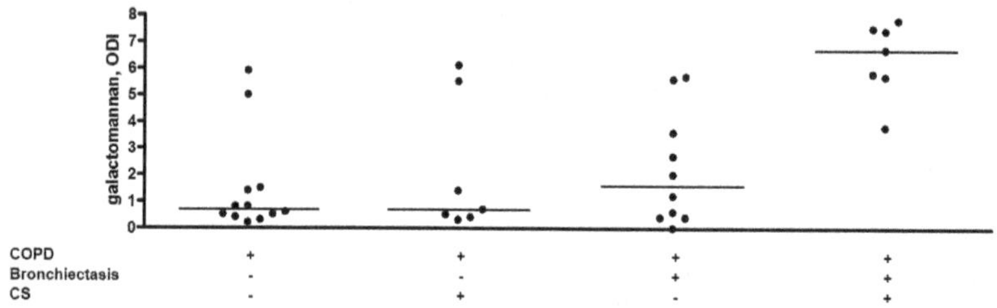

Figure 2. Effect of systemic corticosteroids on sputum galactomannan values. Sputum galactomannan is presented as optical density index. Every dot represents one sample, and the horizontal lines reflect the median values. ODI: optical density index, COPD: chronic obstructive pulmonary disease, CS: systemic corticosteroids in the previous seven days.

Table 3. Associations with sputum galactomannan in COPD patients.

Bivariate Models		
	Estimate	***p*-Value**
CS in COPD without bronchiectasis (n = 19)	0.64	0.54
CS in COPD with bronchiectasis (n = 17)	4.17	**0.0004**
Multivariate Model		
	Estimate	***p*-Value**
Bronchiectasis	0.67	**0.0028**
CS	0.57	**0.0044**
Antibiotics	0.37	0.63
Bronchiectasis–CS interaction	3.43	**0.022**

Two bivariate general linear models were built with galactomannan as exposure: one for patients without and one for patients with bronchiectasis showing that CS were only significant associated with galactomannan in patients having bronchiectasis. One multivariate (two-way analysis of variance) general linear model was built for all patients in which systemic corticosteroids and antibiotics administered in the seven days before sputum induction were considered relevant. CS: systemic corticosteroids, COPD: chronic obstructive pulmonary disease, p-values < 0.05 are shown in bold.

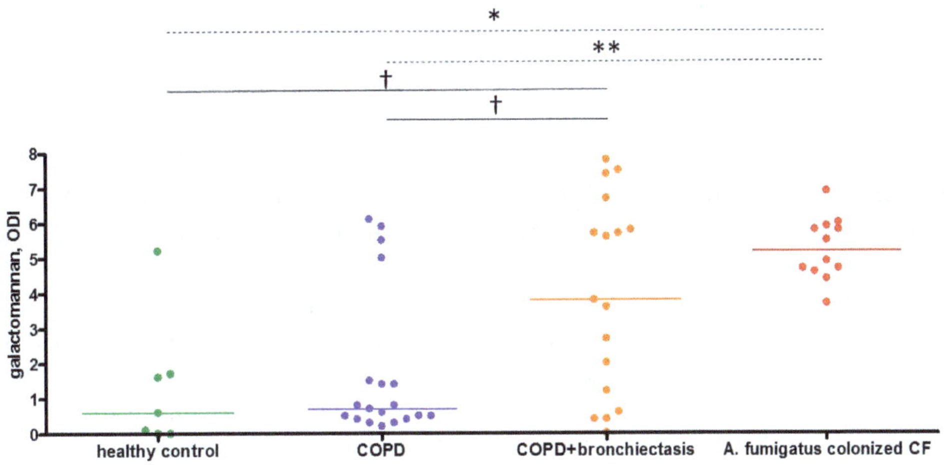

Figure 3. Comparison of COPD sputum galactomannan with healthy and *A. fumigatus*-colonized CF controls. Sputum galactomannan is presented as optical density index. Every dot represents one sample, and the horizontal lines reflect the median values. Kruskal–Wallis test showed an overall significant difference ($p = 0.0012$), with Dunn's post-hoc comparison for multiple testing showing significant differences between groups, indicated with * $p < 0.05$ and ** $p < 0.01$ (dashed lines). The comparison of COPD + bronchiectasis with the other groups using Mann–Withney U-test showed significant differences between groups, indicated with † $p < 0.05$ (solid lines). ODI: optical density index, COPD: chronic obstructive pulmonary disease, CF: cystic fibrosis.

2.5. Sputum A. fumigatus PCR

When automated DNA extraction was used for *A. fumigatus* real-time PCR, only three samples of COPD patients were found to be positive. All of them had high sputum galactomannan levels. All healthy control samples had a negative PCR result, whereas seven out of twelve CF samples with known *A. fumigatus* colonization had a positive PCR result. Five positive control sputum samples were used to compare automated DNA extraction by EasyMAG and manual extraction by MycXtra®. All samples had a positive *A. fumigatus* PCR result after manual DNA extraction compared to only two positive samples after the automated extraction protocol (Table 4). The comparison between sputum galactomannan and *A. fumigatus* PCR is shown in Supplementary Materials Table S2.

Table 4. Comparison of DNA extraction methods in five samples of cystic fibrosis patients with known *A. fumigatus* colonization.

Subject	Sputum Galactomannan, ODI	PCR after EasyMAG Extraction, Ct	PCR after MycXtra® Extraction, Ct
CF1	4.4	negative	positive, 36.7
CF2	3.7	negative	positive, 32.9
CF3	4.7	positive, 29.3	positive, 26.2
CF4	4.6	positive, 30.7	positive, 30.5
CF5	4.7	negative	positive, 33.2

Sputum galactomannan is presented as optical density index. PCR is expressed as negative or positive with the respective Ct value in case of positivity. CF: cystic fibrosis sample, ODI: optical density index, PCR: polymerase chain reaction, Ct: cycle threshold.

3. Discussion

Sputum galactomannan levels suggest a higher load of *A. fumigatus* in COPD-bronchiectasis-overlap patients compared to COPD patients without bronchiectasis. The sputum galactomannan values were particularly higher in COPD-bronchiectasis-overlap patients that received systemic CS.

Fungal culture has a low sensitivity, even in proven aspergillosis, which contributes to an underestimation of fungal presence in the airways [18]. In this study, 16.7% of all COPD patients showed *A. fumigatus* in sputum culture. A positive culture was not associated with clinical characteristics or bronchiectasis. Previous studies reported *A. fumigatus* positive cultures in 14–37% of COPD patients [14,19]. In general, culture procedures are not standardized, and the use of different media and methodologies makes it hard to compare different studies. On the basis of a recent report that emphasized the use of larger inocula for fungal culture, we compared sputum volumes of 10 μL and 100 μL [20]. Indeed, we found a higher *A. fumigatus* culture yield by plating 100 μL of the samples. Nevertheless, the lack of standardization and low sensitivity urges the need for other detection methods.

An attractive, alternative method is the detection of galactomannan on sputum samples. On bronchoalveolar lavage fluid, a galactomannan value of 0.5 is suggestive of the presence of *A. fumigatus*, although this cut-off is under debate. Kimura et al. reported 1.2 as the optimal sputum galactomannan cut-off to diagnose invasive aspergillosis in haematological patients [21], whereas Baxter et al. used the 0.5 cut-off for *Aspergillus* positivity in adult CF sputum samples [22]. Recently, the sputum galactomannan results of patients with chronic pulmonary aspergillosis and allergic bronchopulmonary aspergillosis were found to be much higher, with a cut-off above 6.5 for diagnosis [23]. Our study, which used a comparable homogenization of the samples as the latter, found ODI values in the same range. Furthermore, we validated these results with negative and positive controls, which were confirmed by culture and PCR. Despite the higher median galactomannan ODI in COPD patients with bronchiectasis, our study was not able to define an appropriate cut-off. The median coefficient of variation to evaluate inter-assay difference was acceptable, although we are aware that the inter-assay difference was not optimal for some of our samples.

A. fumigatus PCR after automated DNA extraction was less sensitive than culture and galactomannan detection on COPD sputum samples. Although the performance is good for clear, liquid samples, our in-house protocol was not suitable for sputum samples, as it does not apply mechanical forces prior to fungal DNA extraction. Manual DNA extraction with MycXtra, which includes bead-beating, performed much better in five additionally collected positive control samples. Since this method required a high sample volume, we were not able to apply this on the other, previously collected study samples. Furthermore, manual extraction is labor-intensive and not suited for large laboratories handling many samples on a daily basis. Any protocol for fungal DNA extraction and PCR on sputum needs further optimization prior to its clinical use.

CS temper the innate immune response, thereby permitting *A. fumigatus* to persist and proliferate. In our study, systemic administration of CS was significantly associated with higher sputum galactomannan values, particularly in patients with COPD–bronchiectasis overlap. These findings contrast with the study of Huerta et al. in which no association was found between *Aspergillus* cultures and oral CS [14]. Differences in the studied population or in the dose of CS administered prior to the analysis may explain these discrepancies. As the large majority of our study subjects on CS received high doses in the context of acute exacerbation (40 mg prednisolone), dose–response relationships could not be studied. Together, our data suggest that systemic CS induce a pronounced and rapid growth of residing *A. fumigatus* in the airways, which may predispose to sensitization, bronchiectasis development, or fungal infection. A local deposition of CS via inhalation may have similar effects. Bafadhel et al. found that COPD patients with *A. fumigatus*-positive culture were on higher doses of inhaled CS compared with culture-negative patients [19]. However, the significance of this association was weak and could not be confirmed by others [14] nor by our analysis.

Although this study does not allow us to attribute causality, our findings support the hypothesis that *A. fumigatus* contributes to the development and/or progression of bronchiectasis in COPD. We recently showed that the sensitization to specific *A. fumigatus* allergens was associated with the presence of bronchiectasis in COPD [5]. Next to an upregulation of the Th2 pathway, *Aspergillus* proteases may play an important role through enhanced mucus production and airway remodeling [24,25]. So far, studies that explored these relationships are solely based on fungal cultures, which may explain some of the inconclusive results. Sputum galactomannan seems to provide a more sensitive marker for *A. fumigatus* detection in the airways of COPD patients. This advantage may serve new longitudinal observational studies or even intervention trials in this area.

4. Materials and Methods

4.1. Study Design and Subjects

This academic, single-center study included COPD patients prospectively during hospitalization or an outpatient visit. The inclusion criteria were an established diagnosis of COPD based on a post-bronchodilator forced expiratory volume in 1 s (FEV1)/forced vital capacity (FVC) ratio < 0.7, smoking history of at least 10 pack-years, available CT images of the thorax, and an FEV1 $\geq$ 30% (safety measure for sputum induction). The exclusion criteria were ventilation (mechanical and noninvasive), respiratory diagnosis other than COPD, mycobacterial disease, immunosuppression other than CS, active cancer treatment, history of lung, tracheal, or laryngeal surgery, history of chest radiotherapy, and presence of other inflammatory diseases such as rheumatoid arthritis and inflammatory bowel disease. Investigators were blinded to the results of previous sputum cultures. None of the included patients had a history of allergic or chronic bronchopulmonary aspergillosis, nor invasive *Aspergillus* disease. The presence of bronchiectasis was assessed on CT scans of the lungs. All hospitalized patients received standard therapy for an exacerbation: CS and antibiotics if indicated. They were included after sufficient recovery from the acute event. Oral or intravenous CS and antibiotics administered in the seven days before sputum induction were considered relevant. The study was approved by the local Ethics Committee (Medical Ethical Board of the University Hospitals Leuven, Belgium—M11223) and all patients signed informed consent before enrollment.

4.2. Pulmonary Function and Questionnaires

Post-bronchodilator spirometry was measured using standardized equipment (Whole Body Plethysmograph, Vyaire, Vilvoorde, Belgium), according to the American Thoracic Society/European Respiratory Society guidelines [26]. Diffusion capacity was measured by the single-breath carbon monoxide gas transfer method [27]. The results are reported as percentages predicted of reference values. The post-bronchodilator FEV1 was used to classify the patients according to the Global Initiative for Chronic Obstructive Lung Disease (GOLD) classification. The patients completed the modified Medical Research Council (mMRC) breathlessness scale [28], COPD Assessment Test (CAT™) [29], and Saint Georges Respiratory Questionnaire (SGRQ), a self-administered health-related quality of life measure.

4.3. CT Thorax

All subjects had a high-resolution CT (HRCT) of the thorax at least one year before enrollment. All patients had inspiratory images with 1 mm slices. Bronchiectasis were defined based on Naidich's descriptions: bronchoarterial ratio > 1, lack of tapering, and presence of bronchus within 1 cm of the costal pleura or abutting the mediastinal pleura [30]. All images were blinded to the other data and scored using the modified Reiff score, assessesing the number of involved lobes (the lingula considered separately) and the degree of bronchodilation (1 = tubular, 2 = varicose, and 3 = cystic) [31].

4.4. Eosinophils, Total IgE, *A. fumigatus* Sensitization, and *A. fumigatus*-Specific IgG

Blood samples were collected, and white blood cell count and differentiation were performed by fluorescence flow cytometry (Sysmex XE-5000, Kobe, Japan). Total IgE, IgE against *A. fumigatus* extract, recombinant antigens (rAsp f1-f4 and f6), and *A. fumigatus* IgG were determined by ImmunoCAP fluoroenzyme-immunoassay (Phadia AB, Uppsala, Sweden). The skin prick test with crude *A. fumigatus* extract (ALK, Almere, The Netherlands) was performed according to the guidelines [32].

4.5. Sputum Collection, Homogenization, and Culture

In all COPD patients, sputum was induced by inhalation of hypertonic saline (concentration 3%, 4%, and 5% for 5 min each) generated by an Ultra-Neb ultrasonic nebulizer (DeVilbiss, Port Washington, NY, USA) after pretreatment with 400 μg of inhaled salbutamol. The patient was asked to rinse the mouth thoroughly with water and spit the sputum into a collection tube [33]. As negative and positive control samples, induced sputum samples of 7 healthy controls and spontaneous samples of 12 CF patients with known *A. fumigatus* colonization were collected, respectively. All samples were immediately stored at −80 °C. For homogenization, an equal volume of Sputasol® (Oxoid, Thermo Fisher, Hampshire, UK, 1.4% dithiothreitol) was added to each sample. The samples were subsequently incubated at 37 °C for 30 min and shaken every 10 min. Two volumes of each sample, 10 and 100 μL, were inoculated on Sabouraud agar plates (Sabouraud with chloramphenicol (Bio-Rad, Marnes-la-Coquette, France). The culture plates were incubated at 42 °C for 1 day and subsequently at 30 °C for 1 week. For each sample, an additional plate without inoculation was incubated as a control. The growth was checked daily and the colonies were identified by microscopy.

4.6. Sputum Galactomannan Assay

Of the homogenized sputum, 300 μL was transferred to a sterile tube. An enzyme immunoassay (Platelia™ *Aspergillus* Ag, Bio-Rad, Marnes-la-Coquette, France) was used to detect galactomannan. The results are expressed as optical density index (ODI), the ratio of the optical density of the sample to the mean cut-off control optical density. To exclude false positivity, galactomannan was determined in Sputasol® and in the sterile water we used to prepare the Sputasol® solution. Furthermore, three vials from different batches of amoxicillin clavulanate were tested, as some of the hospitalized patients received this antibiotic, known to influence galactomannan results in previous reports [34]. Moreover, 13 sputum samples were retested to confirm the results.

4.7. Aspergillus PCR on Sputum

A. fumigatus real-time PCR was done following an in-house method with excellent performance in European *Aspergillus* PCR Initiative (EAPCRI) evaluations. Nucleic acid extraction was semi-automatically performed with EasyMAG (Biomérieux, Marcy l' Etoile, France) using NucliSens reagents as recommended by the manufacturer. Briefly, 500 μL of sputum samples was lysed in the presence of magnetic silica beads and subsequently eluted. This method was compared with a manual extraction method using MycXtra® (Myconostica, Cambridge, UK) in five additionally collected CF sputum samples with known *A. fumigatus* colonization. The fungal DNA was extracted as recommended by the manufacturer. Briefly, 1 mL of the homogenized sample was used for extraction, then lysis, bead beating, and purification were performed to remove inhibiting substances with reagents provided by the manufacturer. The nucleic acid extracts where used for real-time PCR (Quantstudio™, Thermo Fisher Life technologies, Carlsbad, CA, USA). The comparative cycle threshold was used to normalize data after running through 45 cycles. The used reagents are shown in the online Supplementary Materials Table S3.

4.8. Statistical Analysis

Statistical analysis was performed using GraphPad Prism 4 (GraphPad Software, La Jolla, CA, USA) and SAS software version 9.4 (SAS Institute, Cary, NC, USA). Non-parametric tests were used for analyses. Univariate comparisons were performed by Mann–Withney U-test and presented as median ± interquartile range. The proportions of discrete variables were compared with χ^2 test and presented as absolute numbers and percentages. The comparison of four groups was performed with the Kruskal–Wallis and post-hoc Dunn's tests for multiple comparison. A multivariate model was built for two-way analysis of variance to study the association between sputum galactomannan, bronchiectasis, and CS. After performing bivariable models with sputum galactomannan as exposure, potential confounders of the association between sputum galactomannan and bronchiectasis were included in the final model if they (1) changed the estimate of the multivariable model ≥10% or (2) the variable was significantly associated with galactomannan and bronchiectasis. The interaction between bronchiectasis and CS was included in the model. p-Values < 0.05 were considered significant in all analyses.

Acknowledgments: Study supported by Belgian Astra Zeneca chair in respiratory pathophysiology and KU Leuven (C2). Wim Janssens and Lieven Dupont are senior clinical investigators of Fond Wetenschappelijk Onderzoek Vlaanderen . Stephanie Everaerts and Kristina Vermeersch are supported as doctoral candidates by Fond Wetenschappelijk Onderzoek Vlaanderen and the Flemisch Government Agency for Innovation by Science and Technology, respectively.

Author Contributions: Wim Janssens, Katrien Lagrou, Lieven J. Dupont, Bart M. Vanaudenaerde, and Stephanie Everaerts conceived and designed the experiments, Stephanie Everaerts performed the experiments, Stephanie Everaerts analyzed the data, Stephanie Everaerts, Kristina Vermeersch, and Wim Janssens wrote the paper.

References

1. Vogelmeier, C.F.; Criner, G.J.; Martinez, F.J.; Anzueto, A.; Barnes, P.J.; Bourbeau, J.; Celli, B.R.; Chen, R.; Decramer, M.; Fabbri, L.M.; et al. Global Strategy for the Diagnosis, Management, and Prevention of Chronic Obstructive Lung Disease 2017 Report. GOLD Executive Summary. *Am. J. Respir. Crit. Care Med.* **2017**, *195*, 557–582. [CrossRef] [PubMed]
2. Martínez-García, M.-A.; de la Rosa Carrillo, D.; Soler-Cataluña, J.-J.; Donat-Sanz, Y.; Serra, P.C.; Lerma, M.A.; Ballestín, J.; Sánchez, I.V.; Selma Ferrer, M.J.; Dalfo, A.R.; et al. Prognostic Value of Bronchiectasis in Patients with Moderate-to-Severe Chronic Obstructive Pulmonary Disease. *Am. J. Respir. Crit. Care Med.* **2013**, *187*, 823–831. [CrossRef] [PubMed]
3. Jairam, P.M.; van der Graaf, Y.; Lammers, J.-W.J.; Mali, W.P.T.M.; de Jong, P.A. PROVIDI Study group Incidental findings on chest CT imaging are associated with increased COPD exacerbations and mortality. *Thorax* **2015**, *70*, 725–731. [CrossRef] [PubMed]
4. Da Silva, S.M.D.; Paschoal, I.A.; de Capitani, E.M.; Moreira, M.M.; Palhares, L.C.; Pereira, M.C. COPD phenotypes on computed tomography and its correlation with selected lung function variables in severe patients. *Int. J. Chronic Obstr. Pulm. Dis.* **2016**, *11*, 503–513. [CrossRef] [PubMed]
5. Everaerts, S.; Lagrou, K.; Dubbeldam, A.; Lorent, N.; Vermeersch, K.; Van Hoeyveld, E.; Bossuyt, X.; Dupont, L.J.; Vanaudenaerde, B.M.; Janssens, W. Sensitization to *Aspergillus fumigatus* as a risk factor for bronchiectasis in COPD. *Int. J. Chronic Obstr. Pulm. Dis.* **2017**, *12*, 2629–2638. [CrossRef] [PubMed]
6. Quint, J.K.; Millett, E.R.C.; Joshi, M.; Navaratnam, V.; Thomas, S.L.; Hurst, J.R.; Smeeth, L.; Brown, J.S. Changes in the incidence, prevalence and mortality of bronchiectasis in the UK from 2004 to 2013: A population-based cohort study. *Eur. Respir. J.* **2016**, *47*, 186–193. [CrossRef] [PubMed]
7. McDonnell, M.J.; Aliberti, S.; Goeminne, P.C.; Restrepo, M.I.; Finch, S.; Pesci, A.; Dupont, L.J.; Fardon, T.C.; Wilson, R.; Loebinger, M.R.; et al. Comorbidities and the risk of mortality in patients with bronchiectasis: An international multicentre cohort study. *Lancet Respir. Med.* **2016**, *4*, 969–979. [CrossRef]
8. Du, Q.; Jin, J.; Liu, X.; Sun, Y. Bronchiectasis as a Comorbidity of Chronic Obstructive Pulmonary Disease: A Systematic Review and Meta-Analysis. *PLoS ONE* **2016**, *11*, e0150532. [CrossRef]
9. Cole, P.J. Inflammation: A two-edged sword—The model of bronchiectasis. *Eur. J. Respir. Dis. Suppl.* **1986**, *147*, 6–15. [PubMed]
10. Agbetile, J.; Fairs, A.; Desai, D.; Hargadon, B.; Bourne, M.; Mutalithas, K.; Edwards, R.; Morley, J.P.; Monteiro, W.R.; Kulkarni, N.S.; et al. Isolation of filamentous fungi from sputum in asthma is associated with reduced post-bronchodilator FEV1. *Clin. Exp. Allergy J. Br. Soc. Allergy Clin. Immunol.* **2012**, *42*, 782–791. [CrossRef] [PubMed]
11. Amin, R.; Dupuis, A.; Aaron, S.D.; Ratjen, F. The effect of chronic infection with *Aspergillus fumigatus* on lung function and hospitalization in patients with cystic fibrosis. *Chest* **2010**, *137*, 171–176. [CrossRef] [PubMed]

12. Fairs, A.; Agbetile, J.; Hargadon, B.; Bourne, M.; Monteiro, W.R.; Brightling, C.E.; Bradding, P.; Green, R.H.; Mutalithas, K.; Desai, D.; et al. IgE sensitization to *Aspergillus fumigatus* is associated with reduced lung function in asthma. *Am. J. Respir. Crit. Care Med.* **2010**, *182*, 1362–1368. [CrossRef] [PubMed]
13. Shah, A.; Panjabi, C. Allergic aspergillosis of the respiratory tract. *Eur. Respir. Rev. Off. J. Eur. Respir. Soc.* **2014**, *23*, 8–29. [CrossRef] [PubMed]
14. Huerta, A.; Soler, N.; Esperatti, M.; Guerrero, M.; Menendez, R.; Gimeno, A.; Zalacaín, R.; Mir, N.; Aguado, J.M.; Torres, A. Importance of *Aspergillus* spp. isolation in Acute exacerbations of severe COPD: Prevalence, factors and follow-up: The FUNGI-COPD study. *Respir. Res.* **2014**, *15*, 17. [CrossRef] [PubMed]
15. Guinea, J.; Torres-Narbona, M.; Gijón, P.; Muñoz, P.; Pozo, F.; Peláez, T.; de Miguel, J.; Bouza, E. Pulmonary aspergillosis in patients with chronic obstructive pulmonary disease: Incidence, risk factors, and outcome. *Clin. Microbiol. Infect.* **2010**, *16*, 870–877. [CrossRef] [PubMed]
16. Barberán, J.; García-Pérez, F.-J.; Villena, V.; Fernández-Villar, A.; Malmierca, E.; Salas, C.; Giménez, M.-J.; Granizo, J.-J.; Aguilar, L. working group on Infectious Diseases from the Spanish Society of Internal Medicine Development of *Aspergillosis* in a cohort of non-neutropenic, non-transplant patients colonised by *Aspergillus* spp. *BMC Infect. Dis.* **2017**, *17*, 34. [CrossRef]
17. Pashley, C.H. Fungal culture and sensitisation in asthma, cystic fibrosis and chronic obstructive pulmonary disorder: What does it tell us? *Mycopathologia* **2014**, *178*, 457–463. [CrossRef] [PubMed]
18. Pashley, C.H.; Fairs, A.; Morley, J.P.; Tailor, S.; Agbetile, J.; Bafadhel, M.; Brightling, C.E.; Wardlaw, A.J. Routine processing procedures for isolating filamentous fungi from respiratory sputum samples may underestimate fungal prevalence. *Med. Mycol.* **2012**, *50*, 433–438. [CrossRef] [PubMed]
19. Bafadhel, M.; Mckenna, S.; Agbetile, J.; Fairs, A.; Desai, D.; Mistry, V.; Morley, J.P.; Pancholi, M.; Pavord, I.D.; Wardlaw, A.J.; et al. *Aspergillus fumigatus* during stable state and exacerbations of COPD. *Eur. Respir. J.* **2014**, *43*, 64–71. [CrossRef] [PubMed]
20. Fraczek, M.G.; Kirwan, M.B.; Moore, C.B.; Morris, J.; Denning, D.W.; Richardson, M.D. Volume dependency for culture of fungi from respiratory secretions and increased sensitivity of *Aspergillus* quantitative PCR. *Mycoses* **2014**, *57*, 69–78. [CrossRef] [PubMed]
21. Kimura, S.; Odawara, J.; Aoki, T.; Yamakura, M.; Takeuchi, M.; Matsue, K. Detection of *sputum Aspergillus galactomannan* for diagnosis of invasive pulmonary aspergillosis in haematological patients. *Int. J. Hematol.* **2009**, *90*, 463–470. [CrossRef] [PubMed]
22. Baxter, C.G.; Rautemaa, R.; Jones, A.M.; Webb, A.K.; Bull, M.; Mahenthiralingam, E.; Denning, D.W. Intravenous antibiotics reduce the presence of *Aspergillus* in adult cystic fibrosis sputum. *Thorax* **2013**, *68*, 652–657. [CrossRef] [PubMed]
23. Fayemiwo, S.; Moore, C.B.; Foden, P.; Denning, D.W.; Richardson, M.D. Comparative performance of *Aspergillus galactomannan* ELISA and PCR in sputum from patients with ABPA and CPA. *J. Microbiol. Methods* **2017**, *140*, 32–39. [CrossRef] [PubMed]
24. Oguma, T.; Asano, K.; Tomomatsu, K.; Kodama, M.; Fukunaga, K.; Shiomi, T.; Ohmori, N.; Ueda, S.; Takihara, T.; Shiraishi, Y.; et al. Induction of mucin and MUC5AC expression by the protease activity of *Aspergillus fumigatus* in airway epithelial cells. *J. Immunol.* **2011**, *187*, 999–1005. [CrossRef] [PubMed]
25. Namvar, S.; Warn, P.; Farnell, E.; Bromley, M.; Fraczek, M.; Bowyer, P.; Herrick, S. *Aspergillus fumigatus* proteases, Asp f 5 and Asp f 13, are essential for airway inflammation and remodelling in a murine inhalation model. *Clin. Exp. Allergy J. Br. Soc. Allergy Clin. Immunol.* **2015**, *45*, 982–993. [CrossRef] [PubMed]
26. Miller, M.R.; Hankinson, J.; Brusasco, V.; Burgos, F.; Casaburi, R.; Coates, A.; Crapo, R.; Enright, P.; van der Grinten, C.P.M.; Gustafsson, P.; et al. ATS/ERS Task Force Standardisation of spirometry. *Eur. Respir. J.* **2005**, *26*, 319–338. [CrossRef] [PubMed]
27. Rosenberg, E. The 1995 update of recommendations for a standard technique for measuring the single-breath carbon monoxide diffusing capacity (transfer factor). *Am. J. Respir. Crit. Care Med.* **1996**, *154*, 827–828. [CrossRef] [PubMed]
28. Bestall, J.C.; Paul, E.A.; Garrod, R.; Garnham, R.; Jones, P.W.; Wedzicha, J.A. Usefulness of the Medical Research Council (MRC) dyspnoea scale as a measure of disability in patients with chronic obstructive pulmonary disease. *Thorax* **1999**, *54*, 581–586. [CrossRef] [PubMed]
29. Jones, P.W.; Harding, G.; Berry, P.; Wiklund, I.; Chen, W.-H.; Kline Leidy, N. Development and first validation of the COPD Assessment Test. *Eur. Respir. J.* **2009**, *34*, 648–654. [CrossRef] [PubMed]

30. Naidich, D.P.; McCauley, D.I.; Khouri, N.F.; Stitik, F.P.; Siegelman, S.S. Computed tomography of bronchiectasis. *J. Comput. Assist. Tomogr.* **1982**, *6*, 437–444. [CrossRef] [PubMed]
31. Chalmers, J.D.; Goeminne, P.; Aliberti, S.; McDonnell, M.J.; Lonni, S.; Davidson, J.; Poppelwell, L.; Salih, W.; Pesci, A.; Dupont, L.J.; et al. The Bronchiectasis Severity Index. An International Derivation and Validation Study. *Am. J. Respir. Crit. Care Med.* **2014**, *189*, 576–585. [CrossRef] [PubMed]
32. Heinzerling, L.; Mari, A.; Bergmann, K.-C.; Bresciani, M.; Burbach, G.; Darsow, U.; Durham, S.; Fokkens, W.; Gjomarkaj, M.; Haahtela, T.; et al. The skin prick test—European standards. *Clin. Transl. Allergy* **2013**, *3*, 3. [CrossRef] [PubMed]
33. Paggiaro, P.L.; Chanez, P.; Holz, O.; Ind, P.W.; Djukanović, R.; Maestrelli, P.; Sterk, P.J. Sputum induction. *Eur. Respir. J. Suppl.* **2002**, *37*, 3s–8s. [PubMed]
34. Mattei, D.; Rapezzi, D.; Mordini, N.; Cuda, F.; lo Nigro, C.; Musso, M.; Arnelli, A.; Cagnassi, S.; Gallamini, A. False-positive *Aspergillus* galactomannan enzyme-linked immunosorbent assay results in vivo during amoxicillin-clavulanic acid treatment. *J. Clin. Microbiol.* **2004**, *42*, 5362–5363. [CrossRef] [PubMed]

Chronic Respiratory Infection in Patients with Chronic Obstructive Pulmonary Disease: What is the Role of Antibiotics?

Marc Miravitlles [1] and Antonio Anzueto [2,3,*]

1 Pneumology Department, Hospital Universitari Vall d'Hebron, Ciber de Enfermedades Respiratorias (CIBERES), 08035 Barcelona, Spain; mmiravitlles@vhebron.net
2 Department of Medicine, Division of Pulmonary Diseases/Critical Care Medicine, The University of Texas Health Science Center at San Antonio, San Antonio, TX 78229, USA
3 Pulmonary Section, The South Texas Veterans Health Care System, Audie L. Murphy Memorial Veterans Hospital Division, Pulmonary Diseases Section (111E), 7400 Merton Minter Boulevard, San Antonio, TX 78229, USA
* Correspondence: anzueto@uthscsa.edu

Academic Editor: Francesco B. Blasi

Abstract: Chronic infections are associated with exacerbation in patients with chronic obstructive pulmonary disease (COPD). The major objective of the management of these patients is the prevention and effective treatment of exacerbations. Patients that have increased sputum production, associated with purulence and worsening shortness of breath, are the ones that will benefit from antibiotic therapy. It is important to give the appropriate antibiotic therapy to prevent treatment failure, relapse, and the emergence of resistant pathogens. In some patients, systemic corticosteroids are also indicated to improve symptoms. In order to identify which patients are more likely to benefit from these therapies, clinical guidelines recommend stratifying patients based on their risk factor associated with poor outcome or recurrence. It has been identified that patients with more severe disease, recurrent infection and presence of purulent sputum are the ones that will be more likely to benefit from this therapy. Another approach related to disease prevention could be the use of prophylactic antibiotics during steady state condition. Some studies have evaluated the continuous or the intermittent use of antibiotics in order to prevent exacerbations. Due to increased bacterial resistance to antibiotics and the presence of side effects, several antibiotics have been developed to be nebulized for both treatment and prevention of acute exacerbations. There is a need to design long-term studies to evaluate these interventions in the natural history of the disease. The purpose of this publication is to review our understanding of the role of bacterial infection in patients with COPD exacerbation, the role of antibiotics, and future interventions.

Keywords: chronic respiratory infections in COPD; exacerbations of chronic obstructive pulmonary disease; antibiotics; bacteria; prevention; colonization

---

1. Introduction

It is important to determine the role of bacteria and other pathogens in chronic obstructive pulmonary disease (COPD) patients with stable disease and during exacerbations. In these COPD patients, the isolation of "potentially pathogenic microorganisms" (PPMs) in respiratory samples ranges between 20% and 60% of cases [1–3]. The most common PPMs seen in COPD patients are *Hemophilus influenza, Moraxella catharralis, Streptococcus pneumonia, Pseudomonas* etc. [1–3]. The bacterial infection is predominantly found in the lower airway of these patient but can also be responsible for upper airway infections such as acute sinusitis. Some studies have suggested that these bacteria contribute to chronic airway inflammation leading to COPD progression [1,2,4]. Therefore, it has been suggested that the term chronic bronchial infection would be more appropriate when addressing the presence of significant concentrations of PPMs in the lower airways of stable COPD patients [2,5]. Patients with chronic bronchial infection may constitute a subgroup of individuals that may be called "infective phenotype" [2]. Our ability to identify bacteria by analysis of conserved 16S rRNA in bacteria has allowed the identification of the lung microbiota (present in the upper airway, sinus, bronchial tree etc.) [6]. We now recognize that the human's airway is covered by a large variety of bacterial species that we were not able to culture using conventional methods [6]. The number of studies examining the microbiome of the lower airways is limited and there is some overlap between bacteria seen in COPD and healthy individuals [7]; however, a recent study has reported a significantly different bacterial community in patients with very severe COPD compared with nonsmokers, smokers and patients with cystic fibrosis [8]. Studies are clearly needed to understand the role of these microbiomes in healthy individuals and COPD patients and how to recognize that an "acute infection" is present; furthermore, we need to understand the impact of antibiotics—given for either acute exacerbations, or chronic long-term administration—on these bacterial communities.

The use of antibiotics in chronically infected patients may be associated with a reduction of bacterial load, and prevention of acquisition of a new bacterial strain; all these effects are associated with a reduction in the frequency and severity of COPD exacerbations. The role of prophylactic antibiotics for the prevention of COPD exacerbations was first studied during the 1950s and 1960s. The problem with these studies was that, at the time, we did not have an adequate definition of COPD; we had a small number of patients; we used narrow-spectrum antibiotics, and not well-defined end-points. After completion of these studies, there was increased concern regarding the development of bacterial resistance; therefore, no new studies were conducted for several years [9]. It was not until the late 1990s, with the availability of new classes of antibiotics and better understanding on the pathophysiology of COPD exacerbation, that new long-term antibiotic studies were conducted.

The most common causes of COPD exacerbations (ECOPD) are infections that are produced by bacteria (40–60%), viruses (about 30%) and atypical bacteria (5–10%) [10,11]. For the last 25 years, the clinical criteria described by Anthonisen et al. [12] have been incorporated in clinical guidelines to help in selecting patients that require empiric antibiotic therapy [13]. More recent studies have identified a change in color, for example, purulence is a good surrogate marker for the presence of bacterial infection [14–16]. Furthermore, only a change in sputum color was identified as a predictor of good response to antibiotics in a placebo-controlled clinical trial in patients with mild to moderate COPD [17]. Therefore, change in sputum color or increased purulence are the only clinical features that help clinicians to decide whether to use an antibiotic in ambulatory ECOPD. The purpose of this publication is to review the role of bacterial infection in patients with COPD both in stable conditions and exacerbation, as well as the role of antibiotics, and what other interventions can impact patients.

2. Molecular Aspects of Antibiotics Activity

There is an increased incidence of antibiotic resistance that is driven largely by inappropriate use of large volumes of antibiotics in animals, food and humans. The increased volume of antibiotics use results in increased selective pressure on bacteria which contributes to the development of resistance. There is a need to develop novel agents that work via different pathways to help overcome bacteria resistance. Recent studies have looked into novel agents of other pathways such as reactive oxygen species (ROS) and oxygen radicals, as an antimicrobial mechanism that may be effective in treating infections [17]. ROS have high antimicrobial activity against Gram-positive and Gram-negative bacteria, viruses and fungi; they also prevent and break down biofilm. ROS include superoxide anion (O^{2-}), peroxide $O_2{}^{-2}$, hydrogen peroxide (H_2O_2), hydroxyl radicals (OH), and hydroxyl ions (OH^-) [18]. ROS act as antimicrobials through a complex mechanism, i.e., hydrogen peroxide appears to directly elicit ROS's antimicrobial action by its activity in thiol groups in enzymes and proteins, DNA and bacterial cell membrane. These compounds possess concentration-dependent activity and toxicity; and their half-life can be short. ROS can be delivered to the site of infection in various ways such as ROS gels allowing sustained continuous release of ROS to target sites [19]. Therefore, ROS can be used to treat local infections such as cavities, prosthetic devices and, by other delivery systems, to the respiratory and urinary epithelium. These functions make ROS highly suitable for chronic inflammatory conditions, where antibiotics are frequently overused and relatively ineffective, such as lung infections in patients with chronic lung diseases such as COPD. The first entirely novel antimicrobial agent to reach early clinical use employing ROS a mechanism has been developed for wound management [20]. ROS agents are also effective at preventing the formation of, and disrupting existing biofilm. These mechanisms can also have important application in respiratory conditions such as in patients undergoing mechanical ventilation [21].

Polysulfides are another substance that has recently been recognized for signaling ROS. Sulfites have been found to have a great role in the origin of life and are an important regulator and modulator of metabolism and signaling in all species including bacteria, and fungus [22]. Stepwise oxidation produces hydrogen persulfide radicals which can be oxidized to intermediate reactive sulfide species that work very similarly to ROS [23]. The "next frontier" of sulfide biology will be the understanding on these molecules and their effect in bacterial cell metabolism [24]. Therefore, the development of these novel antibacterial compounds using ROS could also have an important role in infection prevention and antimicrobial stewardship in chronic lung conditions.

COPD exacerbation is defined as an acute worsening of patients' respiratory symptoms that results in additional therapy; these events can be precipitated by several factors; the most common cause is respiratory infections [25]. Compared to stable COPD, during ECOPD, a much larger percentage of patients have PPMs in addition to significantly higher concentrations of bacteria in the airways [26]. Treatment with appropriate antibiotics significantly decreases the bacterial burden by eradicating bacteria—reducing clinical failure and risk of progression to more severe infections, such as pneumonia [25,27].

While the increased airway inflammation present during ECOPD is reduced following antibiotic treatment, this resolution has been shown to be dependent on bacterial eradication [28]. Patients that have a relapse of their symptoms and/or required re-hospitalization could attribute this to persistent bacterial infection.

Among the major goals of COPD treatment in the current guidelines is the prevention of acute exacerbations [29]. Clinical studies have shown that long-term continuous or intermittent use of antibiotics has a beneficial effect of reducing exacerbation frequency and extending the time to the next exacerbation [30,31]. The mechanism underlying this improvement is unclear. The benefit of long-term antibiotic treatment could be related to changes in bacteria flora and changes in airway inflammation, but there are no clinical studies that support these hypotheses. Macrolides are known to have antibacterial and anti-inflammatory activity; recent data also suggested that they have antiviral activity and possibly disrupt biofilm formation in the airway. In 1987, Anthonisen, et al. [12] reported the results of a large-scale placebo-controlled trial designed to determine the efficacy of antibiotics in ECOPD. In this study, 173 COPD patients (mean FEV1(%) = 33%) were monitored for 3.5 years. Patients were classified based on their symptoms: Type 1 ECOPD patients had increased shortness of breath, increased sputum production, and change in sputum purulence and received any of the following antibiotics (amoxicillin, trimethoprim-sulfamethoxazole, co-trimoxazole, or doxycycline). In these patients, there was a significant improvement in symptoms as compared with placebo; there was no significant difference in the success rates between antibiotics and placebo in patients that had only one of these symptoms (called Type 3). Patients treated with antibiotics had a more rapid improvement in peak flow and a greater percentage of clinical success. In addition, the length of their illness was two days shorter for the antibiotic-treated group. The major limitation of this study was the lack of microbiology data; these investigators assumed that all antibiotics that they used for treating their patients were equivalent. It is important to point out that this study was conducted in the 1980s; since that time, we have seen significant changes in bacterial resistance and also in patients' demographic characteristics. Allegra et al. [32] found a significant benefit using amoxicillin-clavulanate therapy compared with placebo in patients with moderate to severe disease. There was a significant success rate at day 5 in the antibiotics treated group (86% versus 50% in the placebo group, $p < 0.01$) and lower frequency of recurrent exacerbations. Another publication compared the efficacy of amoxicillin-clavulanate versus placebo in patients with mild and moderate COPD (patients with spirometry values FeV1 50–80%) that confirmed the findings of Allegra et al. [32]. These studies demonstrated the superiority of using antibiotics in these patients. Furthermore, the median time to the next exacerbation was also significantly prolonged in patients receiving antibiotics compared to placebo (233 days compared with 160 days, $p < 0.05$). Interestingly, this study demonstrated that sputum purulence was the most reliable marker of clinical failure in the placebo group [25]. A more recent study—a randomized, placebo-controlled trial—investigated the efficacy of doxycycline in addition to systemic corticosteroids in the treatment of hospitalized patients with ECOPD. This study showed that patients treated with doxycycline were not different to those in the placebo group regarding the primary end-point (clinical success at day 30) but showed superior results in some of the secondary end-points (clinical cure on day 10, microbiological success, open-label use of antibiotics and symptoms resolution). Although some of these outcomes are not clinically relevant, the antibiotic treatment was superior in patients with higher plasma levels of C-reactive protein [33]. The poor results observed with doxycycline at day 30 could be explained by the antibiotic bacteriological spectrum and local bacterial resistance patterns.

During an ECOPD, it has been suggested that antibiotics can reduce the burden of bacteria in the airway and, in some patients, can impact the progression of the event to more severe infections, such as pneumonia. A prospective, randomized, double-blind, placebo-controlled trial, evaluated the use of ofloxacin versus placebo in 90 patients with ECOPD who required mechanical ventilation; it showed that the antibiotic-treated group had a significantly lower in-hospital mortality rate (4% vs. 22%, $p = 0.01$) and reduced length of hospital stay (14.9 vs. 24.5 days, $p = 0.01$) compared with the placebo group. In addition, the ofloxacin-treated patients were less likely to develop pneumonia, especially during the first week of mechanical ventilation [27].

Antibiotic Resistance

It has recently been recognized that antibiotic resistance is a major public-health problem worldwide, and international efforts are needed to counteract its emergence. Repeated and improper use of antibiotics is increasingly being recognized as the main cause of this emerging resistance [34]. Therefore, the identification of clinical characteristics that identify patients with ECOPD that can be safely treated without antibiotics is extremely important. In the case of mild to moderate ambulatory patients, the absence of sputum purulence and low values of C-reactive protein are associated with high rates of clinical cure without antibiotics [35]. Another study in hospitalized patients with ECOPD reported similar short- and long-term outcomes in patients with purulent sputum treated with antibiotics compared with patients with non-purulent sputum not treated with antibiotics. These data suggested that clinicians can use the presence or absence of changes in sputum color (purulence) as a way to limit the use of antibiotics; it is suggested that the use of antibiotics could be avoided in this latter group [36].

After the decision to initiate empirical antibiotic therapy, the choice of antibiotic must be considered. The reported relapse rates for patients with ECOPD range from 17% to 32%, and differ according to the antibiotics prescribed [37,38]. An international, multicenter study compared moxifloxacin to amoxicillin/clavulanic acid in patients with moderate to severe COPD (mean FEV1(%) = 39%) and clinical risk factors at 8 weeks post-therapy. There were no significant differences in the primary end-point of the study; however, moxifloxacin resulted in significantly lower clinical failure and higher bacteriological eradication in the sub-population of patients with bacterial pathogens isolated from sputum at inclusion [39]. These results suggest that, in confirmed bacterial ECOPD, the choice of antibiotic, particularly in severe patients, may result in different outcomes and justifies antibiotic selection based on patterns of antimicrobial resistance and the clinical characteristics of the patients.

3. Use of Antibiotics to Prevent Chronic Obstructive Pulmonary Disease Exacerbations

One of the unmet needs in the treatment of COPD is the prevention of COPD exacerbations in patients with recurrent bacterial infections. Long-term use of antibiotics has been suggested as a possible approach in these patients. In the last decade, several studies have been published showing the continuous long-term use of antibiotics in COPD patients [30,40–43] and one employing intermittent/pulsed treatment [23]. Suziki et al. [40] reported the first open-label study on erythromycin in the prevention of ECOPD. The investigators reported that the antibiotic-treated group showed a significant decrease in one or more exacerbations (11%) compared to the control group (56%) and less hospitalizations (p 0.007). Another study by Seemugal et al. [41] also showed that using erythromycin over a 12-month period led to a significant reduction in exacerbations but no differences in lung function changes or inflammatory markers. More recent publications showed significant reductions in inflammatory markers at 6 months with azithromycin [44] and erythromycin [43]. The most recent pivotal study evaluated the efficacy of daily azithromycin (250 mg/day) compared with placebo in a 12-month prospective trial in the prevention of COPD exacerbation [30]. These investigators reported that the use of antibiotics was associated with a 27% decrease in the frequency of exacerbation and significantly prolonged median time to an exacerbation. These investigators also reported that patients with moderate COPD, who were current smokers and had not been treated with long-acting bronchodilators were the most likely to benefit from the antibiotic therapy. More recently, Pomares et al. [42], in a retrospective study, showed significant reduction in exacerbations, hospitalizations and length of stay. The main concern related to the use of prophylactic antibiotics has been the development of bacterial resistance and the impact on the normal microbiota [37]. Another approach recently published by Sethi et al. [31] is on the intermittent use of antibiotics. In this study, the investigators use moxifloxacin given once daily for 5 days; the treatment was repeated every 8 weeks for a total of six courses of therapy. Although the study's primary end-point was not met—a 25% reduction in exacerbations in the per-protocol population—in a post-hoc analysis, patients with moderate-severe COPD and with purulent or muco-purulent sputum at baseline showed a 45% decrease in exacerbations. It is also important to highlight that this study was not associated with increased bacterial resistance, but we do not know whether the investigators prolonged the clinical study to determine an association with the development of resistance [31]. Therefore, there is a need for long-term studies and also with different antibiotics to understand the efficacy of prophylactic therapy and the risk bacteria resistance.

The main issue that we will need to understand before we can recommend the "routine" use of antibiotics to prevent ECOPD is what is the impact on patients' normal microbiota. For example, in the study by Albert et al. [30], patients that received azithromycin showed increased incidence of macrolide-resistant pathogens in nasopharyngeal swabs. Clearly, this intervention was affecting the individual's normal microbiota [45].

4. Dosing Strategies of Antibiotics

There are no standard procedures that determine the dose and duration of antibiotic treatment in patients with ECOPD. The standard duration of antibiotic administration in ECOPD used to be 10 days. A shorter duration of therapy has very important advantages such as reduction of exposure that will result in decreased bacterial resistance and decreased side effects. Fallagas et al. [46] published a meta-analysis that included seven randomized controlled trials that demonstrated, in over 3083 patients, that short duration of antibiotics was as effective and safe as longer-therapy. Another study that included 21 double-blind studies showed that short-term antibiotics demonstrated clinical cure rates at both early and long-term follow-up; bacteriological response was also similar to that achieved with conventional therapy in patients with mild-moderate COPD exacerbations [47].

Therefore, these data demonstrate that short-term antibiotic use is associated with enhanced compliance, decreased resistance and costs. Furthermore, more recent studies demonstrated that a short course of antibiotics for 5 days using quinolones therapy was similar to long-term antibiotic treatment in patients with COPD exacerbation, as indicated by the clinical and bacteriological outcomes [48]. Similar findings were reported using high-dose quinolones with more rapid resolution of symptoms and faster recovery rates compared with traditional therapy with non-quinolones therapy [49].

5. Combination of Antibiotics and Systemic Corticosteroids

In severe COPD patients, the development of exacerbations is common in the use of both antibiotics and systemic corticosteroids. There is no clear data on whether antibiotics have additional benefits when given to patients that have also been treated with systemic corticosteroids. Sachs and colleagues [50] suggested that antibiotics did not provide additional clinical benefit when corticosteroids were given. These findings were irrespective of patients' clinical characteristics such as sputum color or bacterial involvement. It is important to point out that this study had several limitations including a small sample size ($n = 71$), a mild population, and enrolled COPD and asthma patients. In a study by Daniels et al. [33], the lack of an effect with doxycycline in addition to systemic corticosteroids (the primary end-point being clinical success on day 30) may be related to the scarce antibacterial activity of doxycycline against pathogens such as *S. pneumoniae* and *H. influenza*; however, treatment with corticosteroids could help in patients with a more inflammatory response such as those with high C-reactive protein. More recent studies suggest that there are different phenotypes of COPD exacerbations, and systemic corticosteroids may be beneficial in those with predominant eosinophilic inflammation [51]. The different inflammatory profile of COPD exacerbations will need to be taken into consideration in the design of clinical trials examining the efficacy of antibiotics and/or corticosteroids in this disease. Today, we can only assess the host inflammatory response by non-specific markers such as C-reactive protein. It will be very interesting to design future clinical studies that take into consideration the host response in the randomization process to the presence or absence of antibiotics.

6. Measuring Effects and Outcomes

Clinical and microbiological end-points in clinical trials of antibiotic treatment of ECOPD are not well defined. Microbiological results depend on the production of a good quality sputum sample, which results in a positive sputum culture in only 20–50% of the patients. Clinical results are still based on the definition of Chow et al. [52]: "End-points are defined as cure (a complete resolution of signs and symptoms associated with the exacerbation) or improvement (a resolution or reduction of the symptoms and signs without new symptoms and signs associated with the exacerbation)". "Clinical success is considered when either cure or improvement is observed". "Failure is defined as incomplete resolution, persistence or worsening of symptoms that require a new course of antibiotics and/or oral corticosteroids or hospitalization". Evaluation is usually performed at the end-of-therapy visit (days 9–14). This short time frame may not allow the identification of clinical relapses if they occur after initial improvement. Some antibiotics may decrease bacterial load sufficiently to produce an improvement in symptoms that can be perceived as a clinical success at the end of treatment, but when treatment is discontinued, the remaining microorganisms will increase in number and produce recurrent symptoms of exacerbation [53].

In patients with COPD, it is difficult to evaluate their symptoms both during stable conditions and exacerbations. In order to improve the recognition of patients' symptoms, there is growing interest in the use of diary cards and standardized questionnaires to evaluate these conditions. The use of symptom-based diary cards may allow the quantification of the intensity and duration of patient symptoms over time and could be used to assess treatment outcomes [54–56]. There is a recent initiative, funded by regulatory agencies as well as pharmaceutical companies, called the Exacerbations of Chronic Pulmonary Disease Tool (EXACT) [57]. This is a new patient-reported outcome (PRO) diary that was developed to quantify patients' daily symptoms before and after an exacerbation.

The EXACT is a validated instrument that will aid in the quantification of the frequency, severity, and duration of exacerbations. It consists of 14 items that can be incorporated in the form of an e-diary, with scores ranging from 0 to 100 and higher scores indicating a more severe exacerbation. Some standardized quality-of-life questionnaires have been proven to be responsive to changes in health status during or after an exacerbation. The Saint George's Respiratory Questionnaire (SGRQ) has been shown to be useful in monitoring recovery from ECOPD [58]. There is a derivative of the SGRQ that is called COPD Assessment Test (CAT), a short 8-item questionnaire that has been proven to provide a reliable score of patients' symptoms both during stable conditions and exacerbation. The CAT score may also help to quantify the symptoms' severity during exacerbations [59,60]. The generic European quality-of-life scale (EQ-5D) has been proven to be responsive to recovery from ECOPD [61,62] and is a good predictor of treatment failure [62]. The COPD Severity Score (COPDSS) is a severity scale developed by Eisner et al. [63] that is responsive to recovery from exacerbations and provides better predictive value for clinical success than that provided by the usual physiologic and clinical variables [51]. However, these quality-of-life or disease severity questionnaires have not been adequately tested in comparative clinical trials of therapies for ECOPD. In conclusion, the use of antibiotics in patients with COPD exacerbation should be limited to those patients with severe disease that have frequent exacerbations that required prior antibiotics use and or hospitalizations. It is important to point out that these patients should be treated with long-acting bronchodilators and anti-inflammatory therapy.

7. Clinical Guidelines

The current clinical guidelines of antibiotic treatment in ECOPD are based on the Anthonisen disease severity criteria [12] and recommend the use of antibiotics in those patients that have all three key symptoms (increased cough, purulence, and shortness of breath). In addition, antibiotics are also recommended in patients with severe ECOPD or hospitalized patients with only two of the three symptoms (increased purulence of sputum) and/or in patients that require invasive or non-invasive ventilation [13]. The Canadian Respiratory Society guidelines was the first publication to suggest the use of antibiotics based on the patient's risk factors for poor outcome and correlated these findings with the most likely pathogens involved (Table 1) [64,65].

Table 1. Chronic obstructive pulmonary disease exacerbation risk classification based on patients' clinical characteristics and most frequent microorganism.

Severity Classification	FEV1 (% Predicted)	Most Frequent Microorganisms
Mild to moderate COPD without risk factors	>50%	*H. influenzae* *M. catarrhalis* *S. pneumoniae* *C. pneumoniae* *M. pneumoniae*
Mild to moderate COPD with risk factors	>50%	*H. influenzae* *M. catarrhalis* PRSP
Severe COPD	30–50%	*H. influenzae* *M. catarrhalis* PRSP Enteric Gram negatives
Very severe COPD	<30%	*H. influenzae* PRSP Enteric Gram negatives *P. aeruginosa*

Risk factors include: age, use of prior antibiotics within the last 4–6 weeks, prior exacerbations. FEV1: forced expiratory volume in one second. PRSP: penicillin-resistant *S. pneumoniae*. Modified from ref. [64,65].

In general, COPD guidelines do not recommend the use of long-term antibiotics for the prevention of exacerbations. However, evidence of the efficacy of macrolides and, to a lesser extent, quinolones, has been accumulating over recent years. More recent guidelines have included, for the first time, a recommendation related to the long-term use of antibiotics in a specific subgroup of severe COPD patients that have chronic bronchitis, and or bronchiectasis [64,66]. These patients should have an early follow-up to evaluate side effects, such as deafness, and frequent sputum cultures to monitor bacteria resistance patterns. This treatment must be monitored closely for the possible development of side effects and/or changes in the patterns of bacterial resistance.

8. Future Developments of Antibiotics for COPD

Inhaled antibiotics have been developed to deliver lower doses that can obtain higher tissue concentration, maximizing pharmacodynamic parameters and minimizing systemic exposures. Inhaled antibiotics are widely used in the treatment of a number of respiratory tract infections, including cystic fibrosis (CF) [67] and bronchiectasis [68,69].

To date, there has been only one report investigating the use of inhaled antibiotics in patients with COPD. The study, conducted by Dal Negro et al. [70], reported the effect of nebulized tobramycin solution given for 14 days, twice daily, in patients with severe COPD. These investigators evaluated the clinical outcomes and inflammatory markers in patients that were colonized with multidrug-resistant *Pseudomonas aeruginosa*. This study demonstrated that two-week treatment with nebulized tobramycin resulted in a 42% decrease in the incidence of exacerbations compared with the prior 6 months and substantial reduction in pro-inflammatory markers. Ongoing and future trials using inhaled powder formulation of antibiotics (quinolones) will provide information on whether inhaled antibiotics are a useful therapeutic option in the prevention of ECOPD. Multiple clinical trials have been conducted (*clinicaltrials.gov*) on the use of inhaled antibiotics in patients with other chronic lung infections such as cystic fibrosis, and bronchiectasis; or as a prevention of infection in patients receiving mechanical ventilation; however, there are no studies that evaluate the use of inhaled antibiotics in COPD patients with exacerbations.

9. Conclusions

Chronic infections are associated with exacerbation in patients with COPD. Prevention and effective treatment of exacerbations are major objectives in the management of these patients. COPD exacerbations are associated with accelerated decline in lung function, worsening quality of life, increased morbidity, and mortality. Antibiotics are recommended for patients with severe COPD with an acute exacerbation that includes the presence of key clinical signs (increased sputum purulence and worsening shortness of breath). The use of antibiotics in COPD patients with an exacerbation and the presence of these symptoms is associated with clinical benefit, but treatment failure and relapse rates can also be high—mainly in cases of inadequate antibiotic therapy. Therefore, it is important to identify the patients at greatest risk of poor outcomes, since they are the patients who will likely derive the greatest benefits from early treatment with the most potent antibiotic therapy.

The long-term use of antibiotics remains controversial. While several studies showed beneficial effects—reducing frequency of exacerbations/hospitalizations and extending time to the next exacerbations—there are also concerns related to side effects and the development of bacterial resistance. Patients with frequent exacerbations and severe underlying disease will benefit from systemic antibiotic treatment during the exacerbation. In the future, more studies will also show that inhaled and/or nebulized routes will be effective.

References

1. Sethi, S.; Murphy, T.F. Infection in the pathogenesis and course of chronic obstructive pulmonary disease. *N. Engl. J. Med.* **2008**, *359*, 2355–2365. [CrossRef] [PubMed]
2. Matkovic, Z.; Miravitlles, M. Chronic bronchial infection in COPD. Is there an infective phenotype? *Respir. Med.* **2013**, *107*, 10–22. [CrossRef] [PubMed]
3. Miravitlles, M.; Marin, A.; Monsó, E.; Vilà, S.; de la Roza, C.; Hervás, R.; Esquinas, C.; García, M.; Millares, L.; Morera, J.; et al. Color of sputum is a marker of bacterial colonization in COPD. *Respir. Res.* **2010**, *11*, 58. [CrossRef] [PubMed]
4. Wilkinson, T.M.A.; Patel, I.S.; Wilks, M.; Donaldson, G.C.; Wedzicha, J.A. Airway bacterial load and FEV1 decline in patients with chronic obstructive pulmonary disease. *Am. J. Respir. Crit. Care Med.* **2003**, *167*, 1090–1095. [CrossRef] [PubMed]
5. Sethi, S. Infection as a comorbidity of COPD. *Eur. Respir. J.* **2010**, *35*, 1209–1215. [CrossRef] [PubMed]
6. Beasley, V.; Joshi, P.V.; Singanayagam, A.; Molyneaux, P.L.; Johnston, S.L.; Mallia, P. Lung microbiology and exacerbations in COPD. *Int. J. Chronic Obstr. Respir. Dis.* **2012**, *7*, 555–569.
7. Sze, M.A.; Dimitriu, P.A.; Hayashi, S.; Elliott, M.; McDonough, J.C.; Gosselink, J.V.; Cooper, J.; Sin, D.D.; Mohn, W.W.; Hogg, J.C. The lung tissue microbiome in chronic obstructive pulmonary disease. *Am. J. Respir. Crit. Care Med.* **2012**, *185*, 1073–1080. [CrossRef] [PubMed]
8. Erb-Downward, J.R.; Thompson, D.L.; Han, M.K.; Freeman, C.M.; McCloskey, L.; Schmidt, L.A.; Young, V.B.; Toews, G.B.; Curtis, J.L.; Sundaram, B.; et al. Analysis of the lung microbiome in the "healthy" smoker and in COPD. *PLoS ONE* **2011**, *6*, e16384. [CrossRef] [PubMed]
9. Staykova, T.; Black, P.; Chacko, E.; Ram, F.S.F.; Poole, P. Prophylactic antibiotic therapy for chronic bronchitis (Cochrane Review). *Cochrane Database Syst. Rev.* **2003**, CD009764. [CrossRef]
10. Sethi, S. Infectious etiology of acute exacerbations of chronic bronchitis. *Chest* **2000**, *117*, 380S–385S. [CrossRef] [PubMed]
11. Papi, A.; Bellettato, C.M.; Braccioni, F.; Romagnoli, M.; Casolari, P.; Caramori, G.; Fabbri, L.M.; Johnston, S.L. Infections and airway inflammation in chronic obstructive pulmonary disease severe exacerbations. *Am. J. Respir. Crit. Care Med.* **2006**, *173*, 1114–1121. [CrossRef] [PubMed]
12. Anthonisen, N.R.; Manfreda, J.; Warren, C.P.; Hershfield, E.S.; Harding, G.K.M.; Nelson, N.A. Antibiotic therapy in acute exacerbation of chronic obstructive pulmonary disease. *Ann. Intern. Med.* **1987**, *106*, 196–204. [CrossRef] [PubMed]
13. Woodhead, M.; Blasi, F.; Ewig, S.; Garau, J.; Huchon, G.; Ieven, M.; Ortqvist, A.; Schaberg, T.; Torres, A.; van der Heijden, G.; et al. Guidelines for the management of adult lower respiratory tract infections. *Clin. Microbiol. Infect.* **2011**, *17*, E1–E59. [CrossRef] [PubMed]
14. Stockley, R.A.; O'Brien, C.; Pye, A.; Hill, S.L. Relationship of sputum color to nature and outpatient management of acute exacerbations of COPD. *Chest* **2000**, *117*, 1638–1645. [CrossRef] [PubMed]
15. Miravitlles, M.; Kruesmann, F.; Haverstock, D.; Perroncel, R.; Choudhri, S.; Arvis, P. Sputum colour and bacteria in chronic bronchitis exacerbations: A pooled analysis. *Eur. Respir. J.* **2012**, *39*, 1354–1360. [CrossRef] [PubMed]
16. Soler, N.; Agustí, C.; Angrill, J.; Puig de la Bellacasa, J.; Torres, A. Bronchoscopic validation of the significance of sputum purulence in severe exacerbations of chronic obstructive pulmonary disease. *Thorax* **2007**, *62*, 29–35. [CrossRef] [PubMed]
17. Dreyden, M. Reactive oxygen therapy: A novel therapy in soft tissue infection. *Curr. Opin. Infect. Dis.* **2017**, *30*, 143–149. [CrossRef] [PubMed]
18. Dunnil, C.; Patton, T.; Brennan, J.; Barrett, J.; Dryden, M.; Cooke, J.; Leaper, D.; Georgopoulos, N.T. Reactive oxygen species (ROS) and wound healing: The functional role of ROS and emerging ROS-modulating technologies for augmentation of the healing process. *Int. Wound J.* **2015**, *14*, 89–96. [CrossRef] [PubMed]
19. Cooke, J.; Dreyden, M.; Patton, T.; Brennan, J.; Barrett, J. The antimicrobial activity of prototype modified honeys that generate reactive oxygen species (ROS) hydrogen peroxide. *BMC Res. Notes* **2015**, *8*, 20. [CrossRef] [PubMed]
20. Dreyden, M.; Dickinson, A.; Brooks, J.; Hudgell, L.; Saeed, K.; Cutting, K.F. A multicenter clinical evaluation of reactive oxygen topical wound gel in 114 wounds. *J. Wound Care* **2016**, *25*, 140–146. [CrossRef] [PubMed]

21. Halstead, F.B.; Webber, M.A.; Rauf, M.; Burt, R.; Dryden, M.; Oppenheim, B.A. In Vitro activity of an engineered honey, medical-grade honeys, and antimicrobial wound dressings against biofilm-producing clinical bacterial isolates. *J. Wound Care* **2016**, *25*, 93–102. [CrossRef] [PubMed]
22. Barton, L.L.; Fauque, G.D. Biochemistry, physiology and biotechnology of sulfate-producing bacteria. *Adv. Appl. Microbiol.* **2009**, *68*, 41–98. [PubMed]
23. Winterbourn, C.C. The biological chemistry of hydrogen peroxide. *Methods Enzymol.* **2013**, *528*, 3–25. [PubMed]
24. Olson, K.R.; Straub, K.D. The Role of Hydrogen Sulfide in Evolution and the Evolution of Hydrogen Sulfide in Metabolism and Signaling. *Physiology* **2016**, *31*, 60–72. [CrossRef] [PubMed]
25. Llor, C.; Moragas, A.; Hernández, S.; Bayona, C.; Miravitlles, M. Efficacy of antibiotic therapy for acute exacerbations of mild to moderate COPD. *Am. J. Respir. Crit. Care Med.* **2012**, *186*, 716–723. [CrossRef] [PubMed]
26. Monso, E.; Ruiz, J.; Rosell, A.; Manterola, J.; Fiz, J.; Morera, J.; Ausina, V. Bacterial infection in chronic obstructive pulmonary disease. A study of stable and exacerbated outpatients using the protected specimen brush. *Am. J. Respir. Crit. Care Med.* **1995**, *152*, 1316–1320. [CrossRef] [PubMed]
27. Nouira, S.; Marghli, S.; Belghith, M.; Besbes, L.; Elatrous, S.; Abroug, F. Once daily oral ofloxacin in chronic obstructive pulmonary disease exacerbation requiring mechanical ventilation: A randomized placebo-controlled trial. *Lancet* **2001**, *358*, 2020–2025. [CrossRef]
28. White, A.J.; Gompertz, S.; Bayley, D.L.; Hill, S.L.; O'Brien, C.; Unsal, I.; Stockley, R.A. Resolution of bronchial inflammation is related to bacterial eradication following treatment of exacerbations of chronic bronchitis. *Thorax* **2003**, *58*, 680–685. [CrossRef] [PubMed]
29. Vogelmeier, C.F.; Criner, G.J.; Martínez, F.J.; Anzueto, A.; Barnes, P.J.; Bourbeau, J.; Celli, B.R.; Chen, R.; Decramer, M.; Fabbri, L.M.; et al. Global Strategy for the Diagnosis, Management, and Prevention of Chronic Obstructive Lung Disease 2017 Report: GOLD Executive Summary. *Arch. Bronconeumol.* **2017**, *53*, 128–149. [CrossRef] [PubMed]
30. Albert, R.K.; Connett, J.; Bailey, W.C.; Casaburi, R.; Cooper, A.D., Jr.; Criner, G.J.; Curtis, J.F.; Dransfield, M.T.; Han, M.K.; Lazarus, S.C.; et al. Azithromycin for prevention of exacerbations of COPD. *N. Engl. J. Med.* **2011**, *365*, 689–698. [CrossRef] [PubMed]
31. Sethi, S.; Jones, P.W.; Theron, M.S.; Miravitlles, M.; Rubinstein, E.; Wedzicha, J.A.; Wilson, R.; PULSE Study Group. Pulsed moxifloxacin for the prevention of exacerbations of chronic obstructive pulmonary disease: A randomized controlled trial. *Respir. Res.* **2010**, *11*, 10. [CrossRef] [PubMed]
32. Allegra, L.; Blasi, F.; de Bernardi, B.; Cosentini, R.; Tarsia, P. Antibiotic treatment and baseline severity of disease in acute exacerbations of chronic bronchitis: A re-evaluation of previously published data of a placebo-controlled randomized study. *Pulm. Pharmacol. Ther.* **2001**, *14*, 149–155. [CrossRef] [PubMed]
33. Daniels, J.M.A.; Snijders, D.; de Graaff, C.S.; van der Werf, T.S.; Boersma, W.G. Antibiotics in addition to systemic corticosteroids for acute exacerbations of chronic obstructive pulmonary disease. *Am. J. Respir. Crit. Care Med.* **2010**, *181*, 150–157. [CrossRef] [PubMed]
34. Goosens, H.; Ferech, M.; Stichele, R.V.; Elseviers, M.; ESAC Project Group. Outpatient antibiotic use in Europe and association with resistance: A cross-national database study. *Lancet* **2005**, *365*, 579–587. [CrossRef]
35. Miravitlles, M.; Moragas, A.; Hernández, S.; Bayona, C.; Llor, C. Is it possible to identify exacerbations of mild to moderate COPD that do not require antibiotic treatment? *Chest* **2013**, *144*, 1571–1577. [CrossRef] [PubMed]
36. Soler, N.; Esperatti, M.; Ewig, S.; Huerta, A.; Agustí, C.; Torres, A. Sputum purulence-guided antibiotic use in hospitalized patients with exacerbations of COPD. *Eur. Respir. J.* **2012**, *40*, 1344–1353. [CrossRef] [PubMed]
37. Adams, S.; Melo, J.; Luther, M.; Anzueto, A. Antibiotics are associated with lower relapse rates in outpatients with acute exacerbations of chronic obstructive pulmonary disease. *Chest* **2000**, *117*, 1345–1352. [CrossRef] [PubMed]
38. Miravitlles, M.; Murio, C.; Guerrero, T.; DAFNE Study Group. Factors associated with relapse after ambulatory treatment of acute exacerbations of chronic bronchitis. A prospective multicenter study in the community. *Eur. Respir. J.* **2001**, *17*, 928–933. [CrossRef] [PubMed]
39. Wilson, R.; Anzueto, A.; Miravitlles, M.; Arvis, P.; Alder, J.; Haverstock, D.; Trajanovic, M.; Sethi, S. Moxifloxacinvs amoxicillin/clavulanic acid in acute exacerbations of COPD: MAESTRAL study results. *Eur. Respir. J.* **2012**, *40*, 17–27. [CrossRef] [PubMed]

40. Suzuki, T.; Yanai, M.; Yamaya, M.; Satoh-Nakagawa, T.; Sekizawa, K.; Ishida, S.; Sasaki, H. Erythromycin and common cold in COPD. *Chest* **2001**, *120*, 730–733. [CrossRef] [PubMed]
41. Seemungal, T.A.; Wilkinson, T.M.; Hurst, J.R.; Perera, W.R.; Sapsford, R.J.; Wedzicha, J.A. Long-term erythromycin therapy is associated with decreased chronic obstructive pulmonary disease exacerbations. *Am. J. Respir. Crit. Care Med.* **2008**, *178*, 1139–1147. [CrossRef] [PubMed]
42. Pomares, X.; Montón, C.; Espasa, M.; Casabon, J.; Monsó, E.; Gallego, M. Long-term azithromycin therapy in patients with severe COPD and repeated exacerbations. *Int. J. Chronic Obstr. Pulm. Dis.* **2011**, *6*, 449–456. [CrossRef] [PubMed]
43. He, Z.-Y.; Ou, L.-M.; Zhang, J.-Q.; Bai, J.; Liu, G.-N.; Li, M.-H.; Deng, J.-M.; MacNee, W.; Zhong, X.-N. Effect of 6 months of erythromycin treatment on inflammatory cells in induced sputum and exacerbations in chronic obstructive pulmonary disease. *Respiration* **2010**, *80*, 445–452. [CrossRef] [PubMed]
44. Blasi, F.; Bonardi, D.; Aliberti, S.; Tarsia, P.; Confalonieri, M.; Amir, O.; Carone, M.; di Marco, F.; Centanni, S.; Guffanti, E. Long-term azithromycin use in patients with chronic obstructive pulmonary disease and tracheostomy. *Pulm. Phamacol. Ther.* **2010**, *23*, 200–207. [CrossRef] [PubMed]
45. Serisier, D.J. Risks of population antimicrobial resistance associated with chronic macrolide use for inflammatory airway diseases. *Lancet Respir. Med.* **2013**, *1*, 262–274. [CrossRef]
46. Falagas, M.E.; Avgeri, S.G.; Matthaiou, D.K.; Dimopoulos, G.; Siempos, I.I. Short- versus long-duration antimicrobial treatment for exacerbations of chronic bronchitis: A meta-analysis. *J. Antimicrob. Chemother.* **2008**, *62*, 442–450. [CrossRef] [PubMed]
47. El Moussaoui, R.; Roede, B.M.; Speelman, P.; Bresser, P.; Prins, J.M.; Bossuyt, P.M.M. Short-course antibiotic treatment in acute exacerbations of chronic bronchitis and COPD: A meta-analysis of double-blind studies. *Thorax* **2008**, *63*, 415–422. [CrossRef] [PubMed]
48. Wilson, R.; Allegra, L.; Huchon, G.; Izquierdo, J.-L.; Jones, P.; Schaberg, T.; Sagnier, P.-P. Short-term and long-term outcomes of moxifloxacin compared to standard antibiotic treatment in acute exacerbations of chronic bronchitis. *Chest* **2004**, *125*, 953–964. [CrossRef] [PubMed]
49. Anzueto, A.; Miravitlles, M. Short-course fluoroquinolone therapy in exacerbations of chronic bronchitis and COPD. *Respir. Med.* **2010**, *104*, 1396–1403. [CrossRef] [PubMed]
50. Sachs, A.F.; Koeter, G.H.; Groenier, K.H.; van der Waaij, D.; Schiphuis, J.; Meyboom-de Jong, B. Changes in symptoms, peak expiratory flow, and sputum flora during treatment with antibiotics of exacerbations in patients with chronic obstructive pulmonary disease in general practice. *Thorax* **1995**, *50*, 758–763. [CrossRef] [PubMed]
51. Bafadhel, M.; McKenna, S.; Terry, S.; Mistry, V.; Pancholi, M.; Venge, P.; Lomas, D.A.; Barer, M.R.; Johnston, S.L.; Pavord, I.; et al. Blood eosinophils to direct corticosteroid treatment of exacerbations of chronic obstructive pulmonary disease a randomized placebo-controlled trial. *Am. J. Respir. Crit. Care Med.* **2012**, *186*, 48–55. [CrossRef] [PubMed]
52. Chow, A.W.; Hall, C.B.; Klein, J.O.; Kammer, R.B.; Meyer, R.D.; Remington, J.S. Evaluation of new anti-infective drugs for the treatment of respiratory tract infections. Infectious Diseases Society of America and the Food and Drug Administration. *Clin. Infect. Dis.* **1992**, *15*, S62–S88. [CrossRef] [PubMed]
53. Miravitlles, M. Exacerbations of chronic obstructive pulmonary disease: When are bacteria important? *Eur. Respir. J.* **2002**, *20*, 9s–19s. [CrossRef]
54. Moragas, A.; Llor, C.; Gabarrús, A.; Miravitlles, M. Reliability of a self-administered diary of symptoms for assessing the evolution of acute bronchitis. *Arch. Bronconeumol.* **2012**, *48*, 261–264. [CrossRef] [PubMed]
55. Vijayasaratha, K.; Stockley, R.A. Reported and unreported exacerbations of COPD: Analysis by diary cards. *Chest* **2008**, *133*, 34–41. [CrossRef] [PubMed]
56. Llor, C.; Moragas, A.; Miravitlles, M.; ESAB Study. Usefulness of a patient symptom diary card in the monitoring of exacerbations of chronic bronchitis and chronic obstructive pulmonary disease. *Int. J. Clin. Pract.* **2012**, *66*, 711–717. [CrossRef] [PubMed]
57. Leidy, N.K.; Wilcox, T.K.; Jones, P.W.; Roberts, L.; Powers, J.H.; Sethi, S.; EXACT-PRO Study Group. Standardizing measurement of chronic obstructive pulmonary disease exacerbations. Reliability and validity of a patient-reported diary. *Am. J. Respir. Crit. Care Med.* **2011**, *183*, 323–329. [CrossRef] [PubMed]
58. Spencer, S.; Jones, P.W.; GLOBE Study Group. Time course of recovery of health status following an infective exacerbation of chronic bronchitis. *Thorax* **2003**, *58*, 589–593. [CrossRef] [PubMed]

59. Mackay, A.J.; Donaldson, G.C.; Patel, A.R.C.; Jones, P.W.; Hurst, J.R.; Wedzicha, J.A. Usefulness of the chronic obstructive pulmonary disease assessment test to evaluate severity of COPD exacerbations. *Am. J. Respir. Crit. Care Med.* **2012**, *185*, 1218–1224. [CrossRef] [PubMed]
60. García-Sidro, P.; Naval, E.; Martínez Rivera, C.; Bonnin-Vilaplana, M.; García-Rivero, J.L.; Herrejón, A.; Malo de Molina, R.; Marcos, P.J.; Mayoralas-Alises, S.; Ros, J.A.; et al. The CAT (COPD Assessment Test) questionnaire as a predictor of the evolution of severe COPD exacerbations. *Respir Med* **2015**, *109*, 1546–1552. [CrossRef] [PubMed]
61. Goosens, L.M.A.; Nivens, M.C.; Sachs, P.; Monz, B.U.; Rutten-van Mölken, M.P.M.H. Is the EQ-5D responsive to recovery from a moderate COPD exacerbation? *Respir. Med.* **2011**, *105*, 1195–1202. [CrossRef] [PubMed]
62. Miravitlles, M.; Izquierdo, I.; Herrejon, A.; Torres, J.V.; Baró, E.; Borja, J. COPD severity score as a predictor of failure in exacerbations of COPD. The ESFERA study. *Respir. Med.* **2011**, *105*, 740–747. [CrossRef] [PubMed]
63. Eisner, M.D.; Trupin, L.; Katz, P.P.; Yelin, E.H.; Earnest, G.; Balmes, J.; Blanc, P.D. Development and validation of a survey-based COPD Severity Score. *Chest* **2005**, *127*, 1890–1897. [CrossRef] [PubMed]
64. Miravitlles, M.; Soler-Cataluña, J.J.; Calle, M.; Molina, J.; Almagro, P.; Quintano, J.A.; Trigueros, J.A.; Cosío, B.G.; Casanova, C.; Riesco, J.A.; et al. Spanish COPD guidelines (GesEPOC) 2017. Pharmacological treatment of stable chronic obstructive pulmonary disease. *Arch. Bronconeumol.* **2017**, *53*, 324–335. [CrossRef] [PubMed]
65. Balter, M.S.; Hyland, R.H.; Low, D.E.; Mandell, L.; Grossman, R.F.; Chronic Bronchitis Working. Recommendations on the management of chronic bronchitis: A practical guide for Canadian physicians. *Can. Respir. J.* **2003**, *10*, 3B–32B. [CrossRef] [PubMed]
66. Martínez-García, M.A.; Miravitlles, M. Bronchiectasis in COPD patients. More than a comorbidity? *Int. J. Chron Obs. Pulm. Dis.* **2017**, *12*, 1401–1411. [CrossRef] [PubMed]
67. Ramsey, B.; Pepe, M.S.; Quan, J.M.; Otto, K.L.; Montgomery, A.B.; Williams-Warren, J.; Vasiljev-K, M.; Borowitz, D.; Bowman, C.M.; Marshall, B.C.; et al. Intermittent administration of inhaled tobramycin in patients with cystic fibrosis. Cystic Fibrosis Inhaled Tobramycin Study Group. *N. Engl. J. Med.* **1999**, *340*, 23–30. [CrossRef] [PubMed]
68. Drobnic, M.E.; Suñé, P.; Montoro, J.B.; Ferrer, A.; Orriols, R. Inhaled tobramycin in non-cystic fibrosis patients with bronchiectasis and chronic bronchial infection with *Pseudomonas aeruginosa*. *Ann. Pharmacother.* **2005**, *39*, 39–44. [CrossRef] [PubMed]
69. Wilson, R.; Welte, T.; Polverino, E.; de Soyza, A.; Greville, H.; O'Donnell, A.; Alder, J.; Reimnitz, P.; Hampel, B. Ciprofloxacin DPI in non-cystic fibrosis bronchiectasis: A phase II randomized study. *Eur. Respir. J.* **2013**, *41*, 1107–1115. [CrossRef] [PubMed]
70. Dal Negro, R.; Micheletto, C.; Tognella, S.; Visconti, M.; Turati, C. Tobramycin nebulizer solution in severe COPD patients colonized with *Pseudomonas aeruginosa*: Effects on bronchial inflammation. *Adv. Ther.* **2008**, *25*, 1019–1103. [CrossRef] [PubMed]

12

Environmental *Burkholderia cenocepacia* Strain Enhances Fitness by Serial Passages during Long-Term Chronic Airways Infection in Mice

Alessandra Bragonzi [1], Moira Paroni [1,2], Luisa Pirone [3], Ivan Coladarci [4], Fiorentina Ascenzioni [4] and Annamaria Bevivino [3,*]

1. Infections and Cystic Fibrosis Unit, IRCCS San Raffaele Scientific Institute, 20132 Milan, Italy; bragonzi.alessandra@hsr.it (A.B.); moira.paroni@unimi.it (M.P.)
2. Department of Biosciences, University of Milan, 20133 Milan, Italy
3. Territorial and Production Systems Sustainability Department, ENEA, Italian National Agency for New Technologies, Energy and Sustainable Economic Development, Casaccia Research Center, 00123 Rome, Italy; luisapirone77@gmail.com
4. Biology and Biotechnology Department "Charles Darwin", Sapienza University of Rome, 00185 Rome, Italy; ivan.coladarci@gmail.com (I.C.); fiorentina.ascenzioni@uniroma1.it (F.A.)

* Correspondence: annamaria.bevivino@enea.it

Abstract: *Burkholderia cenocepacia* is an important opportunistic pathogen in cystic fibrosis (CF) patients, and has also been isolated from natural environments. In previous work, we explored the virulence and pathogenic potential of environmental *B. cenocepacia* strains and demonstrated that they do not differ from clinical strains in some pathogenic traits. Here, we investigated the ability of the environmental *B. cenocepacia* Mex1 strain, isolated from the maize rhizosphere, to persist and increase its virulence after serial passages in a mouse model of chronic infection. *B. cenocepacia* Mex1 strain, belonging to the *recA lineage* IIIA, was embedded in agar beads and challenged into the lung of C57Bl/6 mice. The mice were sacrificed after 28 days from infection and their lungs were tested for bacterial loads. Agar beads containing the pool of *B. cenocepacia* colonies from the four sequential passages were used to infect the mice. The environmental *B. cenocepacia* strain showed a low incidence of chronic infection after the first passage; after the second, third and fourth passages in mice, its ability to establish chronic infection increased significantly and progressively up to 100%. Colonial morphology analysis and genetic profiling of the Mex1-derived clones recovered after the fourth passage from infected mice revealed that they were indistinguishable from the challenged strain both at phenotypic and genetic level. By testing the virulence of single clones in the *Galleria mellonella* infection model, we found that two Mex1-derived clones significantly increased their pathogenicity compared to the parental Mex1 strain and behaved similarly to the clinical and epidemic *B. cenocepacia* LMG16656^{T}. Our findings suggest that serial passages of the environmental *B. cenocepacia* Mex1 strain in mice resulted in an increased ability to determine chronic lung infection and the appearance of clonal variants with increased virulence in non-vertebrate hosts.

Keywords: *Burkholderia cenocepacia*; mice; environmental; chronic infection; adaptation; lung tissues; *Galleria mellonella*

---

1. Introduction

Cystic fibrosis (CF) is the most common lethal autosomal recessive disease in Caucasians, with an incidence of approximately 1 in 2500 live births and a prevalence of approximately 100,000 CF patients worldwide [1]. The disease is caused by mutations in the cystic fibrosis transmembrane conductance regulator (*CFTR*) gene, that encodes a chloride channel localized in both secretory and absorbing epithelia. CFTR dysfunction results in abnormal transport of sodium and chloride ions across epithelia affecting the composition of secretions in the lung, gastrointestinal tract, pancreas, liver and other secretory glands. In the airways, CFTR mutations result in a dehydrated viscous mucus that compromises mucociliary clearance and predisposes CF patients to chronic bacterial infections and airway inflammation [2,3]. Life expectancy in CF has improved dramatically in the last few decades, with the median predicted survival age of people born between 2012 and 2016 now 43 years [4]; however, pulmonary infections remain the major cause of morbidity and mortality in people with CF [5].

The CF respiratory tract is a highly diverse and complex ecosystem with a high heterogeneity due to the various environmental conditions [6]. As suggested by Conrad and colleagues [7], resources are limited in the CF lung, and ecologically diverse populations can evolve. Typically, after a period of intermittent colonization of the lung, bacterial infections in CF rapidly become chronic with bacteria persisting until the end of the disease. It is thought that bacterial strain(s) adapt to the CF niche by changing their phenotype(s) and genotype(s) [8,9]; in particular, the persisting pathogens can adapt to disease−specific environmental factors such as anaerobic mucus layers [2], the pressure of the innate immune defence system of the immunocompetent host [3], and aggressive antibiotic therapies administered during the chronic phase of the infection [10]. In accordance with this hypothesis, when newly acquired bacterial strains from the environment are re-isolated after a period of infection in CF lungs, their virulence and pathogenicity differ, as demonstrated for *Pseudomonas aeruginosa* [11]. The adaptation process aims to increase the fitness/survival of bacteria in CF lungs and is generated by the activation of a specific genetic program that can guarantee bacterial genetic variability in stressful conditions [12]. This process ultimately results in therapy resistance, a trait that contributes to the progression of the lung disease, the major cause of morbidity and mortality in CF. To date, bacterial adaptation in CF has been widely described for *P. aeruginosa*; this bacterium appears to undergo a characteristic adaptation process resulting in the production of genetically and phenotypically diverse strains [13]. In this context, there is alarming evidence of an increase in transmissible epidemic strains in major European centers with transmission observed between unrelated CF patients [14,15]. Transmission between patients has been widely documented for *B. cenocepacia* [16], however, our knowledge on the generation of transmissible strains is still lacking. Among the *Burkholderia cepacia* complex (Bcc) species, *B. cenocepacia* is especially problematic in CF patients [16–18]. Colonization of the lungs of CF patients by these bacteria is associated with a decrease in long-term survival and, occasionally in a minority of patients, the development of the so-called "cepacia syndrome", that leads to a frequently fatal acute clinical decline [17]. Several studies have revealed that *B. cenocepacia* is widespread in natural habitats such as the rhizosphere of several crop plants, where it represents one of the predominant Bcc species [19–21]. Additionally, it has been reported that *B. cenocepacia* from natural environments are indistinguishable from clinical isolates [22,23] suggesting that humans may acquire Bcc directly from natural environments [21,24]. In support of this hypothesis, candidate determinants related to virulence and transmissibility are not confined solely to clinical *B. cenocepacia* isolates but are also spread among environmental *B. cenocepacia* isolates [25–27]. However, understanding of the adaptation process of environmental *B. cenocepacia* strains to the CF airways is still poor [28]; and whether and how *B. cenocepacia* environmental strains adapt to the airways of CF airways remains to be clarified. No data are available on the ability of environmental *B. cenocepacia* strains to adapt to the CF host. Several years ago, Chung and colleagues [29] showed that *B. cenocepacia* strains convert from a nonpersistent to a persistent phenotype in a mouse model of pulmonary infection. In previous work, we explored the virulence and pathogenic potential of environmental *B. cenocepacia* strains and demonstrated that they do not differ from clinical strains in some pathogenic traits showing a similar capacity to maintain a chronic respiratory infection due to the production of similar virulent factors [26]. Furthermore, although environmental strains appear to be less invasive than the clinical ones in polarized CF epithelial cells, they similarly affect epithelia integrity by modulating the presence and distribution of the tight junction protein ZO-1 [27].

In this work, we investigated the host's role on *B. cenocepacia* adaptation and pathogenicity. We focused our attention on the environmental strain Mex1, belonging to *B. cenocepacia* IIIA. It was collected from the rhizosphere of maize cultivated in a field in Mexico and had previously been characterized for its pathogenicity in vitro and in vivo [26,27]. Notably, in a mouse model of chronic infection, the Mex1 strain caused an extensive inflammatory cell infiltrate in the lung tissues, and has shown a similar capacity to maintain a chronic respiratory infection as the clinical strain LMG16656^T, probably due to production of similar virulent factors in strains of different origin [26]. In view of the fact that *B. cenocepacia* IIIA, among the Bcc species as well as the other *recA* lineages of *B. cenocepacia* species, is particularly problematic for CF patients, we set up a mouse model of chronic infection to investigate the microbe-host interaction of the environmental strain IIIA. Thus, we carried out serial passages of the environmental *B. cenocepacia* Mex1 in mice, with each round of infection lasting 28 days. Next, we evaluated the ability of the rescued bacteria to adapt to the murine lung tissues and to establish new chronic lung infections. Phenotypic analysis, genetic profiling and virulence of the Mex1-derived clones were also investigated.

2. Results

2.1. Characteristics of *B. cenocepacia* Mex1 Strain

The environmental strain Mex1, belonging to *B. cenocepacia* IIIA, was collected from the rhizosphere of maize cultivated in a field in Mexico [26]. Its main characteristics are reported in Table 1. The environmental strain has already shown pathogenic potential in both in vitro and in vivo models [26], a dramatic effect on tight junction integrity and on the presence and distribution of the tight junction protein ZO-1 in CF epithelial monolayers [27]. *B. cenocepacia* Mex 1 strain is also able to form biofilms in nutrient-rich media and can adhere to an abiotic surface as the clinical LMG16656^T strain [30,31].

Table 1. Characteristics of *B. cenocepacia* Mex1 strain.

Isolate Name	Origin	Sequence Type (ST)	Cci-Encoded Genes	CF and Non-CF Epithelial Cells	Transepithelial Resistance (TER)	References
Mex1	maize rhizosphere (Mexico)	423	positive	low-level invasion	strong disruption of tight junction integrity	[26,27]

2.2. Serial Passages of the Environmental *B. cenocepacia* Mex1 in Mice

We established sequential chronic infection in C57Bl/6 mice with *B. cenocepacia* Mex1 strain embedded in agar beads. The schedule of experiments is reported in Figure 1. As previously reported, the agar beads mimic the microaerobic/anaerobic environment that allows bacteria to grow in the form of microcolonies and in the mucus of CF patients [2,32]. Sequential infections were established in two groups of C57Bl/6NCrlBR mice challenged with 1.5×10^7 colony-forming units (CFU)/lung and the infection was followed for almost one month (P1) (Figure 1).

At 28 days from the first challenge (P1), the incidence of chronic *B. cenocepacia* colonization was 30% in the first group of mice and 41.67% in the second group, with no significant difference between the two groups of mice, confirming previous findings [26,30] (Figure 2A). No mortality was observed and the median value of CFU recovered after 28 days was 7.12×10^5 and 1.06×10^5, in the first and second group of mice, respectively (Figure 2B). For the second passage (P2), 192 single colonies recovered from two infected mice (96 colonies for each mice) were re-grown in vitro separately in a 96-well plate. All 96 colonies were pulled for two different agar bead preparations and injected in two groups of mice, respectively. The same procedure for colony isolation and agar beads preparation was followed for the third and the fourth passages of chronic infection (P3 and P4) (Figure 1).

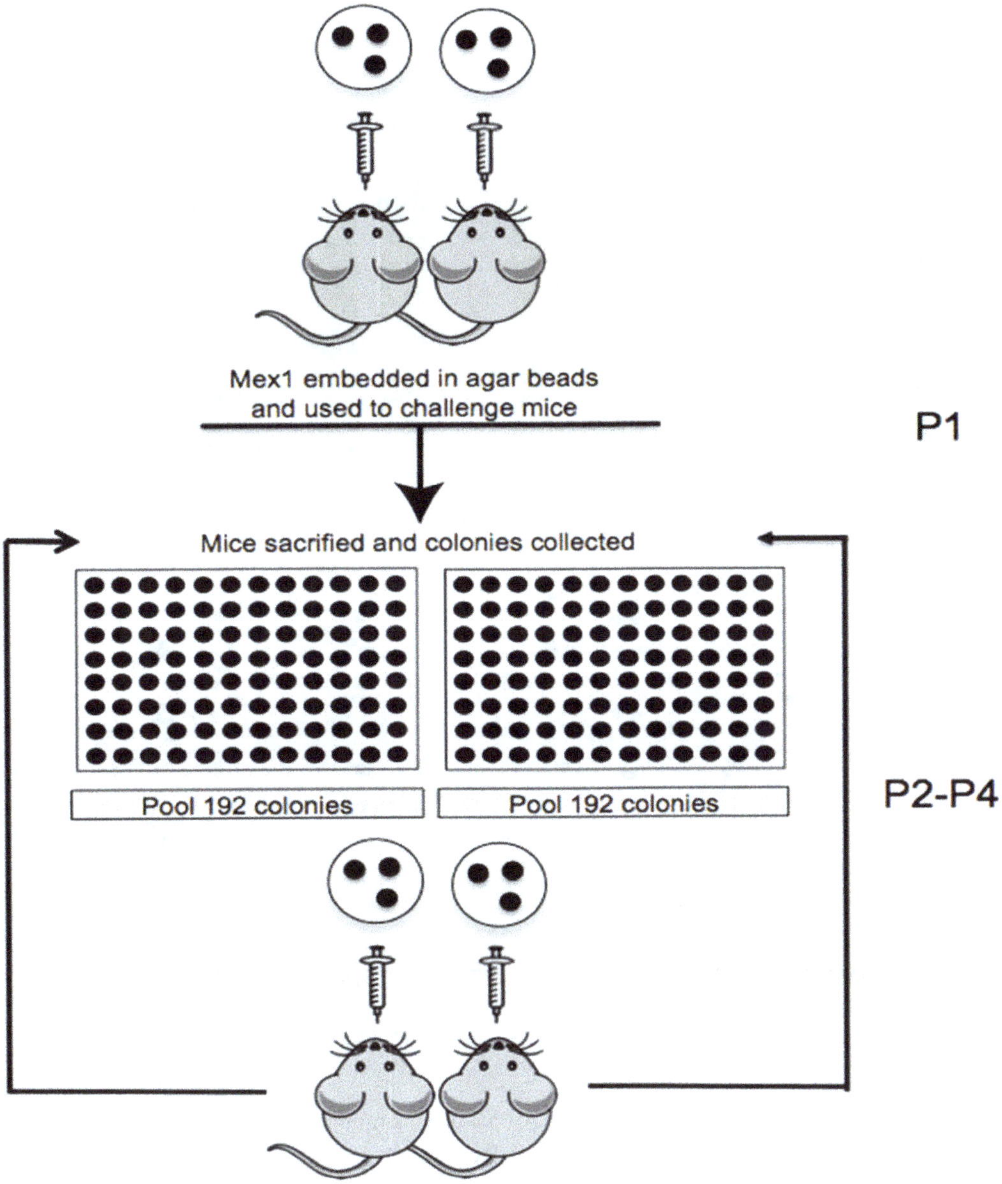

Figure 1. Schedule of sequential chronic *B. cenocepacia* lung infection in mice. Two groups of C57Bl/6NCrlBR mice (n = 8–12) were inoculated with 1.5 × 10^7 CFU/lung of *B. cenocepacia* Mex1 strain embedded in agar beads for 28 days (P1). After 28 days, single colonies were recovered from two groups of infected mice and were re-grown separately; then, they were pulled for two different agar bead preparations and injected in two groups of mice (n = 8–9) (P2). The third and the fourth passages in mice (n = 8–9) (P3 and P4) were carried out as P2 for 28 days each.

At the second serial passage in mice (P2), the percentage of infected mice increased significantly to 89% in one group and 75% in the second group (Fisher exact test: p = 0.0083 P1 vs. P2). Then, the third and fourth passages (P3 and P4) carried out as described above led to an increase in the percentage of infected mice of between 89% and 100%, respectively (Chi-square Test: p = 0.0002 P1 vs. P3; p = 0.0001 P1 vs. P3 and P4) (Figure 2A). There was no significant difference between the median value of CFU recovered from the first to the fourth passages in the sub-group of mice maintaining the infection and ranging between 1.14 × 10^5 and 1.32 × 10^6 CFU/lung (p value = 0.446 P1 vs. P4) (Figure 2B).

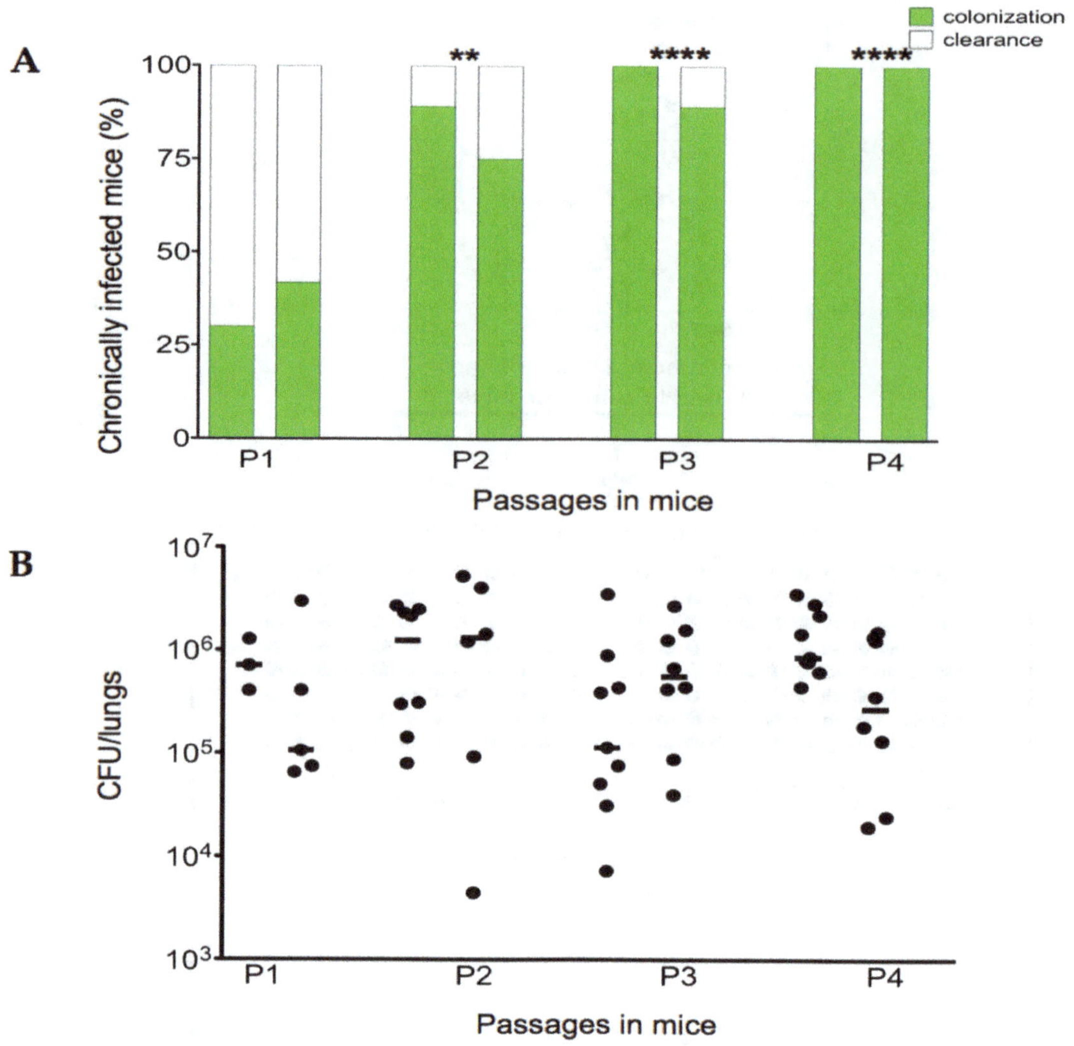

Figure 2. Virulence of *B. cenocepacia* Mex1 after sequential passages in mice. C57Bl/6 mice were infected for four sequential passages by bacteria collected from each passage of 28 days. At each passage mice were sacrificed and evaluated for CFU and percentage of infected mice. (**A**) The percentage of chronically infected mice at different passages. (**B**) The number of CFU of *B. cenocepacia* per lung at different passages. Dots represent individual mice measurements and horizontal lines represent the median values. Two groups of 8–12 mice were analyzed for each passage. Statistical significance is indicated: ** $p < 0.01$, **** $p < 0.0001$.

2.3. Phenotypic and Molecular Characterization of Mex1 Adapted to Murine Lungs

Phenotypic and molecular characterization of bacterial isolates recovered after the fourth passage in mice was carried out, in order to determine whether phenotypic or genetic adaptation occurred. We examined the persistent variants isolated from two groups of eight and nine chronically infected mice after the fourth sequential passages when the percentage of infected mice increased to 100%. Growth on *Burkholderia cepacia* selective agar (BCSA) and genetic profiling by random amplified polymorphic DNA (RAPD) analysis confirmed that the bacteria recovered were genetically indistinguishable from the initially challenged Mex1 strain (Figure 3).

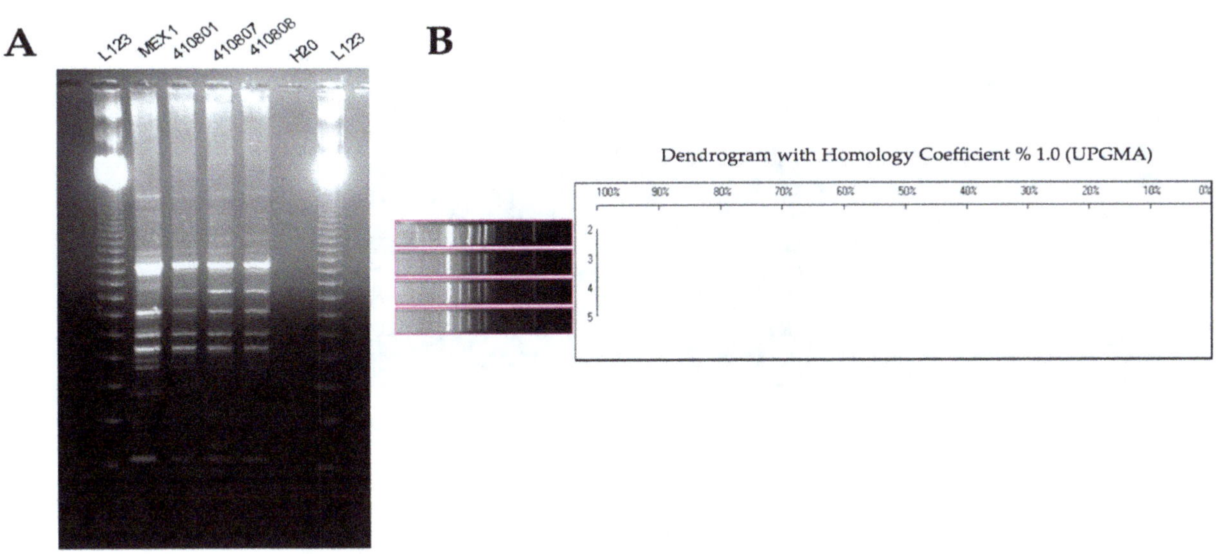

Figure 3. Random amplified polymorphic DNA (RAPD) fingerprints of the *B. cenocepacia* Mex1 challenge and some of its persisting colonies isolated from infected mice. (**A**) The polymorphisms were generated using RAPD primer 270. From left to right: L123, 123-bp molecular size marker ladder; Mex1 strain; clone 410801; clone 410807; clone 410808; negative control. (**B**) The dendrogram showing the clonal relatedness of some persisting colonies, performed with the Unweighted Pair Group Method with Arithmetic mean (UPGMA) by using mathematic averages algorithm programs integral to the Phoretix 1D Pro software. Lanes 2–5: Mex1 strain; clone 410801; clone 410807; clone 41080.

B. cenocepacia Mex1 strain and its derivatives were finally tested by PCR for the presence of the cable pilin subunit gene (*cblA*), encoding the cable pilus. Both the parent and the Mex1 derivative strains were negative for *cblA* gene, while only the clinical *B. cenocepacia* strain LMG 16656 was found positive (data not shown). No differences in biofilm formation (Figure 4) or colonial morphology (Figure 5) between the parental Mex1 and Mex1-derived clones were observed. Indeed, the mucoid colonial morphology, as assessed on yeast extract mannitol (YEM) agar plates, that correlates with higher levels of EPS production, appeared to be a distinct feature of the Mex1 strains as well as their derivative clones.

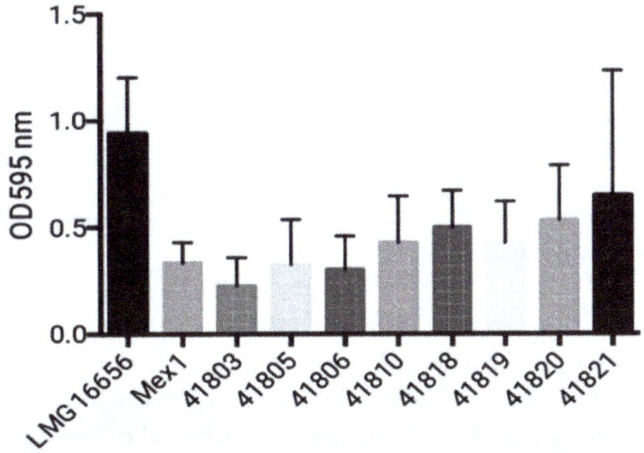

Figure 4. Biofilm formation of Mex1 and some of its derivatives in microtiter plate assay. No significant difference among Mex1 and its derivative clones was found ($p > 0.05$, One-way ANOVA). The clinical LMG16656^{T} formed a higher biofilm in comparison with Mex1 ($p = 0.0311$, Student's t-test). The amount of biofilm was quantified by Crystal Violet staining. Absorbance was measured at 595 nm.

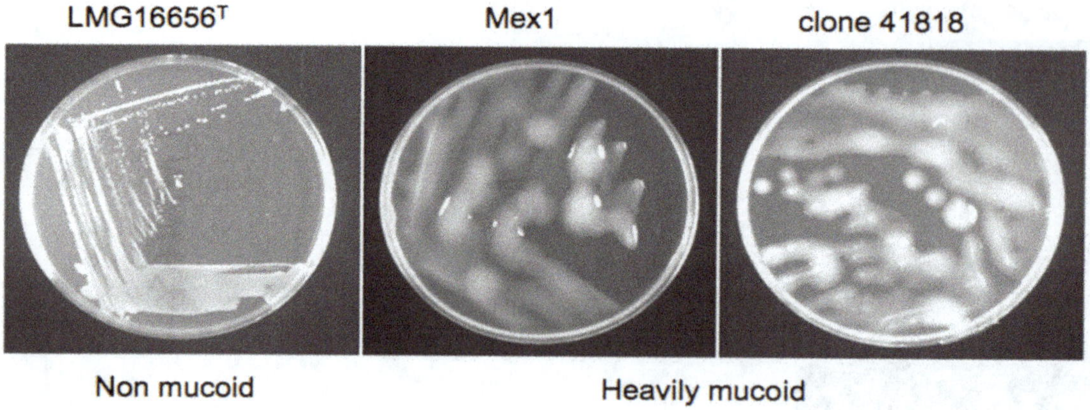

Figure 5. Colonial morphology of Mex1, its derivative (41818 clone as an example) and the clinical *B. cenocepacia* LMG16656^T on YEM agar. Strains were grown at 37 °C for 48 h.

2.4. Survival and Relative Bacterial Loads of Mex1 and Its Derivative Clones in Infected G. mellonella Larvae

The *G. mellonella* model is a valuable experimental system for determining the virulence properties of *B. cepacia* complex genetic mutants [33]. Thus, Mex1 and its derivatives recovered after the fourth passage in mice were screened for their ability to kill *G. mellonella* wax moth larvae. The resulting data were analyzed by determining the percentage survival of the infected larvae (Figure 6) and by the Kaplan-Maier method (Figure 7). As expected, the environmental Mex1 strain was significantly less virulent than LMG16656 as assessed by the log-rank test (p = 0.0106), demonstrating that the *G. mellonella* assays were suitable to identify differences in the virulence of *B. cenocepacia* strains. Overall, most of the Mex1-derived clones were not significantly different from the parental Mex1 strain, with two exceptions—strains 41803 and 41818—that appeared to be more virulent than Mex1 (Figure 6B).

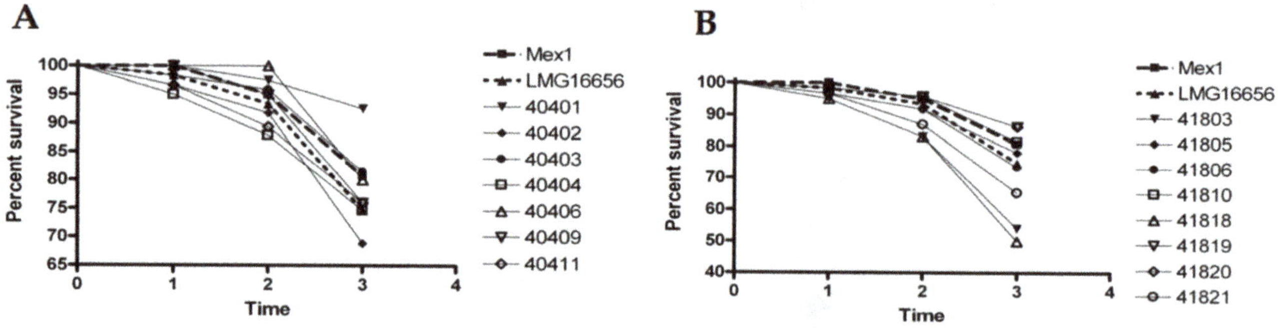

Figure 6. Percent survival of *G. mellonella* following inoculation with Mex1, Mex1-mouse persistent derivatives and the clinical LMG16656^T. The *B. cenocepacia* strains are indicated on the right: Mex1, thick dashed line; LMG16656, thick dotted line. *Y*-axis, percent survival of larvae infected with the indicated bacterial strains; *X*-axis, time post infection (days). Mex1-mouse persistent derivatives were recovered from two groups of eight and 9 C57Bl/6 male mice, and coded as 40 (**A**) and 41 (**B**), respectively.

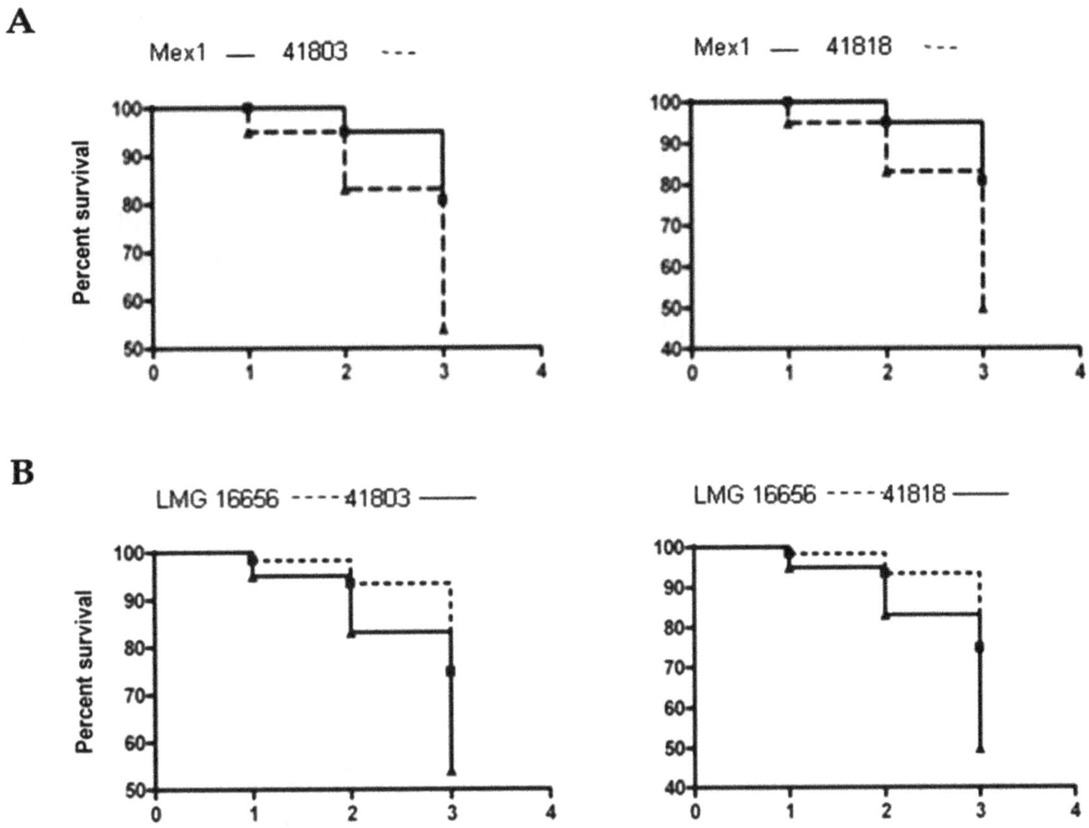

Figure 7. Kaplan-Meier survival plots of larvae injected with the indicated strains. (**A**) The killing ability of Mex1 compared with that of 41803 and 41818 Mex1-derived clones. (**B**) The killing ability of LMG16656 compared with that of 41803 and 41818 Mex1-derived clones. *Y*-axis, percent survival of larvae; *X*-axis, time (days) post infection. Statistical analysis was performed by log-rank test.

Accordingly, the Kaplan-Meier survival and the log-rank test showed a significantly higher virulence of these two strains respect to Mex1, with $p = 0.0156$ and $p = 0.0087$ for 41803 and 41818, respectively, while comparison with LMG16656 revealed no significant differences ($p > 0.05$) (Figure 7). Subsequently, the 50% lethal dose (LD_{50}) causing 50% death of infected larvae was determined. Results indicated that the two reference strains, Mex1 and LMG16656, showed LD_{50} values equal to 250 and 166, respectively. The Mex1-derivatives were more variable with LD_{50} ranging from 25 (41821) to 500 (41819). The clones 41803 and 41818 were characterized by low LD_{50} values, 59 and 38 respectively.

Overall, we have demonstrated that the Mex1 derivative clones showed a different degree of virulence in comparison with the parental strain. In particular, strains 41803 and 41818 were both significantly more virulent than the parental Mex1 strains, with a virulence degree comparable to that of the clinical LMG16656^T strain.

3. Discussion

B. cenocepacia strains occur naturally in a wide range of environments and are able to persist in human hosts, suggesting that the virulence factors needed to colonize animals and other habitats are similar [34]. Among the natural environments, the rhizosphere is a huge reservoir for bacterial species and a source of human pathogens, due to the enhanced biomass and microbial activity as a result of exudation compounds from the roots [35]. In particular, the maize rhizosphere has a strong influence on the specific host—*B. cenocepacia* interactions, and represents a privileged environment of BCC strains [36,37]. It can also be considered as a reservoir for opportunistic human pathogenic bacteria [24]. Interactions with plant roots might pave the way for bacterial adaptation to mammalian and human cells [35]. In this study, we aimed to investigate whether the rhizosphere *B. cenocepacia* Mex1 strain, that showed a low level of virulence in vivo [26], can increase its fitness in mice establishing niche adaptation through serial passages in a murine model.

Among the genetic lineages of *B. cenocepacia* species, *recA* lineage IIIA appears to have global distribution, predominantly among patients with CF, with high transmissibility and a high mortality rate [23,38,39]. Mex1 constitutes a rare environmental *B. cenocepacia* IIIA strain, isolated from the maize rhizosphere in Mexico [26,27]. Mex1 has a unique sequence type (ST), the ST 423, but genetically it is closely related to internationally spread clones as it belongs to the clonal complex 31, the largest clonal complex of all STs reported in the Multi-Locus Sequence Typing (MLST) *B. cepacia* complex database [16]. Until now, the adaptation process of *B. cenocepacia* to the host environment has been investigated for clinical isolates only [40] and, despite the description of several virulent factors, understanding is still poor [41]. Considering environmental *B. cenocepacia* strains, increased fitness of the *B. cenocepacia* HI2424 strain, belonging to the *recA* lineage IIIB, has been shown suggesting the adaptation of a soil isolate to the onion model [42]. In this case, *B. cenocepacia* adaptation was associated with reduced virulence and a loss of pathogenicity to the nematode *C. elegans*. The large, multireplicon genome and the presence of insertion sequences confer genome plasticity that could explain the versatility of *B. cenocepacia* bacteria and their ability to rapidly adapt to new niches [28]. Environmental strains have defense mechanisms that confer to them a survival advantage in this niche and they have been shown to infect various hosts, including mammals, nematodes and plants [43].

This study revealed that the rhizosphere *B. cenocepacia* Mex1 strain, with a low virulence in mice, increased its ability to cause a chronic lung infection following serial passages in mice that adapt to "local environmental" conditions in the murine lung tissues and establish chronic infections in almost all the infected mice. Our results suggest that chemical-physical characteristics of the host play a role in the selection of virulent bacteria. The phenotypic and genotypic tests we performed did not reveal any differences between strains. Colonial morphology revealed that the phenotype of the Mex1-derived clones recovered from infected mice were indistinguishable from the challenge strain. Our findings suggest that the Mex1 strain and its derivative clones were mucoid, in agreement with results obtained by Zlosnik and colleagues [44], who suggested that the capacity to elaborate EPS may be critical for survival in the environment, the natural niche of *B. cepacia* complex bacteria. Serial passages in mice did not determine any phenotypic switching from to nonmucoid to mucoid forms, as that of clinical and virulent *B. cenocepacia* strains. Also, no differences were observed in the genetic fingerprinting of the parental and the Mex1-derived clones. At any rate, RAPD analysis does not exclude the possibility that point mutations, such as SNPs or other point mutations, may have occurred [45].

When we evaluated the virulence of Mex1-derived clones in the *G. mellonella* larvae infection model, two Mex1-derived clones with a virulence degree more similar to that of the clinical and epidemic LMG16656 strain were found, suggesting adaptation to mice and the acquisition or differential expression of virulence factors. *G. mellonella* is an excellent model for assessing the virulence for a range of microorganisms and provides a rapid and cost-effective alternative for screening a large number of bacteria [46]. The wax moth larvae infection model has recently gained popularity in *Burkholderia* research and has been employed to compare virulence among different BCC species [33]. Recently, it was used to assess the efficacy of the combination therapy (tobramycin with econazole or miconazole) for *B. cenocepacia* [47]. From our results, we can speculate that the ability of *B. cenocepacia* to survive and replicate in various growth niches is due to the high genomic plasticity of this bacterial species and to the expression of host specific virulence factors. When properly regulated, this may help it to compete for survival in different settings [41]. As also suggested by Koskiniemi and colleagues [48], following growth inside a host selection can benefit bacterial mutants through an altered expression of virulence genes that better suit the environment of the host.

4. Materials and Methods

4.1. Bacteria and Culture Conditions

The bacterial strain used in this study and its properties are shown in Table 1.

4.2. Ethical Statement

Animal studies adhered strictly to the Italian Ministry of Health guidelines for the use and care of experimental animals. This study was conducted according to protocols approved by the Institutional Animal Care and Use Committee (IACUC, protocol #369 of 28 July 2008) of the San Raffaele Scientific Institute (Milan, Italy).

4.3. Sequential Infection in Mice

Mex1 was included in the agar beads prepared according to the previously described method [26]. Briefly, bacteria were cultured overnight in nutrient broth (NB) at 37 °C to the stationary phase. For agar beads preparation in P2–P4, bacteria isolated from plates were grown in NB broth in a 96-well plate at 37 °C overnight, pooled and centrifuged at 4000 rpm for 10 min. The cells were harvested by centrifugation and re-suspended in 1 mL of PBS (PH 7.4). Bacteria were added to 9 mL of 1.5% NA and subsequently pipetted forcefully into 150 mL of heavy mineral oil, which was kept at 50 °C for bead preparation. The size of the beads was verified microscopically and only those preparations containing beads of 100 μm to 200 μm in diameter were used. The number of *B. cenocepacia* CFU in the beads was determined by plating serial dilutions of the homogenized bacteria-bead suspension on NA plates. The two groups of 8 and 12 C57Bl/6 male mice (Charles River), 6–8 weeks old (20–22 g) were injected with 1.5–2.0 $\times$ 10^7 CFU/lung and the infection was followed for 28 days. Before infection, mice were anesthetized as previously described [30]. After infection, mice were monitored daily for the following clinical signs: coat quality, posture, ambulation, hydration status, and body weight. After 4 weeks, mice were sacrificed, and the lungs were homogenized. Serially diluted lung homogenate samples were plated on NA and the viable cell counts of *B. cenocepacia* were evaluated. Bacterial strains were recovered and the percentage of infected mice was evaluated. Recovery of >1000 CFU from lung cultures was indicative of chronic infection. Next, for the second passage, 192 single colonies recovered after 28 days, from two groups of infected mice were re-grown separately in 96 well plates. Then, they were pooled for two different agar bead preparations and injected in two groups of mice (n = 8–9, respectively). Thereafter, third and fourth passages in mice were carried out as described above.

4.4. Molecular Characterization of Mex1-Derived Clones

4.4.1. Random Amplified Polymorphic DNA (RAPD) Fingerprinting

The environmental *B. cenocepacia* Mex1 strain and its persisting derivatives recovered from infected mice were genetically typed by random amplified polymorphic DNA (RAPD) analysis, as previously described [49]. Each strain was tested in triplicate, and the entire experiment was repeated three times to verify the RAPD reproducibility. The generated fingerprints were analyzed using the Quantity One software package (Bio-Rad Laboratories, Milan, Italy) and Phoretix 1D PRO software (Phoretix International, Newcastle upon Tyne, UK). The Dice coefficient index was used as similarity measure. The dendrogram was created within Phoretix 1D Pro software by using the unweighted pair group method with arithmetic averages (UPGMA) method.

4.4.2. PCR Amplification of *cblA* Gene

The 664-bp *cblA* DNA coding for the cable pilus was amplified with the primers CBL1 and CBL2, according to the procedure described by Clode and colleagues [50].

4.5. Biofilm Formation

Biofilm formation was assessed using the 96-well plate assay and staining the sessile and adherent cells with crystal violet (CV) as described previously [51], with minor modifications [28]. *B. cenocepacia* strains (Mex 1, Mex1-derived clones and the clinical LMG16656^T) were inoculated from pure cultures grown in M9 minimal medium to mid-exponential (OD_{600} ~0.5) phase into at least 6 wells of flat-bottomed 96-well polyvinyl chloride microtiter plates (Greiner Bio-one, Frickenhausen, Germany). Biofilm biomass was quantified by crystal violet staining. Absorbance was measured at 595 nm using a Victor^3 multilabel counter (Perkin-Elmer, Milan, Italy). Each strain was tested in triplicate, and the entire experiment was repeated three times.

4.6. Growth on YEM Yeast Extract-Mannitol (YEM) Agar

Overnight cultures of bacteria were harvested, standardized to an OD590 of 1.0 in PBS, and adjusted to approximately 5×10^6 CFU·mL^{-1}. This bacterial suspension was used to inoculate (via a sterile pipette tip) yeast extract medium (YEM; 0.5 g of yeast extract L^{-1} and 4 g of mannitol L^{-1} supplemented with 15 g of agar L^{-1}) agar plates. Plates were incubated at 37 °C for 48 h prior to measuring the capacities of isolates to elaborate EPS.

4.7. Screening of Mex1-Derived Clones in the G. mellonella Model

The *G. mellonella* infection assay was carried out as described by Uehlinger and colleagues [52] with minor modifications. Overnight bacterial cultures were grown in Luria–Bertani (LB) broth, diluted 1:100 in the same medium and grown to an optical density at 600 nm (OD_{600}) of 0.4. Cultures were pelleted, resuspended in 10 mM $MgSO_4$ plus 1.2 mg/mL ampicillin and adjusted to $OD_{600} = 1$. A 5-µL aliquot (approximately 1×10^6 CFU/mL) was injected into the hindmost left proleg. For 50% lethal dose (LD_{50}) experiments, a series of 10-fold serial dilutions containing from 10^6 to 0 bacteria were injected into *G. mellonella* larvae. Ten to fifteen healthy larvae were injected for each strain and incubated in Petri dishes at 30 °C in the dark. The number of live and dead larvae was scored 24, 48 and 72 h after infection; dead larvae were those that did not move in response to touch. All the tests were performed in triplicate. Control larvae were injected with 5 µL of buffer only.

4.8. Statistical Analysis

In vivo data were statistically analyzed by using GraphPad Prism. Data analysis was performed using a non-parametric two-tailed Mann-Whitney *U*-test for single comparison for CFU counts. Incidences of chronic colonization were compared using Fisher exact test. Differences were considered statistically significant at p values < 0.05.

Biofilm data were analyzed using One-way ANOVA (Prism GraphPad version 6.0 Software Inc., San Diego, CA, USA), considering $p < 0.05$ as the limit of statistical significance.

The Kaplan-Meier curves were used to compare the survival of groups of larvae injected with the *B. cenocepacia* strains. Differences in survival were calculated by using the log-rank test. LD_{50} (CFU) value of each strain was calculated by fitting a linear regression. Survival and LD_{50} were performed using Prism GraphPad version 6.0. A p-value of <0.05 was considered to be statistically significant.

5. Conclusions

The present study evaluated the ability of the environmental *B. cenocepacia* Mex1 strain, isolated from maize-rhizosphere, to persist and increase its virulence by serial passages during long-term chronic airways infection in mice. In conclusion, we found that the environmental *B. cenocepacia* strain increased its capacity to cause a chronic lung infection after serial passages in mice, adapting to the local environmental conditions of murine lung tissues and establishing chronic infection. However, how environmental bacteria adapt in the complex and variable environment of the host is still largely unknown. Clonal variants with increased virulence in non-vertebrate hosts were found. However, in-depth characterization of Mex1 derivative clones by whole-genome sequencing and comparative bioinformatics analysis is necessary to understand whether intraclonal diversification occurred; this could lead to new targets for future anti-*B. cenocepacia* treatment strategies. Understanding the mechanisms of niche specialization of environmental strains and identifying the common targets of adaptation to the lung environment will allow us to evaluate the potential risk of infection with opportunistic pathogens.

Acknowledgments: This work was supported by grants from the Italian Cystic Fibrosis Research Foundation (FFC) (http://www.fibrosicisticaricerca.it/) to Annamaria Bevivino: grant FFC#7/2006 with the contribution of "Delegazione FFC di Latina" and grant FFC#7/2008 with the contribution of "Lega Italiana Fibrosi Cistica, Associazione Siciliana FC". We have dedicated the present article to the memory of Jesús Caballero-Mellado (Centro de Ciencias Genómicas, Universidad Nacional Autónoma de México, Cuernavaca, Morelos, Mexico) who passed away on 16 October 2010, at Cuernavaca, Morelos, Mexico. Jesús was Leader of the Soil Microbiology in Mexico and a great expert on the plant-associated *Burkholderia* species. With Jesus's death, we lost an excellent scientist, a loyal and generous friend, a marvelous speaker, a charming person of the highest sensitivity and nobility. We also acknowledge the Italian CF Foundation for its support and administrative tasks.

Author Contributions: Alessandra Bragonzi, Fiorentina Ascenzioni and Annamaria Bevivino conceived and designed the experiments, contributed reagents, materials and analysis tools, analyzed the data and wrote the paper; Moira Paroni, Luisa Pirone and Ivan Coladarci performed the mouse experiments, molecular characterization and *G. mellonella* infection, respectively.

References

1. Ratjen, F.; Döring, G. Cystic fibrosis. *Lancet* **2003**, *361*, 681–689. [CrossRef]
2. Worlitzsch, D.; Tarran, R.; Ulrich, M.; Schwab, U.; Cekici, A.; Meyer, K.C.; Birrer, P.; Bellon, G.; Berger, J.; Weiss, T.; et al. Effects of reduced mucus oxygen concentration in airway *Pseudomonas infections* of cystic fibrosis patients. *J. Clin. Investig.* **2002**, *109*, 317–325. [CrossRef] [PubMed]
3. Döring, G.; Gulbins, E. Cystic fibrosis and innate immunity: How chloride channel mutations provoke lung disease. *Cell. Microbiol.* **2009**, *11*, 208–216. [CrossRef] [PubMed]
4. Cystic Fibrosis Foundation Patient Registry. Annual Data Report. 2015. Available online: https://www.cff.org/Our-Research/CF-Patient-Registry/2015-Patient-Registry-Annual-Data-Report.pdf (accessed on 1 August 2017).
5. Lyczak, J.B.; Cannon, C.L.; Pier, G.B. Lung infections associated with cystic fibrosis. *Clin. Microbiol. Rev.* **2002**, *15*, 194–222. [CrossRef] [PubMed]
6. Bhagirath, A.Y.; Li, Y.; Somayajula, D.; Dadashi, M.; Badr, S.; Duan, K. Cystic fibrosis lung environment and *Pseudomonas aeruginosa* infection. *BMC Pulm. Med.* **2016**, *16*, 174. [CrossRef] [PubMed]
7. Conrad, D.; Haynes, M.; Salamon, P.; Rainey, P.B.; Youle, M.; Rohwer, F. Cystic fibrosis therapy: A community ecology perspective. *Am. J. Respir. Cell Mol. Biol.* **2013**, *48*, 150–156. [CrossRef] [PubMed]
8. Folkesson, A.; Jelsbak, L.; Yang, L.; Johansen, H.K.; Ciofu, O.; Høiby, N.; Molin, S. Adaptation of *Pseudomonas aeruginosa* to the cystic fibrosis airway: An evolutionary perspective. *Nat. Rev. Microbiol.* **2012**, *10*, 841–851. [CrossRef] [PubMed]
9. Lorè, N.I.; Cigana, C.; De Fino, I.; Riva, C.; Juhas, M.; Schwager, S.; Eberl, L.; Bragonzi, A. Cystic fibrosis-niche adaptation of *Pseudomonas aeruginosa* reduces virulence in multiple infection hosts. *PLoS ONE* **2012**, *7*, e35648. [CrossRef] [PubMed]
10. Döring, G.; Conway, S.P.; Heijerman, H.G.; Hodson, M.E.; Hoiby, N.; Smyth, A.; Touw, D.J. Antibiotic therapy against *Pseudomonas aeruginosa* in cystic fibrosis: A European consensus. *Eur. Respir. J.* **2000**, *16*, 749–767. [CrossRef] [PubMed]
11. Smith, E.E.; Buckley, D.G.; Wu, Z.; Saenphimmachak, C.; Hoffman, L.R.; D'Argenio, D.A.; Miller, S.I.; Ramsey, B.W.; Speert, D.P.; Moskowitz, S.M.; et al. Genetic adaptation by *Pseudomonas aeruginosa* to the airways of cystic fibrosis patients. *Proc. Natl. Acad. Sci. USA* **2006**, *103*, 8487–8492. [CrossRef] [PubMed]
12. Chicurel, M. Can organisms speed their own evolution? *Science* **2001**, *292*, 1824–1827. [CrossRef] [PubMed]

13. Winstanley, C.; O'Brien, S.; Brockhurst, M.A. *Pseudomonas aeruginosa* evolutionary adaptation and diversification in cystic fibrosis chronic lung infections. *Trends Microbiol.* **2016**, *24*, 327–337. [CrossRef] [PubMed]
14. Fothergill, J.L.; Walshaw, M.J.; Winstanley, C. Transmissible strains of *Pseudomonas aeruginosa* in cystic fibrosis lung infections. *Eur. Respir. J.* **2012**, *40*, 227–238. [CrossRef] [PubMed]
15. Parkins, M.D.; Glezerson, B.A.; Sibley, C.D.; Sibley, K.A.; Duong, J.; Purighalla, S.; Mody, C.H.; Workentine, M.L.; Storey, D.G.; Surette, M.G.; et al. Twenty-five-year outbreak of *Pseudomonas aeruginosa* infecting individuals with cystic fibrosis: Identification of the prairie epidemic strain. *J. Clin. Microbiol.* **2014**, *52*, 1127–1135. [CrossRef] [PubMed]
16. Drevinek, P.; Mahenthiralingam, E. *Burkholderia cenocepacia* in cystic fibrosis: Epidemiology and molecular mechanisms of virulence. *Clin. Microbiol. Infect.* **2010**, *16*, 821–830. [CrossRef] [PubMed]
17. Mahenthiralingam, E.; Baldwin, A.; Dowson, C.G. *Burkholderia cepacia* complex bacteria: Opportunistic pathogens with important natural biology. *J. Appl. Microbiol.* **2008**, *104*, 1539–1551. [CrossRef] [PubMed]
18. Courtney, J.M.; Dunbar, K.E.; McDowell, A.; Moore, J.E.; Warke, T.J.; Stevenson, M.; Elborn, J.S. Clinical outcome of *Burkholderia cepacia* complex infection in cystic fibrosis adults. *J. Cyst. Fibros.* **2004**, *3*, 93–98. [CrossRef] [PubMed]
19. Tabacchioni, S.; Bevivino, A.; Dalmastri, C.; Chiarini, L. *Burkholderia cepacia* complex in the rhizosphere: A minireview. *Ann. Microbiol.* **2002**, *52*, 103–117.
20. Pirone, L.; Chiarini, L.; Dalmastri, C.; Bevivino, A.; Tabacchioni, S. Detection of cultured and uncultured *Burkholderia cepacia* complex bacteria naturally occurring in the maize rhizosphere. *Environ. Microbiol.* **2005**, *7*, 1734–1742. [CrossRef] [PubMed]
21. Chiarini, L.; Bevivino, A.; Dalmastri, C.; Tabacchioni, S.; Visca, P. *Burkholderia cepacia* complex species: Health hazards and biotechnological potential. *Trends Microbiol.* **2006**, *14*, 277–286. [CrossRef] [PubMed]
22. LiPuma, J.J.; Spilker, T.; Coenye, T.; Gonzalez, C.F. An epidemic *Burkholderia cepacia* complex strain identified in soil. *Lancet* **2002**, *359*, 2002–2003. [CrossRef]
23. Baldwin, A.; Mahenthiralingam, E.; Drevinek, P.; Vandamme, P.; Govan, J.R.; Waine, D.J.; LiPuma, J.J.; Chiarini, L.; Dalmastri, C.; Henry, D.A.; et al. Environmental *Burkholderia cepacia* complex isolates in human infections. *Emerg. Infect. Dis.* **2007**, *13*, 458–461. [CrossRef] [PubMed]
24. Berg, G.; Alavi, M.; Schmid, M.; Hartmann, A. The rhizosphere as a reservoir for opportunistic human pathogenic bacteria. In *Molecular Microbial Ecology of the Rhizosphere*, 1st ed.; de Bruijn Frans, J., Ed.; John Wiley & Sons, Inc.: Somerset, NJ, USA, 2013; Volume 2, pp. 1209–1216, ISBN 9781118296172.
25. Bevivino, A.; Dalmastri, C.; Tabacchioni, S.; Chiarini, L.; Belli, M.L.; Piana, S.; Materazzo, A.; Vandamme, P.; Manno, G. *Burkholderia cepacia* complex bacteria from clinical and environmental sources in Italy: Genomovar status and distribution of traits related to virulence and transmissibility. *J. Clin. Microbiol.* **2002**, *40*, 846–851. [CrossRef] [PubMed]
26. Pirone, L.; Bragonzi, A.; Farcomeni, A.; Paroni, M.; Auriche, C.; Conese, M.; Chiarini, L.; Dalmastri, C.; Bevivino, A.; Ascenzioni, F. *Burkholderia cenocepacia* strains isolated from cystic fibrosis patients are apparently more invasive and more virulent than rhizosphere strains. *Environ. Microbiol.* **2008**, *10*, 2773–2784. [CrossRef] [PubMed]
27. Bevivino, A.; Pirone, L.; Pilkington, R.; Cifani, N.; Dalmastri, C.; Callaghan, M.; Ascenzioni, F.; McClean, S. Interaction of environmental *Burkholderia cenocepacia* strains with cystic fibrosis and non-cystic fibrosis bronchial epithelial cells in vitro. *Microbiology* **2012**, *158*, 1325–1333. [CrossRef] [PubMed]
28. Vial, L.; Chapalain, A.; Groleau, M.C.; Déziel, E. The various lifestyles of the *Burkholderia cepacia* complex species: A tribute to adaptation. *Environ. Microbiol.* **2011**, *13*, 1–12. [CrossRef] [PubMed]
29. Chung, J.W.; Altman, E.; Beveridge, T.J.; Speert, D.P. Colonial morphology of *Burkholderia cepacia* complex genomovar III: Implications in exopolysaccharide production, pilus expression, and persistence in the mouse. *Infect. Immun.* **2003**, *71*, 904–909. [CrossRef] [PubMed]
30. Bragonzi, A.; Farulla, I.; Paroni, M.; Twomey, K.B.; Pirone, L.; Lorè, N.I.; Bianconi, I.; Dalmastri, C.; Ryan, R.P.; Bevivino, A. Modelling co-infection of the cystic fibrosis lung by *Pseudomonas aeruginosa* and *Burkholderia cenocepacia* reveals influences on biofilm formation and host response. *PLoS ONE* **2012**, *7*, e52330. [CrossRef] [PubMed]
31. Pirone, L. Pathogenicity of Clinical and Environmental *Burkholderia cenocepacia* Strains: Influence of *Pseudomonas aeruginosa* and Cystic Fibrosis Host. Ph.D. Thesis, University of Rome, Rome, Italy, 2009.

32. Bragonzi, A.; Worlitzsch, D.; Pier, G.B.; Timpert, P.; Ulrich, M.; Hentzer, M.; Andersen, J.B.; Givskov, M.; Conese, M.; Döring, G. Nonmucoid *Pseudomonas aeruginosa* expresses alginate in the lungs of patients with cystic fibrosis and in a mouse model. *J. Infect. Dis.* **2005**, *192*, 410–419. [CrossRef] [PubMed]
33. Seed, K.D.; Dennis, J.J. Development of *Galleria mellonella* as an alternative infection model for the *Burkholderia cepacia* complex. *Infect. Immun.* **2008**, *76*, 1267–1275. [CrossRef] [PubMed]
34. Coenye, T.; Vandamme, P. Diversity and significance of *Burkholderia* species occupying diverse ecological niches. *Environ. Microbiol.* **2003**, *5*, 719–729. [CrossRef] [PubMed]
35. Aujoulat, F.; Roger, F.; Bourdier, A.; Lotthé, A.; Lamy, B.; Marchandin, H.; Jumas-Bilak, E. From environment to man: Genome evolution and adaptation of human opportunistic bacterial pathogens. *Genes* **2012**, *3*, 191–232. [CrossRef] [PubMed]
36. Fiore, A.; Laevens, S.; Bevivino, A.; Dalmastri, C.; Tabacchioni, S.; Vandamme, P.; Chiarini, L. *Burkholderia cepacia* complex: Distribution of genomovars among isolates from the maize rhizosphere in Italy. *Environ. Microbiol.* **2001**, *3*, 137–143. [CrossRef] [PubMed]
37. Dalmastri, C.; Baldwin, A.; Tabacchioni, S.; Bevivino, A.; Mahenthiralingam, E.; Chiarini, L.; Dowson, C. Investigating *Burkholderia cepacia* complex populations recovered from Italian maize rhizosphere by multilocus sequence typing. *Environ. Microbiol.* **2007**, *9*, 1632–1639. [CrossRef] [PubMed]
38. Manno, G.; Dalmastri, C.; Tabacchioni, S.; Vandamme, P.; Lorini, R.; Minicucci, L.; Romano, L.; Giannattasio, A.; Chiarini, L.; Bevivino, A. Epidemiology and clinical course of *Burkholderia cepacia* complex infections, particularly those caused by different *Burkholderia cenocepacia* strains, among patients attending an Italian cystic fibrosis center. *J. Clin. Microbiol.* **2004**, *42*, 1491–1497. [CrossRef] [PubMed]
39. Cunha, M.V.; Leitão, J.H.; Mahenthiralingam, E.; Vandamme, P.; Lito, L.; Barreto, C.; Salgado, M.J.; Sá-Correia, I. Molecular analysis of *Burkholderia cepacia* complex isolates from a Portuguese cystic fibrosis center: A 7-year study. *J. Clin. Microbiol.* **2003**, *41*, 4113–4120. [CrossRef] [PubMed]
40. O'Grady, E.P.; Sokol, P.A. *Burkholderia cenocepacia* differential gene expression during host-pathogen interactions and adaptation to the host environment. *Front. Cell. Infect. Microbiol.* **2011**, *1*, 15. [CrossRef] [PubMed]
41. Sousa, S.; Feliciano, J.; Pita, T.; Guerreiro, S.; Leitão, J.H. *Burkholderia cepacia* complex regulation of virulence gene expression: A review. *Genes* **2017**, *8*, 43. [CrossRef] [PubMed]
42. Ellis, C.N.; Cooper, V.S. Experimental adaptation of *Burkholderia cenocepacia* to onion medium reduces host range. *Appl. Environ. Microbiol.* **2010**, *76*, 2387–2396. [CrossRef] [PubMed]
43. Sokol, P.A. *Burkholderia*: Molecular Microbiology and Genomics. In *Burkholderia: Molecular Microbiology and Genomics*; Coenye, T., Vandamme, P., Eds.; Horizon Bioscience; Taylor and Francis, Inc.: Wymondham, UK, 2007; pp. 229–250, ISBN 1904933289.
44. Zlosnik, J.E.A.; Hird, T.J.; Fraenkel, M.C.; Moreira, L.M.; Henry, D.A.; Speert, D.P. Differential mucoid exopolysaccharide production by members of the *Burkholderia cepacia* complex. *J. Clin. Microbiol.* **2008**, *46*, 1470–1473. [CrossRef] [PubMed]
45. Bryant, J.; Chewapreecha, C.; Bentley, S.D. Developing insights into the mechanisms of evolution of bacterial pathogens from whole-genome sequences. *Future Microbiol.* **2012**, *7*, 1283–1296. [CrossRef] [PubMed]
46. Tsai, C.J.-Y.; Loh, J.M.S.; Proft, T. *Galleria mellonella* infection models for the study of bacterial diseases and for antimicrobial drug testing. *Virulence* **2016**, *7*, 214–229. [CrossRef] [PubMed]
47. Van den Driessche, F.; Vanhoutte, B.; Brackman, G.; Crabbé, A.; Rigole, P.; Vercruysse, J.; Verstraete, G.; Cappoen, D.; Vervaet, C.; Cos, P.; et al. Evaluation of combination therapy for *Burkholderia cenocepacia* lung infection in different in vitro and in vivo models. *PLoS ONE* **2017**, *12*, e0172723. [CrossRef] [PubMed]
48. Koskiniemi, S.; Gibbons, H.S.; Sandegren, L.; Anwar, N.; Ouellette, G.; Broomall, S.; Karavis, M.; McGregor, P.; Liem, A.; Fochler, E.; et al. Pathoadaptive mutations in *Salmonella enterica* isolated after serial passage in mice. *PLoS ONE* **2013**, *8*, e70147. [CrossRef] [PubMed]
49. Mahenthiralingam, E.; Simpson, D.A.; Speert, D.P. Identification and characterization of a novel DNA marker associated with epidemic *Burkholderia cepacia* strains recovered from patients with cystic fibrosis. *J. Clin. Microbiol.* **1997**, *35*, 808–816. [PubMed]
50. Clode, F.E.; Kaufmann, M.E.; Malnick, H.; Pitt, T.L. Distribution of genes encoding putative transmissibility factors among epidemic and nonepidemic strains of *Burkholderia cepacia* from cystic fibrosis patients in the United Kingdom. *J. Clin. Microbiol.* **2000**, *38*, 1763–1766. [PubMed]

51. Burmølle, M.; Webb, J.S.; Rao, D.; Hansen, L.H.; Sørensen, S.J.; Kjelleberg, S. Enhanced biofilm formation and increased resistance to antimicrobial agents and bacterial invasion are caused by synergistic interactions in multispecies biofilms. *Appl. Environ. Microbiol.* **2006**, *72*, 3916–3923. [CrossRef] [PubMed]
52. Uehlinger, S.; Schwager, S.; Bernier, S.P.; Riedel, K.; Nguyen, D.T.; Sokol, P.A.; Eberl, L. Identification of specific and universal virulence factors in *Burkholderia cenocepacia* strains by using multiple infection hosts. *Infect. Immun.* **2009**, *77*, 4102–4110. [CrossRef] [PubMed]

13

Synthesized Heparan Sulfate Competitors Attenuate *Pseudomonas aeruginosa* Lung Infection

Nicola Ivan Lorè [1,2,*,†], Noemi Veraldi [3,†], Camilla Riva [1], Barbara Sipione [1], Lorenza Spagnuolo [1], Ida De Fino [1], Medede Melessike [1], Elisa Calzi [3], Alessandra Bragonzi [1], Annamaria Naggi [3] and Cristina Cigana [1,*]

1 Division of Immunology, Transplantation and Infectious Diseases, IRCCS San Raffaele Scientific Institute, Milano 20132, Italy; riva.camilla@hsr.it (C.R.); sipione.barbara@hsr.it (B.S.); lorenza.spagnuolo@quintilesims.com (L.S.); defino.ida@hsr.it (I.D.F.); melessike.medede@hsr.it (M.M.); bragonzi.alessandra@hsr.it (A.B.)
2 Vita-Salute San Raffaele University, Milano 20132, Italy
3 Istituto di Ricerche Chimiche e Biochimiche "G. Ronzoni", Milano 20133, Italy; noemi.veraldi@gmail.com (N.V.); elisacalzi@libero.it (E.C.); naggi@ronzoni.it (A.N.)
* Correspondence: lore.nicolaivan@hsr.it (N.I.L.); cigana.cristina@hsr.it (C.C.);

† These authors contributed equally to this work.

Abstract: Several chronic respiratory diseases are characterized by recurrent and/or persistent infections, chronic inflammatory responses and tissue remodeling, including increased levels of glycosaminoglycans which are known structural components of the airways. Among glycosaminoglycans, heparan sulfate (HS) has been suggested to contribute to excessive inflammatory responses. Here, we aim at (i) investigating whether long-term infection by *Pseudomonas aeruginosa*, one of the most worrisome threat in chronic respiratory diseases, may impact HS levels, and (ii) exploring HS competitors as potential anti-inflammatory drugs during *P. aeruginosa* pneumonia. *P. aeruginosa* clinical strains and ad-hoc synthesized HS competitors were used in vitro and in murine models of lung infection. During long-term chronic *P. aeruginosa* colonization, infected mice showed higher heparin/HS levels, evaluated by high performance liquid chromatography-mass spectrometry after selective enzymatic digestion, compared to uninfected mice. Among HS competitors, an N-acetyl heparin and a glycol-split heparin dampened leukocyte recruitment and cytokine/chemokine production induced by acute and chronic *P. aeruginosa* pneumonia in mice. Furthermore, treatment with HS competitors reduced bacterial burden during chronic murine lung infection. In vitro, *P. aeruginosa* biofilm formation decreased upon treatment with HS competitors. Overall, these findings support further evaluation of HS competitors as a novel therapy to counteract inflammation and infection during *P. aeruginosa* pneumonia.

Keywords: *Pseudomonas aeruginosa* infections; glycosaminoglycans; anti-inflammatory drugs; mouse models; chronic respiratory diseases

---

1. Introduction

Chronic respiratory diseases with different etiology, such as cystic fibrosis (CF), non-CF bronchiectasis, idiopathic pulmonary fibrosis (IPF) and advanced chronic obstructive pulmonary disease (COPD) show common traits such as recurrent and/or persistent infections, together with chronic inflammatory responses and immunopathology [1–3]. In particular, *Pseudomonas aeruginosa* infections are associated with an exaggerated inflammatory response, including neutrophil recruitment, and excessive tissue remodeling. The pathophysiological mechanisms underlying this immunopathological scenario in response to *P. aeruginosa* infections during chronic airway diseases remain to be deciphered.

The lung extracellular matrix represents a highly dynamic complex of fibrous proteins, glycoproteins, and proteoglycans, that composes the non-cellular aspect of tissues and varies in composition according to pathophysiological circumstances. In this context, glycosaminoglycans (GAGs) are long, linear, and heterogeneous polysaccharides formed by repetition of disaccharide units, that not only represent principal components of the extracellular matrix, but are also distributed in the subepithelial tissue, bronchial walls and airway secretions [4]. They include hyaluronic acid, dermatan sulfate (DS), keratan sulfate, heparin and chondroitin sulfate (CS), but the most abundant in the lung parenchyma is heparan sulfate (HS). HS binds several effector molecules, known to be involved in chronic respiratory disease such as COPD and CF. For example, the binding of chemokines to GAGs is thought to favor the generation of the chemotactic gradient [5] responsible for leukocyte recruitment to the site of infection/injury. In addition, HS can bind cytokines and chemokines, such as interferon-(IFN-)γ and interleukin-(IL-)8, protecting them from proteolytic degradation and, thus, increasing their activities [6,7]. Therefore, high neutrophil recruitment in the airways of patients with chronic respiratory diseases may be due not only to increased chemokines expression, but also to their increased stability and prolonged activity when they are bound to HS. This pathological scenario would finally include also tissue remodeling and fibrosis.

Reports indicate that not only the amounts, but also sulfation of GAGs are markedly increased in CF tissues. Secretion of HS is elevated in CF airways, potentially correlating with the exaggerated inflammatory response described in the CF lung [7]. HS levels are increased also in the bronchoalveolar lavage fluid (BALF) of COPD patients with bacterial infections and during exacerbations [8]. In addition, high levels and sulfation of HS have been described also in patients with IPF [9].

Taking into consideration both the increased levels of HS in the context of chronic respiratory diseases and their potential involvement in the pathogenesis, the disruption of the interaction between HS and cytokines/chemokines may impact the inflammatory response. Specific GAG mimetics have been used to target some of these interactions in in vitro models [10]. In this context, we recently tested and characterized several synthesized HS competitors, in particular chemically modified derivatives of heparin with attenuated anticoagulant activity. These HS competitors not only bind to cytokines/chemokines [10], as natural endogenous HS does, but also inhibit the activity of neutrophil elastase (NE), a protease involved in the progression of lung fibrosis and in the sustainment of the inflammatory response in chronic respiratory diseases.

To date, the relevance of HS during *P. aeruginosa* infections, that characterize many chronic respiratory diseases, has not yet been addressed. Here, we utilized mouse models of lung infection to (i) investigate whether chronic *P. aeruginosa* lung infection may impact HS composition, and (ii) explore the potential anti-inflammatory activity of synthesized HS competitors in vivo. We report that: (i) chronic *P. aeruginosa* lung infection increased the levels of specific HS disaccharide building blocks; (ii) two HS competitors, in particular an *N*-acetyl heparin and a glycol-split heparin, named respectively C23 and $C3_{gs20}$, reduced the inflammatory response during acute and chronic *P. aeruginosa* lung infections, and decreased also the bacterial burden in a model of long-term chronic airways colonization.

2. Results

2.1. Evaluation of Specific HS Disaccharides and Their Levels in a Murine Model of Chronic P. aeruginosa Airways Infection

Taking into consideration the increased levels of GAGs in the lungs of mice chronically infected with *P. aeruginosa* for 28 days [11], we evaluated GAG species in this mouse model of chronic airway infection. C57Bl/6NcrlBR mice were inoculated with *P. aeruginosa* AA43 isolate embedded in agar-beads and with sterile agar beads (Ctrl group). After 28 days murine lungs were homogenized, centrifuged and supernatants were separated from pellets to distinguish released GAGs from those present as structural components of the extracellular matrix, respectively. Only lungs from mice that were still infected at 28 days post-challenge were analysed for their GAG content by selective enzymatic digestion [12,13]. High performance liquid chromatography-mass spectrometry (HPLC-MS) profiles of digestion products showed the presence of oligosaccharides from heparin/HS (Figure 1a and Supplementary Figure S1b), but not from other GAGs such as CS or DS. The amount of CS/DS was probably under the limit of detection. Digestion with heparinases lyases produced mainly disaccharides and traces of tetrasaccharides and hexasaccharides. It is known that the presence of the 3-*O*-sulfated glucosamine renders the glycosidic bond between *N*-acetylated, 6-*O*-sulfated glucosamine and the unsulfated glucuronic acid impervious to the action of heparinases [14]. Indeed, we detected tetrasaccharides probably bearing the trisulfated glucosamine residue like Δ4,4,0, but also other tetrasaccharides, i.e., Δ4,3,0 and Δ4,2,1, probably due to a limited efficiency of the enzymatic digestion, despite the excess of enzymes. Thus, we considered the disaccharidic composition, that represents more than the 90% of the digestion products in both infected and uninfected mice. The overall composition of digestion products indicated the presence of HS-like structure rather than heparin, due to the scarce presence of the trisulfated disaccharide (Δ2,3,0) and the high presence of monosulfated or monoacetylated disaccharides (Δ2,1,0 and Δ2,1,1). Indeed, comparing the integrals of HPLC peaks of disaccharides to the sum of the relative integrals (Figure 1b), an increase in digestion products in infected mice when compared to control uninfected mice was observed, with the prevalence of the monosulfated and disulfated disaccharides over the other species detected. More in details, this difference was observed in pellets of lung homogenates (Supplementary Figure S1a), indicating that chronic *P. aeruginosa* lung infection increased the levels of structural HS. Differently, no significant differences were found in the supernatants of infected lungs compared to those of Ctrl uninfected lungs (Supplementary Figure S1a,b).

2.2. Structure and Efficacy of Synthesized HS Competitors in the Mouse Model of Acute P. aeruginosa Airways Infection

We designed and characterized specific heparin derivatives to generate compounds able to act as competitors of endogenous HS in the murine lung. In particular, these HS competitors have been prepared starting from unmodified pig mucosal heparin (PMH) (Table 1) by targeted chemical modification able to strongly diminish/abolish its anticoagulant activity while maintaining the ability to interact with other proteins [10]. The first set of HS competitors included glycol-split heparin $C3_{gs20}$ and *N*-acetyl heparin C23, prepared as described previously [15]. In Figure 2, the major repeating disaccharide unit of heparin derivatives and the structure of the glycol-split uronic acid are shown.

Size is an important parameter that can influence the binding of HS competitors to proteins, especially the minimum length that is required to establish an interaction. For the second set of HS competitors to be tested, two structurally low molecular weight (LMW) analogues of $C3_{gs20}$ and C23 have been prepared by controlled reductive deamination, in order to improve the bio-availability of compounds and to verify the influence of dimensions on the activity of derivatives. In addition, the second set of synthesized HS competitors included compounds MMW $C3_{gs90}$ and MMW $C3_{gs45}$, that have been partially desulfated in order to increase the percentage of non-sulfated uronic acids reactive to the glycol-splitting modification to obtain a higher percentage of flexible joints along the chains. The MW of the first and second sets of compounds prepared (Table 1) ranged from 8 to 17.2 kDa, assuring an interaction with both IL-8 and human NE (12–14-mers for NE and 18-mer for IL-8) [16,17] which are known to be relevant to chronic inflammatory conditions. Notably, under controlled periodate oxidation conditions it is possible to limit the cleavage of glycosidic bonds without significant depolymerization of the HS competitors, as in the case of $C3_{gs20}$. Nevertheless, the combination of desulfation followed by glycol-splitting led to decrease in the MW of MMW $C3_{gs45}$ and MMW $C3_{gs90}$ proportionally to the increase of glycol-splitting, as expected.

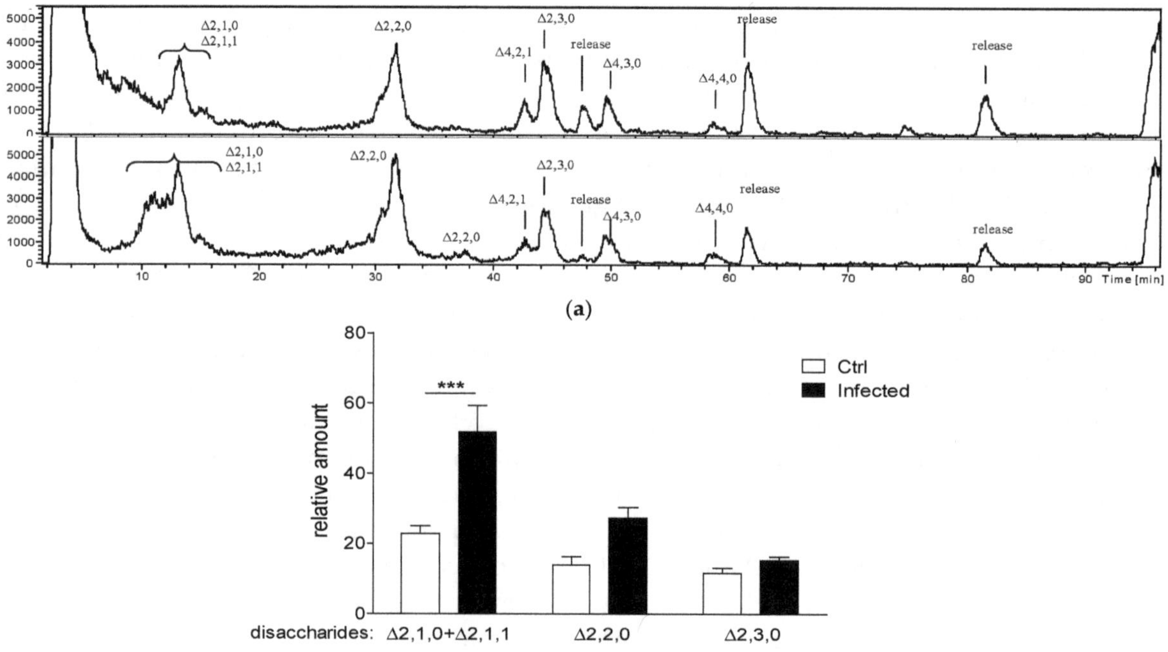

Figure 1. Disaccharide products of the digestion of heparin/HS from murine lungs after chronic *P. aeruginosa* infection. C57Bl/6NcrlBR mice were intratracheally injected with 1–2 × 10^6 colony forming units (CFUs) of *P. aeruginosa* isolate AA43 embedded in agar-beads (Infected) or with sterile agar-beads (Ctrl). After 28 days, lungs were perfused, recovered, homogenized and separated into pellets and supernatants. After removal of proteins, lipids and DNA, the presence of GAGs was verified by NMR. Samples were digested with a cocktail of heparin lyases to selectively degrade heparin/HS and recovered digestion products were desalted and finally analyzed by HPLC-MS. (**a**) Base Peak Chromatogram of digestion products from the pellet of one Ctrl uninfected (**upper** panel) and one infected (**lower** panel) lung homogenate from C57Bl/6NcrlBR mice. The unsaturated bond of the terminal uronic acid is indicated by Δ, and the number of monomers, the number of sulfates and the number of acetyls are reported; (**b**) The graph shows the amount of each disaccharide species detected in the whole lung of an infected and an uninfected Ctrl mouse; 100% is considered the sum of peak areas of one whole lung from infected mouse lungs containing the highest amount of disaccharides. The data are pooled from at least two independent experiments (n = 6–15). Data are the mean ± standard error of the mean (SEM) of at least three samples per type which have been processed independently. Statistical significance is indicated: *** $p < 0.001$.

Table 1. Structural characteristics of synthesized HS competitors originating from PMH (MW 20 kDa, %NAc 15).

HS Competitors	MW (kDa)	*N*-acetyl (%)	Glycol-Split (%)
C23	17.2	100	0
$C3_{gs20}$	16.5	14.6	20
LMW C23	8	91	0
LMW $C3_{gs20}$	8	14.6	18
MMW $C3_{gs45}$	12.6	14.6	45
MMW $C3_{gs90}$	9.6	14.6	90

The average molecular weight (MW), percentage of *N*-acetyl substitution in glucosamine residues and percentage of glycol-split (gs) uronate residues (cleavage by periodate oxidation of vicinal diols in unsubstituted D-GlcA and L-IdoA residues) is reported. Samples MMW $C3_{gs90}$ and MMW $C3_{gs45}$ have been partially desulfated in order to increase the percentage of uronic acids reactive for the glycol-splitting modification. Samples LMW C23 and LMW $C3_{gs20}$ have been obtained by controlled reductive deamination of PMH. LMW, low MW; MMW, medium MW.

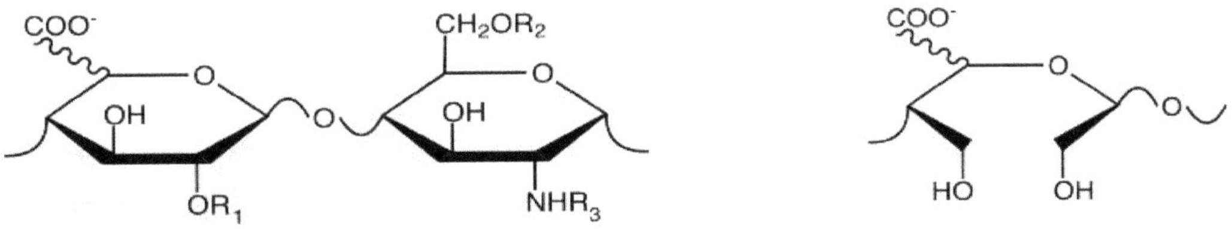

(a) (b)

Figure 2. Structures and characteristics of synthesized HS competitors. The repeating disaccharide unit of compounds (R_1 and R_2 = H/SO_3^-, R_3 = $H/SO_3^-/COCH_3$) is shown. The uronic acid is predominantly in the form L-iduronic acid (L-IdoA and L-IdoA-2-*O*-sulfate; ~80%) with D-glucuronic acid (D-GlcA; ~20%) making up the remainder. (**a**) Structure of the canonical disaccharide building block of heparin; (**b**) The glycol-split uronic acid residue present in compounds $C3_{gs20}$, MMW $C3_{gs90}$ and MMW $C3_{gs45}$.

Heparin derivatives have been shown to exert beneficial effects in inflammation [18]. We thus evaluated the impact of $C3_{gs20}$ and C23 on leukocyte recruitment in the murine BALF following acute *P. aeruginosa* lung infection. Mice were infected with the *P. aeruginosa* AA2 isolate [11,19], known to be highly virulent, and treated subcutaneously with these compounds (30 mg/kg). We found that neither C23 nor $C3_{gs20}$ affected the lung bacterial burden when compared to the vehicle (Figure 3a). C23 significantly reduced the number of total leukocytes in comparison to the vehicle (Figure 3b) and in particular neutrophils (Figure 3c) in the BALF, although the neutrophil percentages were not significantly different between mice treated with the compound and those treated with the vehicle (C23 vs. vehicle p = 0.057). Differently, $C3_{gs20}$ had only moderate inhibitory effects on leukocyte recruitment. C23 significantly reduced also IL-6, IL-12 (p40), granulocyte colony-stimulating factor (G-CSF) and monocyte chemoattractant protein-1 (MCP-1) when compared to the vehicle (Table 2). $C3_{gs20}$ reduced inflammatory mediators but at lower extent and with a statistically significant difference only for IL-6 levels (Table 2). Differently, when the second set of HS competitors, including LMW $C3_{gs20}$, LMW C23, MMW $C3_{gs90}$ and MMW $C3_{gs45}$, were tested in this murine model, they did not affect either the bacterial burden or the recruitment of leukocytes, including neutrophils, in the BALF (Supplementary Figure S2).

Overall, these results indicate C23 and $C3_{gs20}$ as the most promising anti-inflammatory compounds in the mouse model of acute *P. aeruginosa* lung infection.

Table 2. Levels of cytokines and chemokines in murine lungs during acute *P. aeruginosa* lung infection (6 h) and subcutaneous treatment with $C3_{gs20}$ or C23 (30 mg/kg).

Cytokine/Chemokine	Level (pg/500 μg Lung)			*p* Value	
	Vehicle	$C3_{gs20}$	C23	$C3_{gs20}$ vs. Vehicle	C23 vs. Vehicle
IL-4	3.31 ± 0.27	3.54 ± 0.19	3.37 ± 0.63	ns	ns
IL-6	232.9 ± 8.53	176.9 ± 15.95	159.7 ± 7.14	**	***
IL-12p40	10.97 ± 0.79	9.21 ± 0.76	7.86 ± 0.68	ns	*
IL-12p70	83.98 ± 3.46	93.98 ± 9.67	87.04 ± 6.45	ns	ns
IL-13	124.68 ± 8.49	140.26 ± 6.32	114.37 ± 5.33	ns	ns
IL-17A	6.77 ± 0.78	6.85 ± 0.21	6.66 ± 0.99	ns	ns
Eotaxin	353.62 ± 22.52	450.79 ± 33.85	341.3 ± 71.56	ns	ns
G-CSF	542 ± 10.56	465.8 ± 37.58	426.9 ± 36.53	ns	*
IFN-γ	538.19 ± 15.12	525.13 ± 72.72	462.34 ± 54.04	ns	ns
MCP-1	1327 ± 89.7	1239 ± 111.1	864.2 ± 118.6	ns	*
MIP-1β	1302.61 ± 124.2	1308.63 ± 142.3	1003.01 ± 191.9	ns	ns
RANTES	195.83 ± 19.19	247.57 ± 39.04	248.55 ± 46.88	ns	ns

Data are expressed as mean ± SEM. Statistical significance is indicated: * $p < 0.05$, ** $p < 0.01$, *** $p < 0.001$. ns: not significant. MIP-1β, macrophage inflammatory protein-1β; RANTES, regulated on activation normal T expressed and secreted.

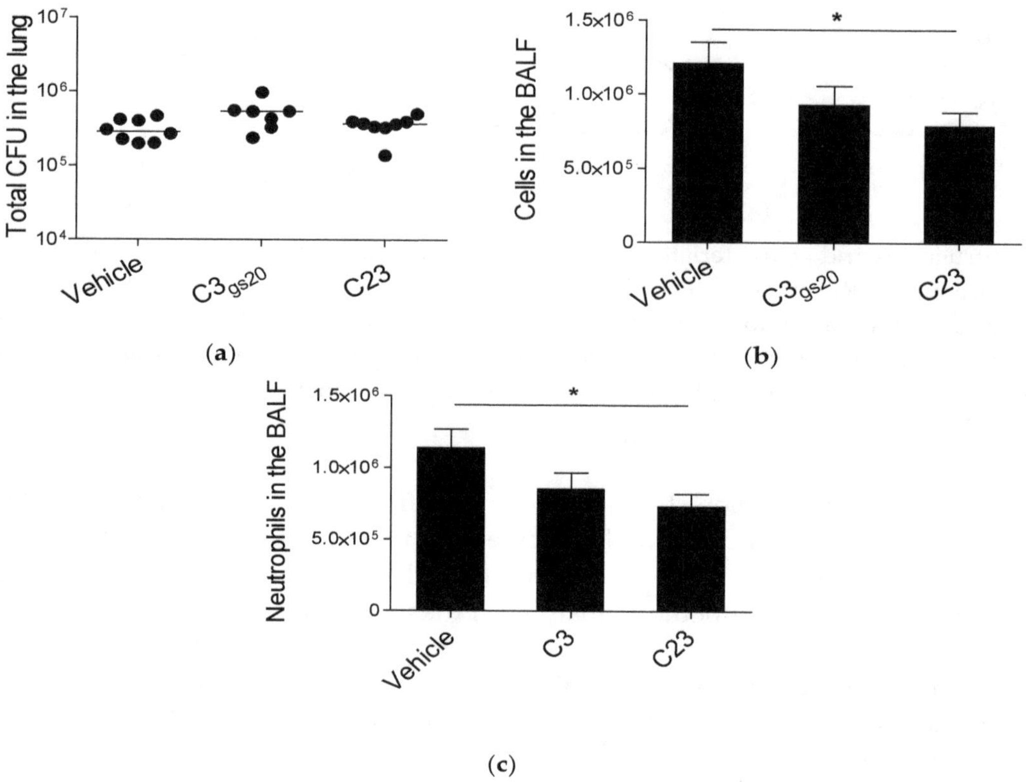

Figure 3. Modulation of the host response by synthesized HS competitors in a mouse model of acute *P. aeruginosa* lung infection. C57Bl/6NcrlBR mice were intratracheally injected with 5×10^6 CFUs of the highly virulent *P. aeruginosa* isolate AA2. Mice were subcutaneously treated with HS competitors (30 mg/kg) or their vehicle two hours before and two hours after the challenge and sacrificed 6 h post-infection. BALF and lung were recovered. (**a**) Total CFUs in the lungs were evaluated; (**b**) Total cell and (**c**) neutrophil recruitment was analyzed in BALF. The data are pooled from at least two independent experiments (n = 7–8). CFUs in individual mice are represented as dots and horizontal lines represent median values. Cells are represented as mean ± SEM. Statistical significance is indicated: * $p < 0.05$.

2.3. Efficacy of Synthesized HS Competitors in Mouse Models of Chronic P. aeruginosa Airways Infection

Next, we tested the ability of HS competitors to reduce inflammation during the development and the course of chronic *P. aeruginosa* lung infection. First, we evaluated the effect of $C3_{gs20}$ and C23 in an agar-beads mouse model of chronic lung infection running for 14 days. C57Bl/6NcrlBR mice were chronically infected with *P. aeruginosa* AA43 isolate, known to persist in the lung with an incidence of colonization around 30–40% [11], and treated subcutaneously with $C3_{gs20}$ and C23 starting from the day of infection. We found that the incidence of chronic lung colonization was reduced in mice infected with $C3_{gs20}$ when compared to those treated with the vehicle (13% for $C3_{gs20}$ and 33% for C23 vs. 33% for vehicle; Figure 4a), although this difference did not reach statistical significance. We also observed a trend to a decrease in lung CFUs in mice treated with $C3_{gs20}$ in comparison to vehicle (Figure 4b). In addition, C23 significantly reduced the recruitment of total leukocytes, including neutrophils, in comparison to vehicle (Figure 4c,d). A similar trend was observed also for $C3_{gs20}$.

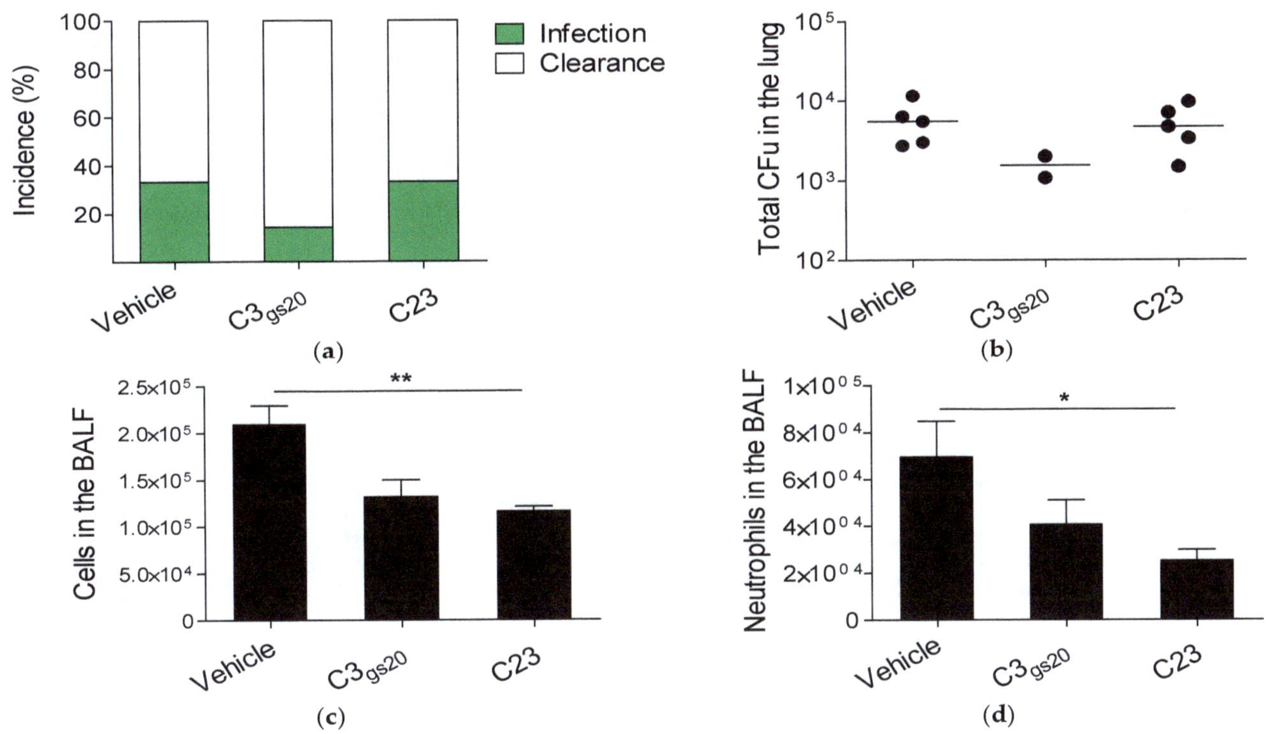

Figure 4. Modulation of the host response by synthesized HS competitors in a mouse model of chronic *P. aeruginosa* lung infection (14 days). C57Bl/6NcrlBR mice were intratracheally injected with 1–2 × 10^6 CFUs of the *P. aeruginosa* isolate AA43 embedded in agar-beads. Mice were treated subcutaneously with HS competitors (30 mg/kg) or vehicle every day starting from the day of infection for 14 days. At the sacrifice, BALF and lung were recovered. (**a**) Bacterial clearance (white) and incidence of colonization (green) were determined; (**b**) CFUs were evaluated in total lung of mice still infected at the sacrifice. Total cell (**c**) and neutrophil (**d**) recruitment was analyzed in BALF. The data are pooled from two independent experiments (n = 14–15). CFUs in individual mice are represented as dots and horizontal lines represent median values. Cells are represented as mean ± SEM. Statistical significance is indicated: * $p < 0.05$, ** $p < 0.01$.

We then investigated whether $C3_{gs20}$ and C23 also impacted an established chronic *P. aeruginosa* lung infection. Thus, we extended the *P. aeruginosa* chronic infection for 28 days and started the treatment with HS competitors and vehicle after ten days from the infection, once chronic infection is well-established [20]. We previously showed that this mouse model of *P. aeruginosa* persistence is highly stable in terms of incidence of colonization and bacterial burden up to three months, and reproduces detectable chronic inflammation and tissue damage for long-term [11,20]. By using this schedule of treatment, the incidence of chronic *P. aeruginosa* lung colonization was not affected by HS competitors and remained stable (percentages of mice still colonized after 28 days: vehicle, 30.4%; $C3_{gs20}$, 30%; C23, 30.8%). However, $C3_{gs20}$ and C23 significantly increased murine body weights when compared with the vehicle, indicating that they promoted a better health status (Figure 5a). In addition, $C3_{gs20}$ and C23 significantly decreased the bacterial burden in the lung in comparison to the vehicle (Figure 5b). $C3_{gs20}$ significantly decreased the infiltration of leukocytes, including neutrophils, in the BALF (Figure 5c,d), and the levels of inflammatory mediators, such as IL-1β, IL-12p70, IL-17A, G-CSF and KC in comparison to the vehicle (Table 3). C23 showed a similar trend, although only the differences of leukocyte infiltration and IL-17A level reached a statistical significance (Figure 5c and Table 3). Other markers were not affected by these compounds as shown in Table 3.

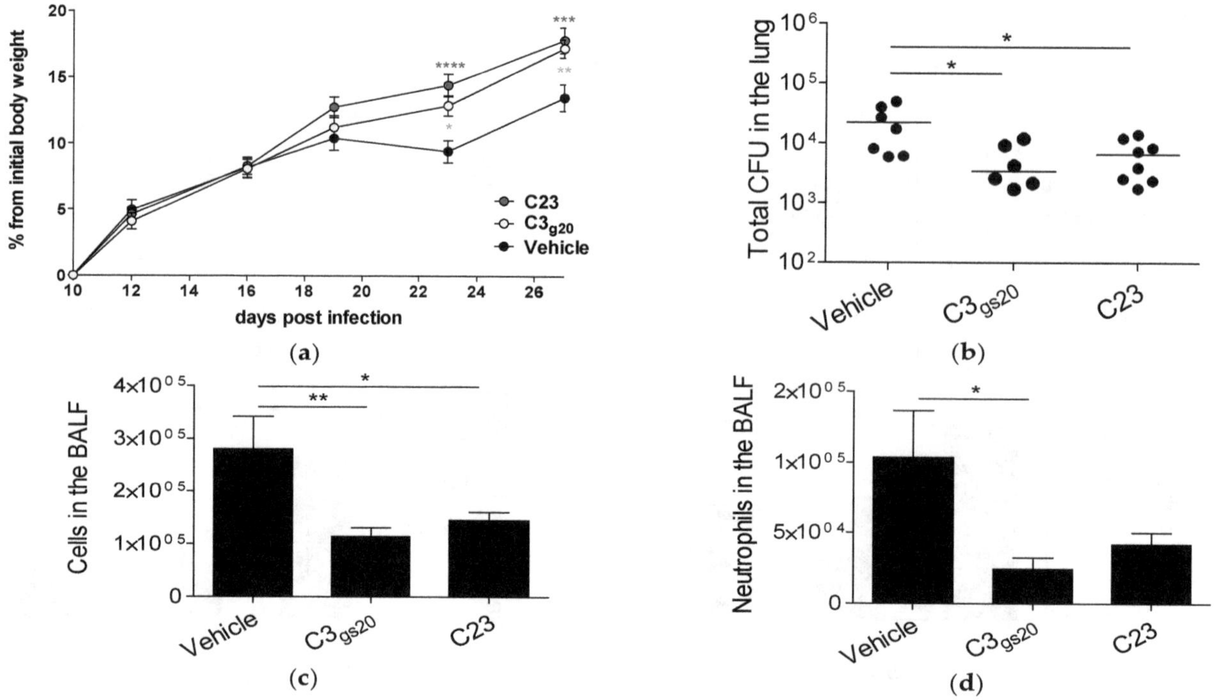

Figure 5. Modulation of the host response by synthesized HS competitors in a mouse model of long-term chronic *P. aeruginosa* lung infection (28 days). C57Bl/6NcrlBR mice were intratracheally injected with 1–2 × 10^6 CFUs of the *P. aeruginosa* isolate AA43 embedded in agar-beads. Mice were treated subcutaneously with HS competitors (30 mg/kg) or vehicle every day starting from ten days post-infection. At the sacrifice, BALF and lung were recovered. (**a**) Changes from initial body weight were calculated for each group of mice at regular intervals. (**b**) Total CFUs in the lungs were evaluated. (**c**) Total cell and (**d**) neutrophil recruitment was analyzed in BALF. The data are pooled from at least two independent experiments (n = 20–26). CFUs in individual mice are represented as dots and horizontal lines represent median values. The other parameters are represented as mean ± SEM. Statistical significance is indicated: * $p < 0.05$, ** $p < 0.01$, *** $p < 0.001$, **** $p < 0.0001$.

Table 3. Levels of cytokines and chemokines in murine lungs during chronic *P. aeruginosa* lung infection (28 days) and subcutaneous treatment with $C3_{gs20}$ or C23 (30 mg/kg).

Cytokine/Chemokine	Level (pg/500 μg Lung)			*p* Value	
	Vehicle	$C3_{gs20}$	C23	$C3_{gs20}$ vs. Vehicle	C23 vs. Vehicle
IL-1α	26 ± 3.14	6.91 ± 0.47	7.75 ± 0.75	ns	ns
IL-1β	24.04 ± 4.92	10.42 ± 2.11	15.93 ± 2.63	*	ns
IL-2	4.49 ± 1.10	nd	nd	n/a	n/a
IL-5	2.96 ± 0.37	2.85 ± 1.03	3.52 ± 0.60	ns	ns
IL-9	99.56 ± 12.57	132.10 ± 24.21	116.00 ± 19.28	ns	ns
IL-10	3.89 ± 0.25	3.10 ± 0.84	3.19 ± 0.47	ns	ns
IL-12p40	11.27 ± 1.07	10.15 ± 1.13	10.20 ± 0.49	ns	ns
IL-12p70	8.93 ± 1.17	4.62 ± 1.19	5.74 ± 0.90	*	ns
IL-13	98.20 ± 14.41	76.03 ± 14.45	98.11 ± 14.37	ns	ns
IL-17A	7.94 ± 1.27	3.29 ± 0.66	4.41 ± 0.90	**	*
Eotaxin	264.20 ± 30.39	135.20 ± 49.53	237.40 ± 34.22	ns	ns
G-CSF	4.62 ± 0.95	2.57 ± 0.54	3.89 ± 0.21	*	ns
GM-CSF	29.95 ± 2.66	nd	28.82 ± 10.48	n/a	ns
IFN-γ	5.22 ± 0.71	3.90 ± 1.03	6.13 ± 0.79	ns	ns
KC	13.92 ± 2.64	7.91 ± 0.69	11.71 ± 1.47	*	ns
MCP-1	84.93 ± 9.12	70.74 ± 12.04	67.41 ± 7.78	ns	ns
MIP-1β	16.94 ± 1.99	15.80 ± 2.38	16.04 ± 2.05	ns	ns
RANTES	6.95 ± 0.59	6.86 ± 1.04	8.47 ± 1.07	ns	ns
TNF-α	6.59 ± 0.33	4.44 ± 0.63	7.55 ± 0.81	ns	ns

Data are expressed as mean ± SEM. Statistical significance is indicated: * $p < 0.05$, ** $p < 0.01$. ns: not significant; nd: not detectable; n/a: not applicable. GM-CSF, granulocyte-macrophage colony-stimulating factor; KC, keratinocyte chemoattractant, TNF-α, tumor necrosis factor alpha.

When we tested the impact of other HS competitors on the host response in this mouse model of chronic lung infection, we found that neither MMW $C3_{gs90}$ nor MMW $C3_{gs45}$ affected either bacterial burden or leukocytes recruitment (Supplementary Figure S3).

Overall these results indicated that $C3_{gs20}$ and C23 have a dual effect: on inflammation, containing leukocyte recruitment in the site of infection, and on infection, reducing the bacterial load.

Taking into consideration the effect of $C3_{gs20}$ and C23 on *P. aeruginosa* bacterial burden in the mouse model of chronic *P. aeruginosa* infection, we asked whether $C3_{gs20}$ and C23 could have any anti-bacterial activity. We did not find any change in minimum inhibitory concentrations after challenge with up to 512 μg/mL. When we investigated the effect on biofilm formation, both $C3_{gs20}$ and C23 induced a statistically significant reduction of AA43 sessile fraction in a dose-dependent fashion (Figure 6). These data suggest an inhibitory effect exerted by $C3_{gs20}$ and C23 on *P. aeruginosa* biofilm formation.

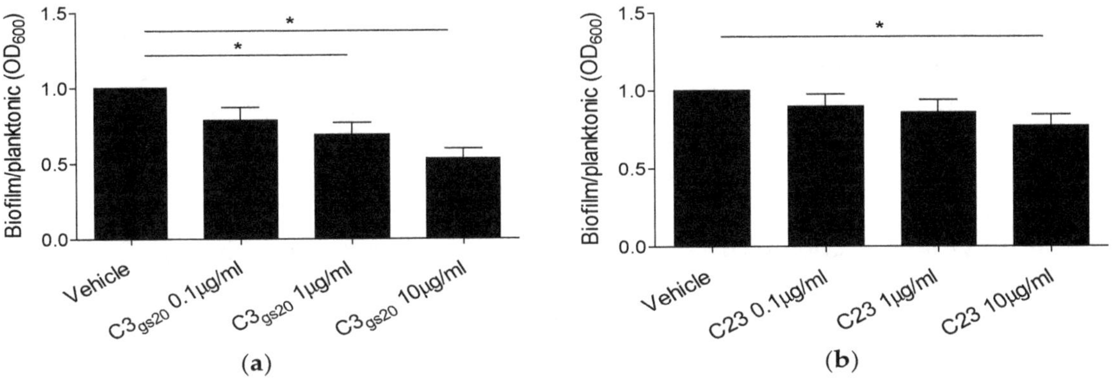

Figure 6. Effect of synthesized HS competitors on *P. aeruginosa* biofilm formation. *P. aeruginosa* strain AA43 was grown for 24 h at 37 °C either in the absence or presence of different concentrations of $C3_{gs20}$ (**a**) and C23 (**b**). Biofilm biomass was quantified by staining with crystal violet and absorbance measurements at OD_{600}. Absorbance of planktonic bacteria in the culture medium was measured at OD_{600}. Results are expressed as the ratio between biofilm absorbance and planktonic bacteria absorbance normalized on the value obtained for AA43 treated with isotonic saline (vehicle). The data derive from three independent experiments in triplicate. Values represent the mean ± SEM. Statistical significance is indicated: * $p < 0.05$.

3. Discussion

Increased levels of GAGs including HS, the most abundant in the lung parenchyma, are common to several chronic respiratory diseases, including CF, COPD and IPF [1,2,5]. Whether *P. aeruginosa* infections may contribute to the increase of HS is still an open question. Clinical data are difficult to interpret due to the large number of confounding variables. Here, using mouse models of lung infection, we demonstrated that long-term chronic *P. aeruginosa* lung infection induces structural changes in HS as shown by increased amounts of specific HS disaccharide building blocks. In addition, our results indicate that two synthesized HS competitors, in particular *N*-acetyl heparin and glycol-split heparin, named respectively C23 and $C3_{gs20}$, competing with endogenous HS, dampen the inflammatory response induced by *P. aeruginosa* and reduce the bacterial burden.

To our knowledge, despite several reports indicating increased levels of highly sulfated HS in the airways of patients affected by chronic respiratory diseases, there are no studies analyzing specifically the impact of bacterial infections on HS levels and composition in the lung. We previously demonstrated that *P. aeruginosa* persistence was associated with a progressive increase of sulfated GAGs in murine lungs [11]. Here, we focused on HS composition and found that long-term chronic *P. aeruginosa* lung colonization led to an increase of specific HS disaccharides, in particular mono- and di-sulfated ones, in the pellet of murine lungs. This finding suggests that *P. aeruginosa* infection increases mainly structural HS, rather than contributing to released HS. In this regard, HS has been detected also in the BALF in COPD patients [8] and in the sputum sol of patients with bronchiectasis [21] indicating HS degradation. However, no reports indicate a correlation between HS levels in airway secretions and bacterial infection. Future clinical studies should determine a potential correlation between bacterial infections/colonization, including by *P. aeruginosa*, and the levels and sulfation of HS in the lungs of patients with chronic respiratory diseases. In addition, we analyzed the HS composition in the lung of C57Bl/6NcrlBR mice. Since the murine genetic background determines infection outcomes [22–24], it would be interesting to clarify whether it can also affect the composition of the extracellular matrix by using different inbred and outbred murine lines.

Besides maintaining lung tissue structure, HS may modulate the behavior of cells by binding growth factors and by interacting with cell surface receptors [4,25]. In addition, it can interact with proteases and cytokines/chemokines impacting on immunopathology. Taking into consideration these evidences and our findings on the increase of HS during chronic *P. aeruginosa* lung infection, we explored a HS inhibitory strategy in mouse models of infection. We chose to chemically modify heparin to synthesize competitors of the endogenous HS, thanks to its structural similarity to HS and its commercial availability; moreover, it is commonly used in hospitals as an anticoagulant drug and considered to be safe. Recently, these synthesized HS competitors with low or absent anticoagulant activity have been shown to bind to IL-8 and TNF-α and to inhibit the activity of NE in vitro [10], suggesting that these compounds could preserve the connective tissues and limit inflammation in vivo. When tested in murine models, C23 and $C3_{gs20}$ reduced neutrophilic recruitment and cytokines/chemokines production both in acute and chronic *P. aeruginosa* lung infection. These results support the finding that HS binding to chemokines may contribute to leukocyte recruitment in the site of infection/injury by generating the chemotactic gradient as well as increasing pro-inflammatory activities of chemokines by protecting them from proteolytic degradation [5–7]. It can be hypothesized that synthesized HS competitors may reduce levels of endogenous HS, thus reducing the chemotactic gradient. In this regard, a HS reduction secondary to decreased inflammation and infection may be plausible after long-term chronic lung infection. However, it would be unlikely that these compounds can directly reduce HS, taking into account their effects after short-term acute *P. aeruginosa* infection. Differently, we speculate that synthesized HS competitors could have competed with endogenous HS for the binding to cytokines/chemokines, thus leading to their degradation/elimination. Further studies to elucidate these mechanisms are necessary, in particular to evaluate the amount of chemokines still bound to endogenous HS during treatment with synthesized HS competitors in vivo. Anyhow, the reduction of neutrophilic recruitment could lead to a decreased immunopathology by itself, since it implies lower levels of neutrophil proteases, including NE. In addition, taking into consideration that HS competitors inhibit NE activity [10], reduced tissue remodeling and fibrosis could be expected. In fact, NE, a protease described as abundant in the airways of patients affected by chronic respiratory diseases [26], degrades several components of the extracellular matrix, including elastin [27], thus contributing to the tissue remodeling and fibrosis [4], and ultimately aggravating the immunopathology. In this context, several attempts to inhibit NE have been carried out, also in clinical studies on patients with respiratory diseases, although with contrasting results [26].

One of the off-target effects of anti-inflammatory treatments is the impairment of the host defense that can lead to the exacerbation of the infection [20,28–30]. However, we did not observe an increase in *P. aeruginosa* burden in the model of acute lung infection. Next, we set-up two schedules of treatment in the mouse model of chronic lung infection. In the 14-day-lasting model of chronic lung colonization, mice had been treated starting from the day of infection. In such a model, synthesized HS competitors could interfere in particular with the early immune response, thus impacting the development and the progression of chronic lung infection. Differently, in the 28-day-lasting model of chronic lung colonization, mice were treated starting from ten days post-infection to evaluate effects of HS competitors on well-established chronic lung infection. In both schedules, we adopted the *P. aeruginosa* AA43 isolate, which can establish chronic infection in C57Bl/6NcrlBR mice with an incidence of colonization around 30–40% [11] starting from seven days post-infection. This choice is fundamental when the aim is determining the impact of anti-inflammatory treatment on the host defense, since an increase in the number of mice still colonized after long-term or in *P. aeruginosa* load could be observed. For instance, using this isolate we recently demonstrated that the IL-17A pathway impairment increased both the incidence of colonization and bacterial burden [20]. Unexpectedly, $C3_{gs20}$ and C23 impacted *P. aeruginosa* infection and, in particular, they reduced the bacterial burden in murine lungs after long-term chronic lung infection.

When administered in different schedules of *P. aeruginosa* lung infection and treatment, $C3_{gs20}$ and C23 showed slight differences: C23 was more potent in inhibiting the inflammatory response in the model of acute lung infection, while $C3_{gs20}$ was more effective in the model of long-term chronic infection, where it decreased the bacterial burden, and it was more potent in hampering in vitro *P. aeruginosa* biofilm formation. We may speculate that these different activities may be addressed to the structures of synthesized HS competitors. Indeed, C23 is a *N*-acetyl heparin, with charge density and distribution similar to that of HS. Therefore, it is potentially able to mimic HS in its interactions and to compete by sequestering cytokines/chemokines from endogenous HS, thus rendering them more susceptible to degradation. Differently from C23, $C3_{gs20}$ maintains the negative charge density of PMH and displays chain flexibility thanks to the glycol-split modification. In this context, its more potent anti-biofilm activity could be due to several interactions: (i) because of its negative charges, it could bind Ca^{++}, known to form a bridge between polyanionic alginate molecules that stabilizes biofilms [31]; (ii) it could interact with biofilm polysaccharides, impeding their binding; (iii) it could counteract the binding between single *P. aeruginosa* cells. However, there could be other explanations to the decrease of *P. aeruginosa* burden after long-term chronic lung colonization following treatment with C23, and in particular $C3_{gs20}$. In fact, HS has been found to be a cell receptor for *P. aeruginosa* and a binding site for bacterial flagella, and this could suggest another role during infection [32,33]. Further studies based on additional structural modifications of these compounds could provide new insights into their biological activities during host–pathogen interplay. Moreover, the reduction of the bacterial burden by HS competitors during *P. aeruginosa* pneumonia suggests that the potential synergy between these compounds and antibiotics currently used in clinics should be investigated.

4. Materials and Methods

4.1. Ethics Statement

Animal studies strictly followed the Italian Ministry of Health guidelines for the use and care of experimental animals. This study was performed following protocols approved by the Institutional Animal Care and Use Committee (IACUC, protocols #502 of 14 July 2011 and #812 of 28 July 2016) of the San Raffaele Scientific Institute (Milan, Italy). Research with *P. aeruginosa* clinical strains has been approved by the responsible physician at the CF Center at Hannover Medical School, Germany. Additional information is available in the Supplementary Materials.

4.2. Bacterial Strains

Sequential *P. aeruginosa* isolates (AA2 and AA43) were recovered from CF patients and previously characterized for genotypic and phenotypic traits, and virulence [19,34,35]. AA2, expressing several virulence factors, including swimming motility, twitching motility and protease secretion, was isolated at the onset of chronic infection. Differently, AA43, a variant with adaptive phenotypes, including mucoidy, absence of swimming motility, low twitching motility and production of protease, was collected after seven years of chronic colonization. AA2 has previously been shown to induce high in vitro and in vivo acute virulence, while AA43 has been shown to be attenuated, but capable of developing chronic lung infection [11,19,36].

4.3. Mouse Strain

C57Bl/6NcrlBR (Charles River, Calco, Lecco, Italy), 8 to 10 weeks old, were maintained in specific pathogen-free conditions at the San Raffaele Scientific Institute (Milan, Italy).

4.4. HS Competitors Synthesis and Characterization

Compounds are HS competitors obtained by chemical modification of PMH in order to reduce the anticoagulant activity whilst maintaining the anti-inflammatory potential. In particular, the *N*-acetyl heparin C23 and glycol-split heparin derivatives $C3_{gs20}$, MMW $C3_{gs90}$ and MMW $C3_{gs45}$, were generated as previously described [15,37] and characterized by ^{13}C-NMR [10] (Supplementary Figure S4a). Additional information is available in the Supplementary Materials. In addition, two LMW variants of C23 and $C3_{gs20}$ were produced by depolymerization of PMH through reductive deamination with nitrous acid using a $NaNO_2$/heparin ratio of 1:7, as explained in detail in the Supplementary Materials, followed by the same modifications introduced on full-length derivatives. These LMW were characterized by HSQC-NMR (Supplementary Figure S4b). The average MWs were determined at a concentration of 5 mg/mL employing Viscotek HP-SEC-TDA as previously described [38].

4.5. Mouse Models of Acute and Chronic *P. aeruginosa* Infection

In the acute infection model, mice were injected intratracheally with 5×10^6 CFUs of planktonic *P. aeruginosa* AA2 isolate, following established procedures [11,19,39]. Mice were treated subcutaneously with 30 mg/kg of synthesized HS competitors [40–42] or with vehicle (isotonic saline) two hours before and two hours after infection, and sacrificed six hours post-infection.

In the chronic infection model, mice were injected intratracheally with $1–2 \times 10^6$ CFUs of *P. aeruginosa* AA43 isolate, embedded in agar beads, following established procedures [11,30,39]. The bacterial load was previously set-up as the minimum inoculum to establish chronic infection [43]. Another group of mice (Ctrl) was intratracheally injected with sterile beads. For the analysis of HS/heparin levels, one batch of infected mice and the Ctrl group were sacrificed after 28 days from the infection, lungs were perfused with isotonic saline to avoid the contamination by circulating HS/heparin, recovered, homogenized and centrifuged. Pellets and supernatants were separated and lyophilized. For the analysis of HS competitor efficacy, one batch of infected mice was treated once a day as described above starting from the day of infection and sacrificed 14 days post-infection. Another batch of mice was treated once a day as described above starting from ten days post-infection and sacrificed 28 days post-infection.

BALF and lung were recovered and processed, and total/differential cell count and bacterial burden evaluated, as previously described [39]. Further information on the procedures are present in the Supplementary Materials.

4.6. HS/heparin Analysis in Murine Lungs

Samples were defatted by washing with chloroform/methanol, then with ethyl ether and freeze-dried, recovered in dPBS with 2 mM $CaCl_2$ and subjected first to proteolytic cleavage with Proteinase K at 55 °C for 48 h, then to DNase I digestion at 37 °C for 48 h. After boiling for 10 min to stop the reaction, samples were filtered on 0.2 μm filters, then purified by 3 kDa ultrafiltration to remove digestion fragments. Purified samples were analyzed by ^{1}H-NMR and eventually subjected to a second protease digestion. Digestion of CS by Chondroitinase ABC was carried out in a 50 mM sodium acetate/phosphate buffer (1:1 *v*/*v*), pH 8 at 37 °C for 48 h. After inactivation by boiling for 10 min samples were filtered onto 0.45 μm cut-off filters.

Digestion of heparin and HS with a cocktail of heparin lyases I–II-III (Grampian Enzymes, Aberdeen, UK), was carried out at 37 °C for 48 h, then stopped by boiling for 10 min followed by 0.2 μm filtration. Products were recovered by 3 kDa ultrafiltration, desalted and lyophilized. 100 μL sample solution was prepared for HPLC-MS analysis on a LC system coupled with an ESI-Q-TOF mass-spectrometer (micrOTOFq, Bruker Daltonics, Bremen, Germany). The chromatographic separation was performed using a Kinetex C18 analytical column (100 × 2.1 mm, 2.6 μm particle size, Phenomenex, Torrance, CA, USA) with Security Guard Cartridges Gemini C18 (4 × 2.0 mm, Phenomenex). A binary solvent system was used for gradient elution at 0.1 ml/min of solvent A (10 mM DBA, 10 mM CH_3COOH in water) and solvent B (10 mM DBA and 10 mM CH_3COOH in methanol): t 0′ 10%B, t 35′ 40%B, t 85′ 50%B, t 88′ 90%B, t 95′ 10%B. Disaccharide standards were purchased from Iduron, Manchester, UK. Data were processed by the DataAnalysis software (HyStar Compass, version 3.2, Bruker Daltonics).

4.7. Evaluation of Cytokines/Chemokines

Cytokines/chemokines and growth factors were measured by Bioplex in the lung homogenates, according to the manufacturer's instructions [11].

4.8. Evaluation of P. aeruginosa Biofilm Formation

Biofilm production was evaluated using the method of staining with crystal violet, as previously described [44]. AA43 was grown for 24 h at 37 °C either in the absence or presence of different concentrations of $C3_{gs20}$ and C23 (10 μg/mL, 1 μg/mL and 0.1 μg/mL). Biofilm biomass was quantified by staining with crystal violet and absorbance measurements at OD_{600}. Absorbance of planktonic bacteria in the culture medium was measured at OD_{600}. Results are expressed as the ratio between biofilm absorbance and planktonic bacteria absorbance normalized on the value obtained for AA43 treated with the vehicle. Further details can be found in the Supplementary Materials.

4.9. Statistics

Statistics were performed with GraphPad Prism. Data analysis was performed using one-way ANOVA followed by Dunnett's analysis to correct for multiple comparisons for CFU counts, cellular counts and cytokine/chemokines quantification. Incidences of chronic colonization were compared using Fisher exact test. Two-way ANOVA with Bonferroni's Multiple Comparison test was used to compare changes in body weight. $p < 0.05$ was considered significant.

5. Conclusions

In conclusion, our study shows that chronic *P. aeruginosa* lung infection increased HS levels in the murine lungs, and that interfering with this phenomenon dampened the inflammatory response. We indeed demonstrated that synthesized HS competitors decreased leukocyte recruitment and cytokine/chemokine production both during acute *P. aeruginosa* infection, and during the development and the course of chronic lung infection in mice. In addition, these compounds reduced *P. aeruginosa* infection in the agar-beads mouse model. Overall, these data support further evaluation of HS competitors as novel therapeutic molecules to counteract excessive inflammation induced by *P. aeruginosa* pulmonary infections in patients affected by chronic respiratory diseases.

Acknowledgments: The authors thank Burkhard Tümmler (Medizinische Hochschule Hannover, Germany) for supplying *P. aeruginosa* clinical isolates and Francesco Viviani for his technical support. This study was supported to Cristina Cigana by Italian Cystic Fibrosis Research Foundation (FFC#14/2013 and 18/2016), with the contribution of the Delegazioni FFC di Milano, Palermo, Vittoria, Ragusa e Siracusa, Catania Mascalucia, Messina, and Gruppo di Sostegno FFC di Tremestieri. Barbara Sipione and Noemi Veraldi had been supported by fellowships of the Italian Cystic Fibrosis Research Foundation.

Author Contributions: Cristina Cigana, Nicola Ivan Lorè and Annamaria Naggi conceived and designed the experiments; Cristina Cigana, Nicola Ivan Lorè, Noemi Veraldi, Camilla Riva, Barbara Sipione, Ida De Fino, Lorenza Spagnuolo, Elisa Calzi and Medede Melessike performed the experiments; Cristina Cigana, Nicola Ivan Lorè, Noemi Veraldi, Camilla Riva and Barbara Sipione analyzed the data; Cristina Cigana, Nicola Ivan Lorè, Noemi Veraldi and Annamaria Naggi interpreted the experiments results; Cristina Cigana and Noemi Veraldi prepared the figures; Cristina Cigana and Alessandra Bragonzi contributed reagents/materials/analysis tools; Cristina Cigana and Nicola Ivan Lorè wrote the manuscript. All authors reviewed the manuscript.

References

1. Hassett, D.J.; Borchers, M.T.; Panos, R.J. Chronic obstructive pulmonary disease (COPD): Evaluation from clinical, immunological and bacterial pathogenesis perspectives. *J. Microbiol.* **2014**, *52*, 211–226. [CrossRef] [PubMed]
2. Cohen, T.S.; Prince, A. Cystic fibrosis: A mucosal immunodeficiency syndrome. *Nat. Med.* **2012**, *18*, 509–519. [CrossRef] [PubMed]
3. Suzuki, A.; Kondoh, Y. The clinical impact of major comorbidities on idiopathic pulmonary fibrosis. *Respir. Investig.* **2017**, *55*, 94–103. [CrossRef] [PubMed]
4. Reeves, E.P.; Bergin, D.A.; Murray, M.A.; McElvaney, N.G. The involvement of glycosaminoglycans in airway disease associated with cystic fibrosis. *Sci. World J.* **2011**, *11*, 959–971. [CrossRef] [PubMed]
5. Proudfoot, A.E.; Handel, T.M.; Johnson, Z.; Lau, E.K.; LiWang, P.; Clark-Lewis, I.; Borlat, F.; Wells, T.N.; Kosco-Vilbois, M.H. Glycosaminoglycan binding and oligomerization are essential for the in vivo activity of certain chemokines. *Proc. Natl. Acad. Sci. USA* **2003**, *100*, 1885–1890. [CrossRef] [PubMed]
6. Sadir, R.; Forest, E.; Lortat-Jacob, H. The heparan sulfate binding sequence of interferon-gamma increased the on rate of the interferon-gamma-interferon-gamma receptor complex formation. *J. Biol. Chem.* **1998**, *273*, 10919–10925. [CrossRef] [PubMed]
7. Solic, N.; Wilson, J.; Wilson, S.J.; Shute, J.K. Endothelial activation and increased heparan sulfate expression in cystic fibrosis. *Am. J. Respir. Crit. Care Med.* **2005**, *172*, 892–898. [CrossRef] [PubMed]
8. Papakonstantinou, E.; Klagas, I.; Roth, M.; Tamm, M.; Stolz, D. Acute Exacerbations of COPD Are Associated With Increased Expression of Heparan Sulfate and Chondroitin Sulfate in BAL. *Chest* **2016**, *149*, 685–695. [CrossRef] [PubMed]
9. Westergren-Thorsson, G.; Hedstrom, U.; Nybom, A.; Tykesson, E.; Ahrman, E.; Hornfelt, M.; Maccarana, M.; van Kuppevelt, T.H.; Dellgren, G.; Wildt, M.; et al. Increased deposition of glycosaminoglycans and altered structure of heparan sulfate in idiopathic pulmonary fibrosis. *Int. J. Biochem. Cell Biol.* **2017**, *83*, 27–38. [CrossRef] [PubMed]
10. Veraldi, N.; Hughes, A.J.; Rudd, T.R.; Thomas, H.B.; Edwards, S.W.; Hadfield, L.; Skidmore, M.A.; Siligardi, G.; Cosentino, C.; Shute, J.K.; et al. Heparin derivatives for the targeting of multiple activities in the inflammatory response. *Carbohydr. Polym.* **2015**, *117*, 400–407. [CrossRef] [PubMed]
11. Cigana, C.; Lore, N.I.; Riva, C.; De Fino, I.; Spagnuolo, L.; Sipione, B.; Rossi, G.; Nonis, A.; Cabrini, G.; Bragonzi, A. Tracking the immunopathological response to *Pseudomonas aeruginosa* during respiratory infections. *Sci. Rep.* **2016**, *6*, 21465. [CrossRef] [PubMed]
12. Linhardt, R.J.; Turnbull, J.E.; Wang, H.M.; Loganathan, D.; Gallagher, J.T. Examination of the substrate specificity of heparin and heparan sulfate lyases. *Biochemistry* **1990**, *29*, 2611–2617. [CrossRef] [PubMed]
13. Prabhakar, V.; Capila, I.; Raman, R.; Srinivasan, A.; Bosques, C.J.; Pojasek, K.; Wrick, M.A.; Sasisekharan, R. The catalytic machinery of chondroitinase ABC I utilizes a calcium coordination strategy to optimally process dermatan sulfate. *Biochemistry* **2006**, *45*, 11130–11139. [CrossRef] [PubMed]
14. Yamada, S.; Yoshida, K.; Sugiura, M.; Sugahara, K.; Khoo, K.H.; Morris, H.R.; Dell, A. Structural studies on the bacterial lyase-resistant tetrasaccharides derived from the antithrombin III-binding site of porcine intestinal heparin. *J. Biol. Chem.* **1993**, *268*, 4780–4787. [PubMed]
15. Casu, B.; Guerrini, M.; Guglieri, S.; Naggi, A.; Perez, M.; Torri, G.; Cassinelli, G.; Ribatti, D.; Carminati, P.; Giannini, G.; Penco, S.; et al. Undersulfated and glycol-split heparins endowed with antiangiogenic activity. *J. Med. Chem.* **2004**, *47*, 838–848. [CrossRef] [PubMed]
16. Spencer, J.L.; Stone, P.J.; Nugent, M.A. New insights into the inhibition of human neutrophil elastase by heparin. *Biochemistry* **2006**, *45*, 9104–9120. [CrossRef] [PubMed]
17. Spillmann, D.; Witt, D.; Lindahl, U. Defining the interleukin-8-binding domain of heparan sulfate. *J. Biol. Chem.* **1998**, *273*, 15487–15493. [CrossRef] [PubMed]

18. Casu, B.; Naggi, A.; Torri, G. Heparin-derived heparan sulfate mimics to modulate heparan sulfate-protein interaction in inflammation and cancer. *Matrix Biol.* **2010**, *29*, 442–452. [CrossRef] [PubMed]
19. Lore, N.I.; Cigana, C.; De Fino, I.; Riva, C.; Juhas, M.; Schwager, S.; Eberl, L.; Bragonzi, A. Cystic fibrosis-niche adaptation of *Pseudomonas aeruginosa* reduces virulence in multiple infection hosts. *PLoS ONE* **2012**, *7*, e35648. [CrossRef] [PubMed]
20. Lore, N.I.; Cigana, C.; Riva, C.; De Fino, I.; Nonis, A.; Spagnuolo, L.; Sipione, B.; Cariani, L.; Girelli, D.; Rossi, G.; et al. IL-17A impairs host tolerance during airway chronic infection by *Pseudomonas aeruginosa*. *Sci. Rep.* **2016**, *6*, 25937. [CrossRef] [PubMed]
21. Chan, S.C.; Shum, D.K.; Ip, M.S. Sputum sol neutrophil elastase activity in bronchiectasis: Differential modulation by syndecan-1. *Am. J. Respir. Crit. Care Med.* **2003**, *168*, 192–198. [CrossRef] [PubMed]
22. Spagnuolo, L.; De Simone, M.; Lore, N.I.; De Fino, I.; Basso, V.; Mondino, A.; Cigana, C.; Bragonzi, A. The host genetic background defines diverse immune-reactivity and susceptibility to chronic *Pseudomonas aeruginosa* respiratory infection. *Sci. Rep.* **2016**, *6*, 36924. [CrossRef] [PubMed]
23. De Simone, M.; Spagnuolo, L.; Lore, N.I.; Rossi, G.; Cigana, C.; De Fino, I.; Iraqi, F.A.; Bragonzi, A. Host genetic background influences the response to the opportunistic *Pseudomonas aeruginosa* infection altering cell-mediated immunity and bacterial replication. *PLoS ONE* **2014**, *9*, e106873. [CrossRef] [PubMed]
24. Lore, N.I.; Iraqi, F.A.; Bragonzi, A. Host genetic diversity influences the severity of *Pseudomonas aeruginosa* pneumonia in the Collaborative Cross mice. *BMC Genet.* **2015**, *16*, 106. [CrossRef] [PubMed]
25. Papakonstantinou, E.; Karakiulakis, G. The 'sweet' and 'bitter' involvement of glycosaminoglycans in lung diseases: Pharmacotherapeutic relevance. *Br. J. Pharmacol.* **2009**, *157*, 1111–1127. [CrossRef] [PubMed]
26. Polverino, E.; Rosales-Mayor, E.; Dale, G.E.; Dembowsky, K.; Torres, A. The Role of Neutrophil Elastase Inhibitors in Lung Diseases. *Chest* **2017**, *152*, 249–262. [CrossRef] [PubMed]
27. Walsh, R.L.; Dillon, T.J.; Scicchitano, R.; McLennan, G. Heparin and heparan sulphate are inhibitors of human leucocyte elastase. *Clin. Sci.* **1991**, *81*, 341–346. [CrossRef] [PubMed]
28. Doring, G.; Bragonzi, A.; Paroni, M.; Akturk, F.F.; Cigana, C.; Schmidt, A.; Gilpin, D.; Heyder, S.; Born, T.; Smaczny, C.; et al. BIIL 284 reduces neutrophil numbers but increases *P. aeruginosa* bacteremia and inflammation in mouse lungs. *J. Cyst. Fibros.* **2014**, *13*, 156–163. [CrossRef] [PubMed]
29. Yonker, L.M.; Cigana, C.; Hurley, B.P.; Bragonzi, A. Host-pathogen interplay in the respiratory environment of cystic fibrosis. *J. Cyst. Fibros.* **2015**, *14*, 431–439. [CrossRef] [PubMed]
30. Lore, N.I.; Bragonzi, A.; Cigana, C. The IL-17A/IL-17RA axis in pulmonary defence and immunopathology. *Cytokine Growth Factor Rev.* **2016**, *30*, 19–27. [CrossRef] [PubMed]
31. Guragain, M.; King, M.M.; Williamson, K.S.; Perez-Osorio, A.C.; Akiyama, T.; Khanam, S.; Patrauchan, M.A.; Franklin, M.J. The *Pseudomonas aeruginosa* PAO1 Two-Component Regulator CarSR Regulates Calcium Homeostasis and Calcium-Induced Virulence Factor Production through Its Regulatory Targets CarO and CarP. *J. Bacteriol.* **2016**, *198*, 951–963. [CrossRef] [PubMed]
32. Plotkowski, M.C.; Costa, A.O.; Morandi, V.; Barbosa, H.S.; Nader, H.B.; de Bentzmann, S.; Puchelle, E. Role of heparan sulphate proteoglycans as potential receptors for non-piliated *Pseudomonas aeruginosa* adherence to non-polarised airway epithelial cells. *J. Med. Microbiol.* **2001**, *50*, 183–190. [CrossRef] [PubMed]
33. Bucior, I.; Pielage, J.F.; Engel, J.N. *Pseudomonas aeruginosa* pili and flagella mediate distinct binding and signaling events at the apical and basolateral surface of airway epithelium. *PLoS Pathog.* **2012**, *8*, e1002616. [CrossRef] [PubMed]
34. Cigana, C.; Curcuru, L.; Leone, M.R.; Ierano, T.; Lore, N.I.; Bianconi, I.; Silipo, A.; Cozzolino, F.; Lanzetta, R.; Molinaro, A.; et al. *Pseudomonas aeruginosa* exploits lipid A and muropeptides modification as a strategy to lower innate immunity during cystic fibrosis lung infection. *PLoS ONE* **2009**, *4*, e8439. [CrossRef] [PubMed]
35. Cigana, C.; Lore, N.I.; Bernardini, M.L.; Bragonzi, A. Dampening Host Sensing and Avoiding Recognition in *Pseudomonas aeruginosa* Pneumonia. *J. Biomed. Biotechnol.* **2011**, *2011*, 852513. [CrossRef] [PubMed]
36. Bragonzi, A.; Paroni, M.; Nonis, A.; Cramer, N.; Montanari, S.; Rejman, J.; Di Serio, C.; Doring, G.; Tummler, B. *Pseudomonas aeruginosa* microevolution during cystic fibrosis lung infection establishes clones with adapted virulence. *Am. J. Respir. Crit. Care Med.* **2009**, *180*, 138–145. [CrossRef] [PubMed]
37. Naggi, A.; Casu, B.; Perez, M.; Torri, G.; Cassinelli, G.; Penco, S.; Pisano, C.; Giannini, G.; Ishai-Michaeli, R.; Vlodavsky, I. Modulation of the heparanase-inhibiting activity of heparin through selective desulfation, graded *N*-acetylation, and glycol splitting. *J. Biol. Chem.* **2005**, *280*, 12103–12113. [CrossRef] [PubMed]

38. Bertini, S.; Bisio, A.; Torri, G.; Bensi, D.; Terbojevich, M. Molecular weight determination of heparin and dermatan sulfate by size exclusion chromatography with a triple detector array. *Biomacromolecules* **2005**, *6*, 168–173. [CrossRef] [PubMed]
39. Kukavica-Ibrulj, I.; Facchini, M.; Cigana, C.; Levesque, R.C.; Bragonzi, A. Assessing *Pseudomonas aeruginosa* virulence and the host response using murine models of acute and chronic lung infection. *Methods Mol. Biol.* **2014**, *1149*, 757–771. [PubMed]
40. Yang, Y.; MacLeod, V.; Dai, Y.; Khotskaya-Sample, Y.; Shriver, Z.; Venkataraman, G.; Sasisekharan, R.; Naggi, A.; Torri, G.; Casu, B.; et al. The syndecan-1 heparan sulfate proteoglycan is a viable target for myeloma therapy. *Blood* **2007**, *110*, 2041–2048. [CrossRef] [PubMed]
41. Poli, M.; Asperti, M.; Naggi, A.; Campostrini, N.; Girelli, D.; Corbella, M.; Benzi, M.; Besson-Fournier, C.; Coppin, H.; Maccarinelli, F.; et al. Glycol-split nonanticoagulant heparins are inhibitors of hepcidin expression in vitro and in vivo. *Blood* **2014**, *123*, 1564–1573. [CrossRef] [PubMed]
42. Cassinelli, G.; Lanzi, C.; Tortoreto, M.; Cominetti, D.; Petrangolini, G.; Favini, E.; Zaffaroni, N.; Pisano, C.; Penco, S.; Vlodavsky, I.; et al. Antitumor efficacy of the heparanase inhibitor SST0001 alone and in combination with antiangiogenic agents in the treatment of human pediatric sarcoma models. *Biochem. Pharmacol.* **2013**, *85*, 1424–1432. [CrossRef] [PubMed]
43. Bragonzi, A.; Worlitzsch, D.; Pier, G.B.; Timpert, P.; Ulrich, M.; Hentzer, M.; Andersen, J.B.; Givskov, M.; Conese, M.; Doring, G. Nonmucoid *Pseudomonas aeruginosa* expresses alginate in the lungs of patients with cystic fibrosis and in a mouse model. *J. Infect. Dis.* **2005**, *192*, 410–419. [CrossRef] [PubMed]
44. Baldan, R.; Cigana, C.; Testa, F.; Bianconi, I.; De Simone, M.; Pellin, D.; Di Serio, C.; Bragonzi, A.; Cirillo, D.M. Adaptation of *Pseudomonas aeruginosa* in Cystic Fibrosis airways influences virulence of *Staphylococcus aureus* in vitro and murine models of co-infection. *PLoS ONE* **2014**, *9*, e89614. [CrossRef] [PubMed]

14

Inhaled Antibiotic Therapy in Chronic Respiratory Diseases

Diego J. Maselli [1,2], Holly Keyt [1,2] and Marcos I. Restrepo [1,2,*]

1 Division of Pulmonary Diseases & Critical Care Medicine, South Texas Veterans Health Care System, San Antonio, TX 78229, USA; masellicacer@uthscsa.edu (D.J.M.); keyt@uthscsa.edu (H.K.)
2 University of Texas Health at San Antonio, San Antonio, TX 78240, USA
* Correspondence: restrepom@uthscsa.edu

Academic Editor: Francesco B. Blasi

Abstract: The management of patients with chronic respiratory diseases affected by difficult to treat infections has become a challenge in clinical practice. Conditions such as cystic fibrosis (CF) and non-CF bronchiectasis require extensive treatment strategies to deal with multidrug resistant pathogens that include *Pseudomonas aeruginosa*, Methicillin-resistant *Staphylococcus aureus*, *Burkholderia* species and non-tuberculous *Mycobacteria* (NTM). These challenges prompted scientists to deliver antimicrobial agents through the pulmonary system by using inhaled, aerosolized or nebulized antibiotics. Subsequent research advances focused on the development of antibiotic agents able to achieve high tissue concentrations capable of reducing the bacterial load of difficult-to-treat organisms in hosts with chronic respiratory conditions. In this review, we focus on the evidence regarding the use of antibiotic therapies administered through the respiratory system via inhalation, nebulization or aerosolization, specifically in patients with chronic respiratory diseases that include CF, non-CF bronchiectasis and NTM. However, further research is required to address the potential benefits, mechanisms of action and applications of inhaled antibiotics for the management of difficult-to-treat infections in patients with chronic respiratory diseases.

Keywords: aerosols; cystic fibrosis; bronchiectasis; nontuberculous mycobacteria

---

1. Introduction

Chronic respiratory diseases that produce bronchiectasis are associated with difficult-to-treat infections that create a real challenge in clinical practice. Difficult-to-treat infections due to multidrug-resistant (MDR) pathogens cause great concern for physicians, caregivers and patients, because these infections are associated with high morbidity, mortality and healthcare system cost. One of the cornerstones of the management of serious and difficult-to-treat infections is the use of antibiotics [1–6]. However, the emergence of antimicrobial-resistant pathogens, the lack of newly-developed therapies, and the high cost associated with management of these infections represent major challenges in the care of patients with chronic respiratory diseases.

Patients with chronic respiratory diseases such as cystic fibrosis (CF) and non-CF bronchiectasis may be affected by complex infections by *Pseudomonas aeruginosa*, Methicillin-resistant *Staphylococcus aureus*, *Burkholderia* species and non-tuberculous *Mycobacteria* (NTM) [1–6]. Currently, there are limited alternatives available for the management of patients with these serious infections. Inhaled antibiotics have been used to treat respiratory tract infections for several decades [7]. Advantages of inhaled antibiotic administration include the potential to deliver higher drug concentrations at the site of infection without the systemic adverse effects observed with the use of parenteral or oral antibiotic agents. However, clinical and technical issues have limited the advancement of the science in this area of research. Over the past decades there has been increasing interest in development of inhaled antibiotics that may help with the management of (MDR) pathogens, particularly those that are difficult to eradicate or that have a high chance of recurrence. Adjunctive therapies that combine inhaled and systemic antibiotics may potentially increase the efficacy of these medications in the care of patients with MDR pathogens and chronic respiratory disease. This narrative review will describe the currently available evidence regarding the use of inhaled antibiotics for the treatment of difficult-to-treat infections in patients with chronic respiratory diseases that include CF, non-CF bronchiectasis and NTM pulmonary infections.

2. Cystic Fibrosis

Cystic fibrosis (CF) is a multisystem autosomal recessive disorder affecting approximately 70,000 people worldwide and 30,000 people in the United States (US) [8]. CF is caused by dysfunction of the cystic fibrosis transmembrane conductance regulator (CFTR) protein, an ion channel located on the apical surface of epithelial cells which is responsible for chloride and bicarbonate transport across the cell membrane [9]. The results of CFTR dysfunction are abnormally thick and viscous secretions in the airways and impaired mucociliary clearance. The natural history of CF is characterized by recurrent lower-respiratory tract infections, often caused by drug-resistant pathogens such as *S. aureus*, *P. aeruginosa*, *Burkholderia cepacia* complex, *Stenotrophomonas maltophilia*, and others [8]. Recurrent infections contribute to a cycle of chronic inflammation, airway destruction and the development of bronchiectasis, leading ultimately to progressive decline in lung function.

However, with advances in diagnostic and therapeutic techniques, patients with CF have an increasing life span [10]. In 2014, there were more adults alive with CF than children for the first time. Inhaled antibiotic therapy has significantly contributed to improved survival [8]. Generally, inhaled antibiotics have been shown to improve lung function, delay decline in lung function, prolong time to exacerbations and improve quality of life in people with CF [10]. Despite these improvements, there is more work to be done: CF continues to cause mortality at an early age; the median predicted survival age in the US in 2015 was 41.6 years [8]. The most common cause of death in patients with CF continues to be respiratory/cardiorespiratory disease, mostly related to infectious complications [8].

One of the most prevalent pathogens in the CF airway is *P. aeruginosa* [8]. More than half of patients in the US with CF have at least one strain of *P. aeruginosa*, including MDR *P. aeruginosa*. However, the prevalence of *P. aeruginosa* has declined over the past decades. Advances in delivery and the increased availability of inhaled antibiotics, as well as the widespread implementation of therapy to eradicate initial acquisition of *P. aeruginosa*, has contributed to this decline [1,11]. As the prevalence of *P. aeruginosa* has decreased, there has been a sharp rise in the prevalence of *S. aureus* in CF airways, including methicillin-resistant *S. aureus* (MRSA). *S. aureus* is now the most prevalent organism in the CF airway. From 2000 to 2015, the prevalence of MRSA increased five-fold with most strains being hospital-acquired infections (approximately two-thirds), compared to community-acquired infections (approximately one-third) [8,12–14]. Other common pathogens causing respiratory illness in patients with CF include *Haemophilus influenzae*, which is more common in infants and young patients, *S. maltophilia*, *Achromobacter* species and *B. cepacia* complex [8] (Table 1). More than 10% of patients with CF have cultures positive for mycobacterial species [8].

Table 1. Common pathogens in patients with cystic fibrosis (CF) and median age of first infection (CFFPR 2015).

Pathogen	Percent with Infection	Median Age in Years at First Infection
S. aureus	70.6	3.6
P. aeruginosa	47.5	5.5
methicillin-resistant *S. aureus* (MRSA)	26.0	11.9
H. influenzae	15.5	2.6
S. maltophilia	13.6	10.0
multi-drug resistant *P. aeruginosa* (MDR-PA)	9.2	22.4
Achromobacter sp.	6.1	14.3
B. cepacia complex	2.6	19.9

2.1. *Pseudomonas aeruginosa* and Cystic Fibrosis (CF)

P. aeruginosa is the most common pathogen in the airways of patients with CF and is associated with accelerated decline in lung function as well as higher morbidity and mortality [15,16]. Infections due to *P. aeruginosa* range in severity from colonization without an immunologic response to severe pneumonia. However, once acquired, *P. aeruginosa* is difficult to eradicate and patients frequently become chronically infected [1,17]. Over time *P. aeruginosa* strains undergo a phenotypic change to the mucoid phenotype, characterized by production of alginate and associated with even greater difficulty in eradication of the pathogen [1,17]. The Leeds criteria were developed to help researchers describe *P. aeruginosa* infections in patients [18]. By this system, chronic infection is defined as having more than 50% of cultures positive for *P. aeruginosa* in the prior year. In 2015, 30% of patients in the US had chronic *P. aeruginosa* infection [8]. That same year, 17% of patients had intermittent *P. aeruginosa* infection (<50% of cultures positive for *P. aeruginosa*), 29% were free from *P. aeruginosa* in the prior year, and 18% had never had a positive *P. aeruginosa* culture. Chronic infection is associated with increased morbidity and mortality in patients with CF and the natural history of these infections is punctuated by periods of acute pulmonary exacerbations. Currently, the only US FDA-approved indication for inhaled antibiotics is for chronic *P. aeruginosa* infection in patients with CF.

2.2. Systemic vs. Inhaled Antibiotics

There are several systemic antipseudomonal agents available for use including extended-spectrum penicillins, aminoglycosides, cephalosporins, fluoroquinolones, monobactams, and others. The most commonly used systemic regimens for treatment of *P. aeruginosa* infections consist of intravenous (IV) β-lactams combined with aminoglycosides [19]. The rationale for combined treatment is based on the knowledge that *P. aeruginosa* strains develop resistance to antimicrobial agents relatively easily [15]. There is a lack of high-quality evidence demonstrating a clear benefit of this approach, nonetheless, it is considered to be standard of care in the US and recommended by the CF Pulmonary Guidelines Treatment of Pulmonary Exacerbations [3].

Systemic delivery of antipseudomonal antibiotics exposes patients to the potential for significant toxicity. For example, tobramycin is an aminoglycoside commonly administered IV for treatment of acute exacerbations of CF. However, IV tobramycin does not penetrate well into the sputum, at a peak reaching only approximately 12% of serum levels. Because bactericidal effect can only be reliably produced with concentrations 25 times the minimum inhibitory concentration (MIC), high doses are required to achieve concentrations inhibitory to *P. aeruginosa* in the airway [20]. These high doses increase the risk of systemic adverse events such as nephrotoxicity and ototoxicity [10,21]. IV administration of broad-spectrum antibiotics also disrupts the normal gut flora, increases risk for secondary infections such as *Clostridium difficile*, and may promote drug resistance [22].

The delivery of antibiotics via inhalation poses significant advantages for treating lower airway infections compared to systemic (oral or IV) therapy. Inhaled therapy allows for targeted delivery of high-concentrations of medications directly to intended the site of activity with minimal systemic absorption and toxicity [23]. In the 1980s, administration of tobramycin via inhalation for the treatment of infections caused by *P. aeruginosa* in CF patients resulted in higher concentrations of the drug at the site of activity with minimal systemic absorption [24,25]. Since then, additional antibiotics have been studied in patients with chronic PA infections, including: tobramycin (available as a solution for inhalation (TSI) or dry-powder inhaler (TIP)), aztreonam for inhalation solution (AZLI), colistin, and inhaled fluoroquinolones. With the increase in prevalence of *S. aureus* in the CF airway, there is a burgeoning increase in development of nebulized vancomycin as well.

These aerosolized antibiotics reduce the frequency of exacerbations, reduce airway bacterial density, improve pulmonary function, and improve quality of life in patients with CF [26]. Therefore, these medications are considered to be standard of care as part of chronic management of pulmonary disease associated with CF, and are recommended by the American Thoracic Society (ATS) in their CF Pulmonary Guidelines [2].

2.3. Tobramycin

Tobramycin, an aminoglycoside with activity against *P. aeruginosa*, was one of the first inhaled antibiotics studied in CF (Table 2). Systemic absorption of inhaled tobramycin is low and up to 95% of patients achieve a sputum concentration of drug at least 25 times the MIC, with a median serum/sputum concentration of 0.01 [27]. Such high concentrations are required for effective killing of *P. aeruginosa* because aminoglycosides bind to mucins in sputum and reduce the availability of effective antibiotic [27]. Tobramycin solution for inhalation (TSI) can be administered using the PARI LC PLUS® jet nebulizer and the DeVilbiss Pulmo-Aide® compressor in approximately 20 min or using the PARI eFlow® electronic nebulizer in approximately 7 min [28]. The drug is administered twice daily. It has been well-established that cyclic treatment with TSI is associated with improved pulmonary function, decreased sputum density, fewer hospitalizations and decreased need for systemic antibiotics.

A specific formulation of tobramycin for inhalation was developed in the 1980s and in landmark trials published in the early 1990s, patients with moderate-to-severe lung disease who were treated with TSI had significant improvements in forced expiratory volume in one second (FEV_1), reduced rates of hospitalization, and decreased hospitalization days compared to patients who received placebo [26,29,30]. Follow-up studies in younger patients and those with milder lung disease demonstrated that treatment with TSI twice daily for 28 days was safe and resulted in decreased density of *P. aeruginosa* in the lower airways, decreased rates of pulmonary exacerbations requiring hospitalization, but without significant impact on lung function [31,32].

The initial TSI trials established the practice of the intermittent 28-day "on/off" regimens for inhaled antibiotics. This design was based on the observation that there was minimal additional improvement in lung function after four weeks of therapy in conjunction with the concern for selection of resistant bacteria. However, in an early phase trial, patients treated with continuous tobramycin had improvement in lung function that remained above baseline for 12 weeks [33]. More recently, the use of continuous therapy either with a single agent or as alternating therapy, has increased in an effort to prevent exacerbations and decline in lung function [34]. A 28-week, multicenter, randomized, double-blind, placebo-controlled trial was conducted to evaluate the use of continuous alternating therapy with TSI and aztreonam compared to intermittent TSI alone [35]. The trial faced difficulty with enrolling patients and did not achieve statistical significance but suggested a potential benefit in reduction of pulmonary exacerbations (by 25%), rates of hospitalization (by 35%), treatment with non-study antibiotics and median time to first exacerbation (175 days vs. 140 days). Further studies are needed to determine the optimal duration of therapy and whether there is a benefit with continuous therapy.

The optimal regimen and duration of treatment for a first positive culture for *P. aeruginosa* is also unclear. The ELITE trial, a multicenter, open-label, randomized study was designed to answer this question in patients with newly-acquired *P. aeruginosa* infection [36]. Patients were randomized to 28 or 56 days of treatment with standard doses of TSI administered twice daily. More than 90% of patients had negative cultures for *P. aeruginosa* one month after the end of treatment without significant difference between the two groups. Patients also remained *P. aeruginosa*-free for more than two years after treatment with no significant difference in the median time to recurrence between the two groups [36].

The role of TSI in acute pulmonary exacerbations is unclear. Small retrospective studies have demonstrated no significant difference between treatment with inhaled or IV antipseudomonal antibiotics during acute exacerbations [37–39]. A small pilot study of 20 patients with CF patients chronically infected with *P. aeruginosa* compared 14 days of IV tobramycin vs. TSI 300 mg twice a day [40]. Although the study was small, there was a significant improvement in the time to next exacerbation requiring hospitalization in the TSI group (8.9, mean = 4.7 vs. 4.3, mean = 1.3 months; $p < 0.001$). Patients that received IV therapy developed higher levels of proteinuria and other markers of tubular injury compared to inhaled therapy. Of note, patients in the study were treated with twice- or thrice-daily dosing of IV tobramycin whereas once daily, extended-interval dosing is recommended by CF consensus guidelines based on specific evidence for decreased nephrotoxicity in children. Larger randomized controlled trials are lacking and therefore, current pulmonary guidelines recommend against this treatment approach.

TSI is generally well tolerated; the most common side effects include cough (41–88%), voice alteration (12–16%), and tinnitus (3%) [26,31,32,41]. Symptoms are typically transient and resolve with discontinuation of the medication. However, complaints of tinnitus may be one of the sentinel symptoms of cochlear toxicity and should be carefully evaluated.

Recently, tobramycin inhalation powder (TIP) has been evaluated as an alternative to TSI. The dry powder formulation uses a T-326 inhaler, has shorter administration time and decreases the potential for contamination of the device but with increased side effects and tolerability issues [28]. This type of formulation may be preferred by patients because of the shorter administration duration compared to TSI [42]. With respect to pharmacokinetic properties, similar medication levels were observed with 112 mg of tobramycin powder every 12 h compared to 300 mg of TSI [43]. Konstan et al. reported that TIP formulation was non-inferior to TSI in an open-label study of 553 patients with CF who were over the age of six [44]. Compared to TSI, TIP had similar efficacy in terms of lung function and sputum *P. aeruginosa* density but could be delivered much faster (5.6 min vs. 19.7 min; $p < 0.001$). The rates of cough and overall discontinuation of study drug were much higher in the TIP group, however, despite this, overall satisfaction and quality of life scores were higher in the group of patients who were able to tolerate and were subsequently assigned to the dry-powder formulation [44]. A study evaluated the safety of TIP after one year of exposure (7 cycles) in 62 patients with CF [45]. This presentation of tobramycin was overall well tolerated with no apparent serious adverse events. The most common side effects were cough (15%), impaired hearing (10%) and respiratory tract infections (10%). This safety profile is consistent with prior studies [44,46].

Table 2. Studies of inhaled tobramycin in CF patients with *P. aeruginosa* present in sputum.

Study/Year	Preparation	Dose/Frequency	Duration	Patient Population	Key Outcomes after Treatment
MacLusky 1989 [30]	TSI	80 mg/TID	32 months	$n = 27$	Stability in pulmonary function, controls showed decline
Smith 1989 [33]	TSI	600 mg/TID	12 weeks	$n = 22$	Improved symptoms, decrease in bacterial density
Ramsey 1993 [29]	TSI	600 mg/TID	12 weeks, 28 days on, 28 days off	$n = 71$	Improved pulmonary function
Ramsey 1999 [26]	TSI	300 mg/BID	24 weeks (on/off every 28 days)	$n = 520$	Improved pulmonary function and decreased hospitalizations
Gibson 2003 [31]	TSI	300 mg/BID	28 days	$n = 21$	Treatment reduced lower airway *P. aeruginosa* density
Murphy 2004 [32]	TSI	300 mg/BID	28 days on, 28 days off (7 cycles)	$n = 184$, mild lung disease	Decreased hospitalization rates
Konstan 2011 [44]	TIP or TSI	112 mg/BID or 300 mg/BID	28 days on, 28 days off (3 cycles)	$n = 517$	Comparable efficacy, but greater satisfaction with inhalation powder
Galeva 2013 [46]	TIP	112 mg/BID	28 days on, 28 days off (1 cycle)	$n = 62$	Trend towards improvement in the lung function

BID, twice daily; TID, three times daily; TSI, tobramycin solution for inhalation; TIP, tobramycin inhalation powder.

2.4. Aztreonam

Aztreonam is a monobactam antibiotic delivered intravenously or via inhalation, with activity against *P. aeruginosa* and other Gram-negative pathogens. Early randomized, double-blind, placebo-controlled trials conducted in patients with CF were short-term but demonstrated positive results with the use of aztreonam solution for inhalation compared to placebo (Table 3). McCoy et al. demonstrated in 211 patients with CF receiving intermittent inhaled tobramycin that administration of inhaled aztreonam twice or three times daily using the PARI eFlow (Altera)® electronic nebulizer for 28 days significantly increased time to next respiratory exacerbation compared to placebo (92 days vs. 71 days; $p = 0.002$), improved FEV_1 by 6.3–10.3%, and improved quality of life scores compared to placebo [47]. Retsch-Bogart et al. also demonstrated improvement in FEV_1 and quality of life scores, as well as a decrease in hospital days in patients using inhaled aztreonam compared to placebo (0.5 days vs. 1.5 days; $p = 0.049$) [48].

Given that the use of inhaled antipseudomonal antibiotics for patients with chronic *P. aeruginosa* infection is now well established, long-term, placebo-controlled trials of specific inhaled antibiotics are not feasible. However, a longer, 18-month, open label study in 195 patients with a mean age of 26 years, suggested that long-term use of inhaled aztreonam for 28 days every other month is safe and effective [49]. This study demonstrated improvement in pulmonary function and quality of life scores without an increase in resistance to aztreonam. The findings were more significant with three times a day use compared to twice a day [50]. In addition, a study of 273 individuals with CF aged six years or older demonstrated improved lung function and fewer exacerbations over three 28-day cycles of inhaled aztreonam compared with inhaled tobramycin [51]. These beneficial effects have not been observed in CF patients with other pathogens. For instance, a double-blind, randomized trial evaluated the effects of inhaled aztreonam three times daily for 24 weeks or placebo in 100 CF patients with chronic *B. cepacia* infection [52]. No significant differences were observed in lung function, exacerbation rates, use of antibiotics or hospitalizations. Until further studies are carried out, aztreonam is only recommended for CF patients with *P. aeruginosa* infection.

Inhaled aztreonam is generally well tolerated. The most commonly reported adverse reactions include cough (32–35%), headache (6–11%), bronchospasm (6–10%), nasal congestion (7–10%), nasal congestion (7–10%), and rhinorrhea (7%) [47,48,53]. There are reports of patients having bronchoconstriction with use and, therefore, providers should consider a monitored trial dose particularly in patients with severe lung disease.

Table 3. Studies of inhaled aztreonam in CF patients with *P. aeruginosa* present in sputum (or *Burkholderia* spp.).

Study	Preparation	Dose/Frequency	Duration	Patient Population	Key Outcomes after Treatment
McCoy 2008 [47]	AZLI	75 mg/BID or TID	28 days with 56 days of follow-up	*n* = 211, receiving inhaled tobramycin	Decreased exacerbation rates, improved lung function and respiratory symptoms
Retsch-Bogart 2009 [48]	AZLI	75 mg/TID	28 days	*n* = 164	Improved lung function and quality of life scores, and decreased number of hospital days
Oermann 2010 [49]	AZLI	75 mg/BID or TID	28 days on, 28 days off (up to 9 cycles)	*n* = 195	TID-treated patients demonstrated greater improvements in lung function and respiratory symptoms
Assael 2013 [51]	AZLI or TSI	75 mg/TID (AZLI) or 300 mg/BID (TSI)	28 days on, 28 days off (up to 9 cycles)	*n* = 273	AZLI-treated patients experienced improved lung function compared to TSI
Tullis 2014 [52]	AZLI	75 mg/TID	24 weeks	*n* = 100, *Burkholderia* spp. present in the sputum	No improvement in lung function
Flume (2016) [35]	AZLI + TSI	75 mg/TID + 300 mg/BID	Alternating 28 days of tobramycin, 28 days of aztreonam for 28 weeks	*n* = 90	Trend towards a reduction in exacerbations and hospitalizations

AZLI, aztreonam solution for inhalation; BID, twice a day; TID, three times a day; TSI, tobramycin solution for inhalation.

2.5. Colistin

Colistin belongs to the polymyxin group of antibiotics. It was first discovered in the mid-20th century as a fermentation product of the bacteria *Bacillus colistinus* and acts as a deterrent to interfere with the structure and function of bacterial cell walls [54]. Colistin is bactericidal and active against Gram negative bacteria including *P. aeruginosa*. Nebulized colistin is a preferred inhaled therapy for patients with CF and chronic *P. aeruginosa* in the United Kingdom and has been used for decades in Europe (Table 4). A prospective, double-blind, placebo-controlled study of 40 patients with CF, aged 7–35 years, compared three months of nebulized colistin to placebo and found that patients treated with colistin had improved symptom scores, slower decline in lung function and reduced inflammatory parameters [55]. Hodson et al. compared TSI and colistin in 115 patients with CF who were chronically infected with *P. aeruginosa*. Patients were randomized to receive TSI or colistin twice daily for four weeks [56]. Treatment with TSI resulted in a significant improvement in the primary endpoint of relative change in lung function compared to baseline. There was no significant improvement in the colistin-treated patients but both groups had significant decline in bacterial density [56].

Table 4. Studies of inhaled colistin in CF patients with *P. aeruginosa* present in sputum.

Study	Preparation	Dose/Frequency	Duration	Patient Population	Key Outcomes after Treatment
Jensen 1987 [55]	CSI	1 million units/BID	3 months	$n = 40$	Improvements in symptom scores and slower decline in lung function
Hodson 2002 [56]	CSI or TSI	80 mg/BID(CSI) or 300 mg/BID(TSI)	4 weeks	$n = 115$	TSI improved lung function but CSI did not. Both decreased bacterial load
Schuster 2013 [57]	CDP or TSI	1.6 million units/BID (CDP) or 300 mg/BID (TSI)	28 days on, 28 days off (3 cycles)	$n = 380$	CDP was non-inferior to TSI, but the primary endpoint regarding lung function was not reached

CSI, colistin solution for inhalation; CDP, colistin dry powder; TSI, tobramycin solution for inhalation; BID, twice a day.

Colistin has also been reformulated as a dry powder inhaler and was found to be non-inferior to TSI in a 24-week, randomized, non-blinded trial of 380 patients with CF [57]. However, both study groups failed to reach the primary endpoint of the trial, which was an improvement in FEV_1 [57].

The most significant adverse effect reported in association with nebulized colistin is bronchospasm. Bronchoconstriction with a transient decrease in FEV_1 has been reported in up to 17.7% of patients [56,58–60]. This can be mitigated by administration of a short-acting β-2 agonist prior to treatment. Colistin has not been approved for use in the US due to a report of a patient death associated with inhalation of pre-mixed solution of colistin. After mixing colistin with sterile water, it undergoes conversion to the bioactive form which has a component (polymyxin E1) that is toxic to lung tissue. Premixing colistin into aqueous solution and storing it for more than 24 h results in increased concentrations of polymyxin E1 and increased potential for toxicity [61]. Despite this, colistin is used in CF centers in the US for chronic *P. aeruginosa* infection.

2.6. Fluoroquinolones

Fluoroquinolones are important antipseudomonal antibiotics and inhaled preparations have been studied in CF patients with chronic *P. aeruginosa* infections (Table 5). Inhaled levofloxacin is the most recently introduced and is currently approved for use in Europe for patients with CF and chronic *P. aeruginosa* infection. Early trials compared varying doses of inhaled levofloxacin (120, 240 mg daily, 240 mg twice daily) to placebo in 151 patients and demonstrated a dose-dependent improvement in lung function and significant decrease in the incidence of acute pulmonary exacerbations over 28 days [62]. More recently, a phase 3, open-label randomized trial compared the safety and efficacy of levofloxacin 240 mg inhaled twice daily to standard doses of TSI in 282 patients with CF who were at least 12 years of age. Between the two groups, there was no difference in lung function or adverse effects at 28 days [63]. Flume et al. compared the safety and efficacy of a 28-day course of levofloxacin inhalation solution to placebo in a multinational, randomized, double-blind trial in 330 patients with CF. Although there was an improvement in the relative change in FEV_1 percent predicted from baseline (mean difference 1.31%, $p = 0.01$), there was in the patients randomized to levofloxacin compared to the placebo arm [64]. Possible explanations for these results include insufficient antibiotic concentrations, dissimilarities in the study populations or an inappropriate definition of an exacerbation. The most commonly reported adverse events with levofloxacin administration include cough, taste disturbances, tiredness or weakness. It is contraindicated in pregnant or breastfeeding patients, those with epilepsy and those with a history of tendon disorders related to the use of fluoroquinolone antibiotics.

Ciprofloxacin has been formulated into a dry powder for inhalation (DPI) [65,66] and a liposomal form [21,67], and because of its adequate tolerability profile and minimal systemic exposure it has been considered for the treatment of patients with chronic pulmonary conditions and *P. aeruginosa* infection. The DPI form of ciprofloxacin is delivered via a T-326 inhaler and employs the PulmoShere® technology, which uses an emulsion-based spray-drying process to produce highly dispersible low density particles [68]. Ciprofloxacin DPI has been tested in patients with CF with various results [69–72]. A phase 1, randomized, single-blind, placebo-controlled trial explored the effects of ciprofloxacin DPI in 25 patients with CF and chronic infection with *P. aeruginosa* [69]. Ciprofloxacin was detected at microbiological active concentrations (sputum) and no serious adverse events or changes in pulmonary function were reported. These results led to a phase 2b, randomized, double-blind, controlled trial that studied the effects ciprofloxacin DPI at 32.5 or 48.75 mg twice a day for 28 days or placebo in CF patients colonized with *P. aeruginosa* [71]. Patients treated with ciprofloxacin DPI did not achieve a significant improvement with either dose in FEV_1 from baseline compared to placebo ($p = 0.154$). The density of *P. aeruginosa* was lower after therapy in the treated group compared to placebo; the mean *P. aeruginosa* colony count expressed as $\log_{10}$ CFU/g was 6.73 vs. 7.08 for the 32.5 mg dose ($p < 0.001$) and 6.77 vs. 7.37 for the 48.75 mg dose ($p = 0.002$), but the effects were not sustained after four weeks of therapy. Additional phase 3 studies, with longer treatment duration are required before the role of inhaled ciprofloxacin in CF can be determined. The most common side effects reported with ciprofloxacin DPI are bitter taste (14–94%), bronchospasm (50–67%), headache (17–33%) and cough (3–17%) [69–71].

Table 5. Studies of inhaled fluoroquinolones in CF patients with *P. aeruginosa* present in sputum.

Study	Preparation	Dose/Frequency	Duration	Patient Population	Key Outcomes after Treatment
Geller 2011 [62]	LSI	120 or 240 mg daily or 240 mg BID	28 days	$n = 151$	Dose dependent increase in lung function and decrease in exacerbations
Stuart Elborn 2015 [63]	LSI or TSI	240 mg/BID (CSI) or 300 mg/BID (TSI)	28 days on, 28 days off (3 cycles)	$n = 282$	LSI was non-inferior to TSI with regards to lung function
Flume 2016 [64]	LSI	240 mg/BID	28 days	$n = 330$	Improvement in lung function but no difference in time to next exacerbation
Dorkin 2015 [71]	CiDP	32.5 mg or 48.75 mg/BID	28 days	$n = 286$	No significant improvements in lung function compared to placebo

BID, twice a day; CiDP, ciprofloxacin dry powder; LSI, levofloxacin solution for inhalation; TSI, tobramycin solution for inhalation.

3. Non-Cystic Fibrosis Bronchiectasis

Bronchiectasis is a permanent dilation of the airways often associated with chronic respiratory symptoms such as persistent cough, excessive sputum production and recurrent pulmonary infections [4]. In patients without cystic fibrosis (CF), the presence of bronchiectasis can be secondary to a wide range of conditions. Non-CF bronchiectasis (NCFB) has been linked to autoimmune diseases (i.e., rheumatoid arthritis), impaired secretion clearance (i.e., primary ciliary dyskinesia), immunodeficiency (i.e., common variable immunodeficiency), previous infections (i.e., *Mycobacterium tuberculosis*), preexisting pulmonary conditions (i.e., chronic obstructive pulmonary disease) and others [72]. While NCFB was previously considered a rare disease, in the past decades its prevalence has increased [73]. This is likely due to increased physician recognition and the widespread availability of computed tomography, but other factors such as antibiotic prescription practices, and environmental and geographical factors may be influencing these observations [74,75]. The prevalence of NCFB ranges from 500 to 1100 per 100,000 persons, and is more common among women and older individuals [63,76–78].

The pathophysiology of NCFB has been well characterized. In the susceptible host, an initial pulmonary insult (i.e., infection or inflammation) will result in a permanent dilation of the airways. These changes in the architecture the airways will affect normal airway secretion clearance.

The accumulation of mucus will in turn favor the development of infections, which lead to further inflammation and distortion of the airways. This concept is known as the "vicious cycle" of bronchiectasis [72]. Therefore, pulmonary infections play a pivotal role in the development and worsening of NCBF and their management plays an integral part in the care of these patients. The most common pathogens identified in patients with NCFB are *H. influenzae* (55–29%) and *P. aeruginosa* (28–12%), although in up to a fifth of cases a pathogen cannot be identified [79–83]. Other respiratory pathogens identified in patients with NCFB using cultures, quantitative polymerase chain reaction (PCR) technique, or by ribosomal gene pyrosequencing include *S. maltophilia*, *B. cepacia* complex, *M. catarrhalis*, *S. aureus*, and various species of *Prevotella* and *Veillonella* [81–83]. Most recently, the United States Bronchiectasis Research Registry ($n = 1826$) reported that 63% of the patients included in the cohort had evidence of non-tuberculous mycobacteria (NTM) [84]. The most common NTM isolated was *M. avium* complex, followed by *M abscessus/chelonae*. The patients that participated in this study originated from tertiary referral centers with an interest in NTM, which may explain the difference in the reported prevalence of NTM compared to studies from other parts of the world [84].

The type of organism identified in patients with NCFB has important implications. Patients with positive cultures for *P. aeruginosa* have worse outcomes compared to those with other pathogens [85–88]. For instance, a retrospective study exploring the clinical characteristics and outcomes of 539 patients with NCFB showed that those with positive sputum cultures with *P. aeruginosa* had worse pulmonary function compared to those with other pathogens [85]. Similar findings were reported in a prospective study of 142 patients, in which FEV_1 and diffusion of carbon monoxide were significantly lower in those with positive testing for *P. aeruginosa* [86]. A Spanish, single-center study of 76 patients with NCFB revealed that accelerated lung function decline was independently associated with chronic colonization with *P. aeruginosa* (odds ratio 30.4, 95% confidence interval 3.8 to 39.4, $p = 0.005$) [87]. Exploring the rates of health care utilization, a longitudinal retrospective observational cohort study of 155 patients with NCFB showed that hospital admissions were significantly higher in a *P. aeruginosa* infected group compared to patients infected with *H. influenzae* (1.3 vs. 0.7 admissions per year, $p = 0.035$) [88]. Moreover, the presence of *P. aeruginosa* has been linked to worse quality of life and greater risk for hospitalization [89,90]. There is also a strong association between increased mortality and the identification of *P. aeruginosa* in patients with NCFB [90,91]. Using a phenotypic cluster analysis based on a microbiologic analysis and the sputum production characteristics, a study showed that NCFB patients with chronic infection with *P. aeruginosa* had significantly more exacerbations, worse pulmonary function and quality of life, and increased markers of inflammation [92]. The reasons why *P. aeruginosa* has such a profound effect on patients with NCFB is multifactorial and related to its virulence factors. This pathogen can survive in wide fluctuations of pH, nutrient limitations and resists multiple classes of antibiotics [93,94]. A key feature of this organism is the ability to form a biofilm, which limits its exposure to host defense mechanisms and antibiotics [93,94]. For these reasons, patients with NCFB require cultures during routine visits as surveillance in addition to periods of exacerbation, as these not only may guide therapy, but may also identify patients at risk for poor outcomes [4].

Antimicrobial therapies continue to play a central role in the therapy of NCFB as maintenance and during exacerbations. Systemic antibiotics may have a higher toxicity profile, require intravenous access, and medical personnel are often employed for appropriate and safe delivery. Inhaled antibiotics are an attractive alternative for patients with pulmonary infections. The objective of inhaled antibiotics is to provide the highest concentrations of active drug at the site of infection without risking systemic toxicity. Various inhaled antibiotics have been studied in patients with NCBF with variable results and while both inhaled ciprofloxacin products are completing phase 3 trials, no inhaled antibiotics have been approved.

3.1. Tobramycin

The efficacy of tobramycin in patients with CF and *P. aeruginosa* infections, has led to various studies in NCFB cohorts (Table 6). An initial placebo-controlled, multicenter, double-blind, randomized study explored the efficacy and safety of tobramycin solution in 74 patients with NCFB and *P. aeruginosa* [95]. The patients in the treatment group ($n = 37$) had a significant decreased in the mean *P. aeruginosa* colony forming units (CFU) per gram of sputum compared to no change in the control group ($n = 37$). Additionally, *P. aeruginosa* was eradicated in 35% of patients in the treatment group with substantial improvement in clinical symptoms. No significant differences were observed in the development of tobramycin-resistant strains or in the pulmonary function test results. Patients that received inhaled tobramycin experienced more dyspnea (32% vs. 8%), cough (41% vs. 24%), wheezing (16% vs. 0%) and chest discomfort (19% vs. 0%) compared to placebo, but it did not limit the delivery of therapy. A subsequent study that explored the effects of three cycles of 14 days of tobramycin solution and 14 days off therapy in 41 patients with NCBF and a history of *P. aeruginosa* revealed improvements in the mean pulmonary total symptom severity scores (reduction of 1.5 units, $p = 0.006$) and St. George Respiratory Questionnaire scores (reduction of 9.8 units, $p < 0.001$) [96]. Notably, 22% of the patients withdrew from the study due to adverse events, which more commonly were respiratory: cough (43.9%), dyspnea (34.1%), and increased sputum production (29.3%). A double-blind, placebo-controlled study explored clinical outcomes in 30 patients with NCFB and chronic infection with *P aeruginosa* treated with 300 mg of aerosolized tobramycin or placebo twice daily in two cycles, each for six months, with a one-month washout period [97]. Despite the small sample size of the study, the investigators reported an improvement in the number of admissions (0.15 ± 0.37 vs. 0.75 ± 1.16, $p = 0.038$) and days of admission to the hospital (2.05 ± 5.03 vs. 12.65 ± 21.8, $p = 0.047$) compared to placebo, but no difference was observed in antibiotic use, number of exacerbations, pulmonary function or quality of life markers. Bronchospasm was the most frequently reported adverse event (13%), but responded well to bronchodilator therapy. In addition, inhaled tobramycin has been studied in addition to systemic antibiotics during an acute exacerbation of NCFB. A double-blind, multicenter study evaluated the effects of inhaled tobramycin solution or placebo in addition to oral ciprofloxacin in 53 NCFB patients and known *P. aeruginosa* infection during an acute exacerbation [98]. Patients who received double therapy had a trend towards greater rates of eradication (37.5% vs. 20%, $p = 0.18$) compared to single oral ciprofloxacin, but cure rates and relapse rates were similar in both groups. No systemic adverse reactions were observed, but respiratory adverse events (wheezing) were again reported more frequently in patients that received inhaled tobramycin compared to placebo (50% vs. 15%, $p < 0.01$). Based on the current evidence, the use of inhaled tobramycin cannot be recommended for patients with NCFB on a routine basis or during an exacerbation. Despite improvements in some clinical and microbiologic parameters, the studies have small sample sizes and with relatively short-lived exposures and it remains undetermined if prolonged courses of therapy may induce microbiologic resistance. Respiratory adverse events can be present in up to 50% of the patients and this may limit the use of this therapy, particularly in those patients with reactive airways diseases, such as asthma. Future studies, with larger sample sizes and more prolonged exposures that resemble clinical practice may identify subgroups of patients that have greater benefits while limiting adverse events.

Preliminary data suggest that tobramycin inhalation powder is well tolerated in NCFB, with cough being the most frequently encountered side effect (13%), but larger studies are still needed to evaluate the efficacy and optimal dose of this medication [99].

Table 6. Studies of inhaled tobramycin in NCFB patients with *P. aeruginosa* present in sputum.

Study/Year	Preparation	Dose/Frequency	Duration	Patient Population	Key Outcomes after Treatment
Barker 2000 [95]	TSI	300 mg/BID	28 days	$n = 74$	Decrease in bacterial load
Scheinberg 2005 [96]	TSI	300 mg/BID	14 days on, 14 days off (3 cycles)	$n = 41$	Improvements in respiratory symptoms
Drobnic 2005 [97]	TSI	300 mg/BID	6 months	$n = 30$	Improvement in the number of admissions and days of admission to the hospital
Bilton 2006 [98]	Oral ciprofloxacin or oral ciprofloxacin + TSI	750 mg/BID (ciprofloxacin) 300 mg/BID (TSI)	2 weeks	$n = 53$, with an acute exacerbation	Double therapy resulted in a trend towards greater rates of eradication, but cure rates and relapse rates were similar in both groups

BID, twice a day; TSI, tobramycin solution for inhalation.

3.2. Ciprofloxacin

Inhaled ciprofloxacin, both DPI [100] and liposomal form [101–104], has been studied in NCFB (Table 7). A multicenter, phase 2 study of 124 patients with NCFB and positive respiratory cultures for pre-defined potential pathogens received 28 days of DPI ciprofloxacin 32.5 mg twice a day against placebo [100]. Subjects in the treatment group ($n = 60$) had significantly increased rate of pathogen eradication (35% vs. 8%, $p = 0.001$) and an important reduction in total sputum bacterial load counts compared to placebo ($n = 64$). Importantly, a reduction CFUs was observed in subjects with *P. aeruginosa* and *H. influenzae*, the most common pathogens affecting NCFB patients. Adverse events were comparable in both groups, including bronchospasm, which occurred rarely (5.0% vs. 4.7%, $p = 1.0$).

Table 7. Studies of inhaled ciprofloxacin in NCFB patients with *P. aeruginosa* present in sputum.

Study/Year	Preparation	Dose/Frequency	Duration	Patient Population	Key Outcomes after Treatment
Wilson 2013 [100]	CiDP	32.5 mg/BID	28 days	$n = 24$	Reduction in the bacterial load
Bilton 2010 [101]	ILC	150 mg or 300 mg/daily	28 days	$n = 36$	Both doses resulted in a reduction in the bacterial load
Bilton 2011 [102]	ILC	100 mg or 150 mg/daily	28 days	$n = 96$	Both doses resulted in a reduction in the bacterial load
Serisier 2013 [103]	ILC + CiSI	150 mg (ILC) + 60 mg (CiSI)/daily	28 days on, 28 days off (3 cycles)	$n = 42$	Delayed time to first pulmonary exacerbation and reduction in the bacterial load
Haworth 2017 [104]	ILC + CiSI	150 mg (ILC) + 60 mg (CiSI)/daily	28 days on, 28 days off (6 cycles)	$n = 582$	Increase in the median time to first exacerbation that required antibiotics and a decrease in the annual rate of exacerbations (regardless of the need of antibiotics)

BID, twice daily; CiDP, ciprofloxacin dry powder; CiSI, ciprofloxacin solution for inhalation; ILC, inhaled liposomal ciprofloxacin.

The liposomal form of inhaled ciprofloxacin has potential advantages, including controlled and prolonged release of the drug at the site of action, protection against drug degradation, reduced systemic exposure and augmented cellular uptake [104]. This form of ciprofloxacin is delivered using a PARI LC Sprint® nebulizer and PARI TurboBoy-S® compressor [21,67]. A phase 2 study of 36 patients with NCFB explored the effects of once a day inhaled liposomal ciprofloxacin at two different doses for 28 days [105]. Both doses (150 and 300 mg) were effective at reducing *P. aeruginosa* CFUs in the sputum compared to baseline measures by 3.5 log ($p < 0.001$) and 4.0 log ($p < 0.001$) units, respectively. Patients tolerated the study drug well [101]. Similar findings were observed in a multicenter, randomized, double-blind, placebo-controlled trial (ORBIT-1) of inhaled liposomal ciprofloxacin (100 or 150 mg) for 28 days in 96 NCFB patients [102]. Patients of both treatment arms exhibited significant decrease in *P. aeruginosa* CFUs compared to placebo and the medication was well tolerated. These results lead to the development of a phase 2, multicenter, randomized study (ORBIT-2) testing the effects of inhaled liposomal (150 mg) and free (60 mg) ciprofloxacin or placebo on 42 NCFB patients with more than two bronchiectasis exacerbations in the previous year and positive cultures for *P. aeruginosa* at the time of screening [103]. Compared to placebo ($n = 22$), treatment with inhaled liposomal ciprofloxacin ($n = 20$) delayed time to first pulmonary exacerbation (median 134 vs. 58 days, $p = 0.057$), significantly decreased the sputum bacterial density of *P. aeruginosa* (-4.2 ± 3.7 vs. -0.08 ± 3.8 $\log_{10}$ CFU/g, $p = 0.02$), and had a similar adverse effect profile. Two identical trials, ORBIT-3 and ORBIT-4, that included 582 NCFB patients with chronic infection of *P. aeruginosa*, compared the effects of placebo and 48 weeks of the combination of inhaled liposomal (150 mg) and free ciprofloxacin (60 mg) in a 28 days on and 28 days off regimen for six cycles [99]. Patients treated with the liposomal ciprofloxacin had an increase in the median time to first exacerbation that required antibiotics and a decrease in the annual rate of exacerbations (regardless of the need of antibiotics) compared to placebo [99]. As with previous trials, inhaled liposomal ciprofloxacin was associated with reduction in the bacterial load. No improvements in lung function were observed and the treatment was well tolerated with similar rates of adverse events in both study groups [104]. Taking into consideration the findings of the recent trails, inhaled ciprofloxacin has been associated with reductions in the bacterial load and improvement in important clinical outcomes. Hence, inhaled liposomal ciprofloxacin is an attractive treatment option for NCFB for with chronic infection of *P. aeruginosa*.

3.3. Other Antibiotics

There is a paucity of studies evaluating inhaled antibiotics other than tobramycin and ciprofloxacin in NCFB. A randomized study evaluated the use of nebulized gentamycin (80 mg) twice daily for 12 months compared to placebo in 65 patients with NCFB [106]. Important inclusion criteria were: positive pathogenic bacteria isolated from sputum cultures, at least two exacerbations the prior year, ability to tolerate nebulized gentamicin, and no chronic use of antibiotics [106]. Inhaled gentamycin was studied using gentamicin injectable solution reconstituted for nebulization using 0.9% saline and the Porta-Neb Ventstream® nebulizer. At the end of the study, the treatment group had higher rates of eradication of *P. aeruginosa* and other respiratory pathogens compared to placebo (30.8% vs. 8.7% and 92.8% vs. 38.5%, $p < 0.001$). Additionally, patients treated with gentamycin experienced fewer exacerbations, had an increased time to first exacerbation, and had improvements in symptom scores. Despite these improvements, none of the treatment effects were sustained after three-month treatment-free follow-up period [106].

The use of aztreonam for inhalation solution has been shown to be effective in patients with CF [47,48]. Because of these observations, two identical randomized multicenter phase 3 trials (AIR-BX1 and AIR-BX2) were designed to evaluate the effects of inhaled aztreonam for four weeks or placebo in patients with NCFB [107]. For this study the Altera® Nebulizer System was used to deliver the study drug. All of the 540 patients included in the trials had positive sputum for susceptible Gram-negative pathogens. Although patients exposed to aztreonam had decrease in sputum bacterial density, this did not translate into significant improvements in respiratory symptoms or time to exacerbation. Adverse events were more frequently reported in the aztreonam groups compared to placebo: dyspnea (46% vs. 35%, $p < 0.01$) and fatigue (30% vs. 20%, $p < 0.01$). The discrepancies between the aztreonam CF studies and the results from the AIR-BX1 and AIR-BX2 trials may be due to suboptimal dosing schemes, different airway clearance regimens, and potential overlap with other diseases in older NCFB patients.

Inhaled colistin has gained interest for the treatment of NCFB because of its antipseudomonal properties. A study explored the effects of inhaled colistin (1 million IU twice a day for six months) vs. placebo in 144 NCFB patients and chronic infection with *P. aeruginosa* [108]. Colistin was studied using the I-neb® adaptive aerosol delivery device, which monitors the time and peak flow of the initial three breaths during the nebulization and then delivers therapy intermittently at the start of inspiration to optimize drug delivery [109]. Using this device, therapy is completed in approximately three minutes. The use of inhaled colistin failed to meet the primary endpoint of time to exacerbation versus placebo (165 days vs. 111 days, $p = 0.11$) [108]. In a post-hoc analysis, in those patients considered adherent to therapy, inhaled colistin reduced the median time to exacerbation (168 days vs. 103 days, $p = 0.038$) and improved respiratory symptoms. Adverse events were similar in both study arms (total adverse events: 64% in the colistin group vs. 54% in the placebo group, $p = 0.25$) [108]. In another study, colistin (1 million IU twice a day for 12 months) was compared to conventional therapy in 39 patients with NCFB and chronic infection with *P. aeruginosa* [110]. Patients that received therapy did not experience any improvement in exacerbation rates. Notably, 25% of the patients of the treatment group stopped the therapy due to adverse effects, mainly respiratory. The discrepancies of tolerability between these two studies may be related to the age of the patients included (mean age 59.2 years vs. 77.7 years) and the duration of the study (6 months vs. 12 months) [108,110]. Future, longer duration studies with an emphasis on dose ranging are still needed to understand the potential benefits of inhaled gentamycin, aztreonam and colistin in NCFB. Based on the current evidence these therapies cannot be recommend for routine use in patient with NCFB.

4. Non-Tuberculous Mycobacteria

Nontuberculous mycobacteria (NTM) are common pathogens found in the environment and isolated from many parts of the world [111]. Over past decades increasing rates of human disease secondary to NTMs have been reported [112–114]. NTMs could affect multiple organs, but pulmonary disease is the most common reason for clinical symptoms as a result of NTM inhalation. However, not always the identification of NTMs determine pulmonary disease. Several scientific organizations have published evidence based guidelines for the diagnosis and management of NTM disease [5,6]. The distribution of NTM species varies according to the geographic reasons, but most of the published data are reported from Europe (United Kingdom), North America (United States of America and Canada), Israel and Japan. The most commonly identified NTM that causes lung disease are *Mycobacterium avium* complex (MAC), *M. abscessus* complex (MABSC) and *M. kansasii*. In the US, inhaled antibiotics are used in up to 10% of the patients with NTM infections [84].

NTM infection are commonly found in patients with risk factors such as chronic lung diseases such as COPD, asthma, alpha-1 antitrypsin deficiency, CF, non-CFB, primary ciliary dyskinesia, and allergic bronchopulmonary aspergillosis [112]. However, patients without pre-existing lung disease such as the classic report of "Lady Windermere Syndrome", that occurs in white, tall, thin women with pectum excavatum and mitral valve prolapse has been described. These patients usually present with a middle lobe syndrome with bronchiectasis. In addition, NTM lung disease has been found in conditions such as GERD, immunodeficiency and the use of some medications (e.g., immunosuppressive medications, proton pump inhibitors) [84]. Several studies suggest that patients with CF bronchiectasis managed with inhaled antibiotics may be prone to NTM infection. The exact mechanism is unclear, but microbiome balance may play a role, and changes induced by inhaled antibiotics may promote the emergence of NTM in patients with CF, that were initially suppressed by other bacterial species that competed for the same lung environment. However, a study that included 30 MABSC cases and 60 NTM negative CF patients found no association between inhaled antibiotics and MABSC infection [115].

Treatment of pulmonary NTM, especially *M. abscessus*, is complex, requiring multiple systemic antibiotics for long periods of time. However, there is important toxicity and limited efficacy adds to the level of complexity in patients who do not respond to initial therapy, and who have refractory disease or recurrence. The data regarding the use of inhaled antibiotics for patients with NTM is limited. Olivier et al. identified 20 patients with bronchiectasis treated with inhaled amikacin for refractory NTM lung disease [116]. The dosing scheme selected used consisted of an initial dose of 250 mg once daily, followed by 250 mg twice daily after two weeks if no dysphonia was reported. Patients were then told to increase the dose to 500 mg twice daily after two weeks if tolerated. The patients had positive cultures for *M. abscessus* ($n = 15$) and MAC ($n = 5$). The patients received a median of duration therapy of 60 months (ranges from 6 to 190 months) and a follow-up of 19 months. Forty percent of patients had a least one culture, but only 25% (5/20 patients) had persistent negative cultures throughout the follow up period. Symptomatology improved, unchanged and worsened in 45%, 35% and 20%, respectively. Radiological worsening on chest CT scans was noted in 55%, with improvement in 30% and no change in 15%, respectively. Adverse events limited the continuation of inhaled amikacin in seven patients (35%), mainly due to ototoxicity (10%), hemoptysis (10%), and less commonly nephrotoxicity, persistent dysphonia and vertigo (one patient for each adverse event). This observational study suggests that in patients who fail standard systemic therapy, the use of inhaled amikacin may bring some benefit, but with an important rate of adverse events, that should be explained to the patients [116]. Some experts, recommend inhaled amikacin as a step-down therapy in patients presenting drug toxicity with systemic antibiotics. The British Thoracic Society Guidelines currently available for public consultation recommend that MABSC lung disease patients should receive an initial phase of systemic antibiotic treatment followed by a continuation phase of a combined regimen of inhaled and/or oral antibiotics. The recommendation was graded D based on evidence level 3 or 4 (e.g., non-analytical studies, case series, case reports and expert opinion). In conclusion, inhaled amikacin should be considered in place of IV amikacin when systemic administration is impractical, contraindicated or long-term treatment with aminoglycosides is required, particularly for patients with pulmonary disease due to MABSC, MAC, *M. xenopi*, and *M. malmoense*, For patients with CF, the CF foundation and the ECFS [6] recommend that the continuation phase with oral macrolide therapy should be combined with inhaled amikacin and in addition 2–3 oral antibiotics such as minocycline, clofazimine, moxifloxacin, and linezolid.

Recent hope has been given to a novel formulation of liposomal amikacin that may prevent the adverse events related to free amikacin. Rose et al. investigated the activity of an inhaled formulation of liposomal amikacin in an in vitro and in vivo murine model of NTM infection [117]. Macrophage monolayers were infected with MAC and MABSC and treated with liposomal amikacin vs. free amikacin for four days assessing bacterial survival. The authors found that liposomal amikacin was more effective in eliminating intracellular MAC and MABSC compared to free amikacin [117]. In the in vivo model, inhaled liposomal amikacin showed similar reduction of MAC in the lungs as systemic amikacin and no development of acquired resistance [117]. Olivier KN and collaborators performed a double-blind phase II randomized controlled trial that assessed the efficacy and safety of once-daily (590 mg) inhaled liposomal amikacin for the treatment of MAC and MABSC lung disease compared to placebo [118]. The modified intent-to-treat analysis of 89 patients with MAC or MABSC showed that despite the primary endpoint of baseline to Day 84 change on a semiquantitative mycobacterial growth scale was not achieved. Improvement of other endpoints such as sputum conversion, six-minute-walk distance and limited systemic toxicity were observed among subjects refractory MAC lung disease treated with inhaled liposomal amikacin versus placebo [118].

Most recently, the applications of liposomal ciprofloxacin in NTM have been investigated in pre-clinical studies. The efficacy of two different formulations inhaled liposomal ciprofloxacin, Dual Release Ciprofloxacin for Inhalation (DRCFI) and Ciprofloxacin for Inhalation (CFI), was compared to a non-liposomal ciprofloxacin solution and empty liposomes (control) in mice infected intranasally with MAC subspecies Hominissuis [119]. One week after infection, the different formulations were administered intranasally daily for three weeks. Treatment DRCFI or CFI resulted in significant reduction in CFUs from $(1.1 \pm 0.5) \times 10^7$ to $(2.5 \pm 0.6) \times 10^6$ and $(2.3 \pm 0.4) \times 10^6$, respectively. Treatment with the solution of non-liposomal ciprofloxacin and empty liposomes resulted in no changes in the bacterial load. A subsequent, in vitro study demonstrated that a CFI was able to inhibit MAC subspecies *Hominissuis* microaggregates and biofilm formation on plastic surfaces and cultured epithelial cells, providing further evidence of the antimicrobial properties of this preparation [120]. Similar reductions in biofilm formation after treatment with liposomal ciprofloxacin were observed in macrophage monolayers infected with *M. avium*, *M. abscessus* and MAC subspecies *hominissuis* [121]. These observations are promising and warrant further in vivo study, particularly given the urgent need for therapeutic alternatives in these difficult to eradicate pathogens.

In conclusion, there are limited data regarding the use of inhaled antibiotics for the management of patients with NTM pulmonary infections. However, as suggested previously, clinicians treating NTM pulmonary infections should consider the use of inhaled antibiotics when systemic administration is impractical or impossible, aminoglycosides are contraindicated due to systemic adverse effects, long term therapies are needed or palliation of symptoms is the goal of treatment.

5. Future Directions

The use of inhaled antibiotics has increased over the last decades in respiratory conditions and the scope of their use is still not completely understood in CF, NCFB and NTM pulmonary infections. In CF, there is an increased interest in the applications of inhaled antibiotics to treat Gram-positive infections given the increase rate of these infections [8]. For instance, an ongoing, double-blind, comparator-controlled, randomized study will evaluate the use of nebulized vancomycin vs. placebo in CF patients with chronic infection with MRSA [122]. Another area of interest is the effects of combining different types of antibiotics. Post hoc analyses of a dataset of previous trial of CF patients treated with tobramycin explored the effects of concomitant use oral azithromycin by study subjects on clinical outcomes [123,124]. Azithromycin was shown to potentially reduce the antimicrobial effects of tobramycin possibly by inducing bacterial stress responses [123,124]. These results have important implications as a significant number of patients with CF utilize oral macrolides and inhaled antibiotics. Future studies are still required to elucidate the complex interactions that may occur with the combination of antibiotics.

Although the results of the recent trials regarding the benefit of inhaled antibiotics in NCFB have not led to the routine use of these therapies, there are still areas of uncertainty that deserve further evaluation. NCBF is a heterogeneous disease and further classifying patients beyond the chronic infection (or not) of *P. aeruginosa* might be required to identify better target subgroups [92]. Adverse events may limit the use of some of these antibiotics, particularly in the elderly, so dose ranging studies and better patient selection algorithms are still warranted. There has been success with oral macrolides in the reduction of exacerbation rates patients with NCFB, however it is unclear the effect of these chronic antibiotic administration on the microbiome [125,126]. Future studies may explore the use of inhaled antibiotics in conjunction with oral therapies (possibly at lower doses) to maximize antimicrobial effects while limiting toxicity [98]. It is not clear if the use oral macrolides in NCFB may have a similar impact on the antibacterial properties of inhaled therapies as seen in CF patients. It is imperative to better understand the factors that could explain why some inhaled antibiotics are effective in CF compared to NCFB. Recognition of these disease characteristics may further aid the clinicians in the selection and treatment of appropriate inhalational therapies for these patients with NCFB.

The success in development of liposomal formulations of antibiotics has promoted new avenues of research in the delivery of lung-targeted medications. Their effects on infected macrophages and biofilms have promising applications in CF, NFCF, and pulmonary NTM infections [121]. In addition to lipid nanocarriers, other polymers have shown promise in the controlled delivery of medications via permeabilization through shell hydrolysis and medium dissolution [127,128]. Through these mechanisms it may be possible to better tailor antibiotic release rates improving the duration of the delivery while achieving target peak concentrations [128,129].

Finally, as our understanding of the role of the microbiome in the outcomes of patients with bronchiectasis increases it might be possible to better select antibiotic strategies. There is increasing evidence that bacterial communities interact with one another and the effects of antibiotics in these interactions are incompletely understood. Because patients with CF, NCFB, and NTM infections often receive IV and oral antibiotics in conjunction with inhaled antibiotics, the interactions between the microbial populations are particularly relevant. Newer, more sensitive molecular techniques are able to identify microorganisms that may not be identified with standard methods [82,130]. It is remains unclear how this information may guide the clinician when selecting antibiotic therapy, but might be important in patients in which microbiome studies reveal that *P. aeruginosa* is not the dominant pathogen. Future studies are needed to explore the benefits of inhaled antibiotics in subgroups of patients with bronchiectasis stratified according to microbiome signatures.

6. Conclusions

Great advances have been made in the field of inhaled antibiotics, especially in CF and NCFB. As technology continues to improve the delivery of these medications, clinicians will require balancing the potential benefits of inhaled antibiotics with toxicity and the development of resistance. This is of particular importance in patients with CF, which are now living longer because of the availability of treatments targeting specific gene mutations and will require prolonged antibiotic therapy. Future studies are still required to determine which subgroups of patients with NCFB have the highest likelihood of benefits with inhale antibiotics. The applications of inhaled antibiotics in NTM infections are less understood, and further studies are needed to establish the role of these treatments in this patient population. Combination therapy of oral and inhaled antibiotics may lead to important interactions that are only partially understood. The results of ongoing trials evaluating the use of inhaled antibiotics are eagerly awaited to establish if these can be added to the armamentarium of therapies for patients with CF, NCFB and NTM infections.

References

1. Mogayzel, P.J., Jr.; Naureckas, E.T.; Robinson, K.A.; Brady, C.; Guill, M.; Lahiri, T.; Lubsch, L.; Matsui, J.; Oermann, C.M.; Ratjen, F.; et al. Cystic Fibrosis Foundation pulmonary guideline. Pharmacologic approaches to prevention and eradication of initial *Pseudomonas aeruginosa* infection. *Ann. Am. Thorac. Soc.* **2014**, *11*, 1640–1650. [CrossRef] [PubMed]
2. Mogayzel, P.J., Jr.; Naureckas, E.T.; Robinson, K.A.; Mueller, G.; Hadjiliadis, D.; Hoag, J.B.; Lubsch, L.; Hazle, L.; Sabadosa, K.; Marshall, B. Cystic fibrosis pulmonary guidelines. Chronic medications for maintenance of lung health. *Am. J. Respir. Crit. Care Med.* **2013**, *187*, 680–689. [CrossRef] [PubMed]
3. Flume, P.A.; Mogayzel, P.J.; Robinson, K.A.; Goss, C.H.; Rosenblatt, R.L.; Kuhn, R.J. Cystic fibrosis pulmonary guidelines: Treatment of pulmonary exacerbations. *Am. J. Respir. Crit. Care Med.* **2009**, *180*, 802–808. [CrossRef] [PubMed]
4. Pasteur, M.C.; Bilton, D.; Hill, A.T. British thoracic society guideline for non-CF bronchiectasis. *Thorax* **2010**, *65*, 577. [CrossRef] [PubMed]
5. Griffith, D.E.; Aksamit, T.; Brown-Elliott, B.A.; Catanzaro, A.; Daley, C.; Gordin, F.; Holland, S.M.; Horsburgh, R.; Huitt, G.; Iademarco, M.F.; et al. An official ATS/IDSA statement: Diagnosis, treatment, and prevention of nontuberculous mycobacterial diseases. *Am. J. Respir. Crit. Care Med.* **2007**, *175*, 367–416. [CrossRef] [PubMed]
6. Floto, R.A.; Olivier, K.N.; Saiman, L.; Daley, C.L.; Herrmann, J.L.; Nick, J.A.; Noone, P.G.; Bilton, D.; Corris, P.; Gibson, R.L.; et al. US cystic fibrosis foundation and european cystic fibrosis society consensus recommendations for the management of non-tuberculous mycobacteria in individuals with cystic fibrosis. *Thorax* **2016**, *71*, i1–i22. [CrossRef] [PubMed]
7. Quon, B.S.; Goss, C.H.; Ramsey, B.W. Inhaled antibiotics for lower airway infections. *Ann. Am. Thorac. Soc.* **2014**, *22*, 425–434. [CrossRef] [PubMed]
8. Cystic Fibrosis Foundation Patient Registry: 2015 Annual Data Report; ©2016 Cystic Fibrosis Foundation: Bethesda, 2016; pp. 1–94. Available online: https://www.cff.org/Our-Research/CF-Patient-Registry/2015-Patient-Registry-Annual-Data-Report.pdf (accessed on 16 May 2017).
9. Stoltz, D.A.; Meyerholz, D.K.; Welsh, M.J. Origins of cystic fibrosis lung disease. *N. Engl. J. Med.* **2015**, *372*, 351–362. [CrossRef] [PubMed]
10. Weers, J. Inhaled antimicrobial therpy-barriers to effective treatment. *Adv. Drug Deliv. Rev.* **2015**, *85*, 24–43. [CrossRef] [PubMed]

11. Saiman, L.; Siegel, J.D.; LiPuma, J.J.; Brown, R.F.; Bryson, E.A.; Chambers, M.J.; Downer, V.S.; Fliege, J.; Hazle, L.A.; Jain, M.; et al. Infection prevention and control guideline for cystic fibrosis: 2013 update. *Infect. Control. Hosp. Epidemiol.* **2014**, *35*, S1–S67. [CrossRef] [PubMed]
12. Stone, A.; Quittell, L.; Zhou, J.; Alba, L.; Bhat, M.; DeCelie-Germana, J.; Rajan, S.; Bonitz, L.; Welter, J.J.; Dozor, A.J.; et al. Staphylococcus aureus nasal colonization among pediatric cystic fibrosis patients and their household contacts. *Pediatr. Infect. Dis. J.* **2009**, *28*, 895–899. [CrossRef] [PubMed]
13. Glikman, D.; Siegel, J.D.; David, M.Z.; Okoro, N.M.; Boyle-Vavra, S.; Dowell, M.L.; Daum, R.S. Complex molecular epidemiology of methicillin-resistant *Staphylococcus aureus* isolates from children with cystic fibrosis in the era of epidemic community-associated methicillin-resistant *S. aureus*. *Chest* **2008**, *133*, 1381–1387. [CrossRef] [PubMed]
14. Champion, E.A.; Miller, M.B.; Popowitch, E.B.; Hobbs, M.M.; Saiman, L.; Muhlebach, M.S. Antimicrobial susceptibility and molecular typing of MRSA in cystic fibrosis. *Pediatr. Pulmonol.* **2014**, *9*, 230–237. [CrossRef] [PubMed]
15. Emerson, J.; Rosenfeld, M.; McNamara, S.; Ramsey, B.; Gibson, R.L. *Pseudomonas aeruginosa* and other predictors of mortality and morbidity in young children with cystic fibrosis. *Pediatr. Pulmonol.* **2002**, *34*, 91–100. [CrossRef] [PubMed]
16. Nixon, G.M.; Armstrong, D.S.; Carzino, R.; Carlin, J.B.; Olinsky, A.; Robertson, C.F.; Grimwood, K. Clinical outcome after early *Pseudomonas aeruginosa* infection in cystic fibrosis. *J. Pediatr.* **2001**, *138*, 699–704. [CrossRef] [PubMed]
17. Breidenstein, E.B.; de la Fuente-Núnez, C.; Hancock, R.E. *Pseudomonas aeruginosa*: All roads lead to resistance. *Trends Microbiol.* **2011**, *19*, 419–426. [CrossRef] [PubMed]
18. Lee, T.W.R.; Brownlee, K.G.; Conway, S.P.; Denton, M.; Littlewood, J.M. Evaluation of a new definition for chronic *Pseudomonas aeruginosa* infection in cystic fibrosis patients. *J. Cyst. Fibros.* **2003**, *2*, 29–34. [CrossRef]
19. Smyth, A.; Elborn, J.S. Exacerbations in cystic fibrosis: 3. Management. *Thorax* **2008**, *63*, 180–184. [CrossRef] [PubMed]
20. Shteinberg, M.; Elborn, J.S. Use of inhaled tobramycin in cystic fibrosis. *Adv. Ther.* **2015**, *32*, 1–9. [CrossRef] [PubMed]
21. Cipolla, D.; Blanchard, J.; Gonda, I. Development of liposomal ciprofloxacin to treat lung infections. *Pharmaceutics* **2016**, *8*, 6. [CrossRef] [PubMed]
22. Burke, D.G.; Harrison, M.J.; Fleming, C.; McCarthy, M.; Shortt, C.; Sulaiman, I.; Murphy, D.M.; Eustace, J.A.; ShaWnahan, F.; Hill, C.; et al. Clostridium difficile carriage in adult cystic fibrosis (CF); implications for patients with CF and the potential for transmission of nosocomial infection. *J. Cyst. Fibros.* **2017**, *16*, 291–298. [CrossRef] [PubMed]
23. Wenzler, E.; Fraidenburg, D.R.; Scardina, T.; Danziger, L.H. Inhaled Antibiotics for Gram-Negative Respiratory Infections. *Clin. Microbiol. Rev.* **2016**, *29*, 581–632. [PubMed]
24. Mendelman, P.M.; Smith, A.L.; Levy, J.; Weber, A.; Ramsey, B.; David, R.L. Aminoglycoside penetration, inactivation, and efficacy in cystic fibrosis sputum. *Am. Rev. Respir. Dis.* **1985**, *132*, 761–765. [PubMed]
25. Cipolla, D.; Chan, H.K. Inhaled antibiotics to treat lung infection. *Pharm. Pat. Anal.* **2013**, *2*, 647–663. [CrossRef] [PubMed]
26. Ramsey, B.W.; Pepe, M.S.; Quan, J.M.; Otto, K.L.; Montgomery, A.B.; Williams-Warren, J.; Vasiljev-K, M.; Borowitz, D.; Bowman, C.M.; Marshall, B.C.; et al. Intermittent administration of inhaled tobramycin in patients with cystic fibrosis. *N. Engl. J. Med.* **1999**, *340*, 23–30. [CrossRef] [PubMed]
27. Geller, D.E.; Pitlick, W.H.; Nardella, P.A.; Tracewell, W.G.; Ramsey, B.W. Pharmacokinetics and bioavailability of aerosolized tobramycin in cystic fibrosis. *CHEST J.* **2002**, *122*, 219–226. [CrossRef]
28. Vendrell, M.; Muñoz, G.; de Gracia, J. Evidence of inhaled tobramycin in non-cystic fibrosis bronchiectasis. *Open Respir. Med. J.* **2015**, *9*, 30–36. [CrossRef] [PubMed]
29. Ramsey, B.W.; Dorkin, H.L.; Eisenberg, J.D.; Gibson, R.L.; Harwood, I.R.; Kravitz, R.M.; Schidlow, D.V.; Wilmott, R.W.; Astley, S.J.; McBurnie, M.A.; et al. Efficacy of aerosolized tobramycin in patients with cystic fibrosis. *N. Engl. J. Med.* **1993**, *328*, 1740–1746. [CrossRef] [PubMed]
30. MacLusky, I.B.; Gold, R.; Corey, M.; Levison, H. Long-term effects of inhaled tobramycin in patients with cystic fibrosis colonized with *Pseudomonas aeruginosa*. *Pediatr. Pulmonol.* **1989**, *7*, 42–48. [CrossRef] [PubMed]

31. Gibson, R.L.; Emerson, J.; McNamara, S.; Burns, J.L.; Rosenfeld, M.; Yunker, A.; Hamblett, N.; Accurso, F.; Dovey, M.; Hiatt, P.; et al. Significant microbiological effect of inhaled tobramycin in young children with cystic fibrosis. *Am. J. Respir. Crit. Care Med.* **2003**, *167*, 841–849. [CrossRef] [PubMed]
32. Murphy, T.D.; Anbar, R.D.; Lester, L.A.; Nasr, S.Z.; Nickerson, B.; VanDevanter, D.R.; Colin, A.A. Treatment with tobramycin solution for inhalation reduces hospitalizations in young CF subjects with mild lung disease. *Pediatr. Pulmonol.* **2004**, *38*, 314–320. [CrossRef] [PubMed]
33. Smith, A.L.; Ramsey, B.W.; Hedges, D.L.; Hack, B.; Williams-Warren, J.; Weber, A. Safety of aerosol tobramycin administration for 3 months to patients with cystic fibrosis. *Pediatr. Pulmonol.* **1989**, *7*, 265–271. [CrossRef] [PubMed]
34. Dasenbrook, E.C.; Konstan, M.W.; VanDevanter, D.R. Association between the introduction of a new cystic fibrosis inhaled antibiotic class and change in prevalence of patients receiving multiple inhaled antibiotic classes. *J. Cyst. Fibros.* **2015**, 370–375. [CrossRef] [PubMed]
35. Flume, P.A.; Clancy, J.P.; Retsch-Bogart, G.Z.; Tullis, D.E.; Bresnik, M.; Derchak, P.A. Continous alternating inhaled antibiotics for chronic pseudomonal infection in cystic fibrosis. *J. Cyst. Fibros.* **2016**, 809–815. [CrossRef] [PubMed]
36. Ratjen, F.; Munck, A.; Kho, P.; Angyalosi, G. Treatment of early *Pseudomonas aeruginosa* infection in patients with cystic fibrosis: The ELITE trial. *Thorax* **2010**, *65*, 286–291. [CrossRef] [PubMed]
37. Cooper, D.M.; Harris, M.; Mitchell, I. Comparison of intravenous and inhalation antibiotic therapy in acute pulmonary deterioration in cystic fibrosis. *Am. Rev. Respir. Dis.* **1985**, *131*, A242.
38. Schaad, U.B.; Wedgewood-Krucko, J.; Suter, S.; Kramer, R. Efficacy of inhaled amikacin as adjunct to intravenous combination therapy (ceftazidime and amikacin) in cystic fibrosis. *J. Pediatr.* **1987**, *111*, 599–605. [CrossRef]
39. Stephens, D.; Garey, N.; Isles, A.; Levison, H.; Gold, R. Efficacy of inhaled tobramycin in the treatment of pulmonary exacerbations in children with cystic fibrosis. *Pediatr. Infect. Dis.* **1983**, *3*, 209–211. [CrossRef]
40. Al-Aloul, M.; Nazareth, D.; Walshaw, M. Nebulized tobramycin in the treatment of adult CF pulmonary exacerbations. *J. Aerosol. Med. Pulm. Drug Deliv.* **2014**, *27*, 299–305. [CrossRef] [PubMed]
41. Sommerwerck, U.; Virella-Lowell, I.; Angyalosi, G.; Viegas, A.; Cao, W.; Debonnett, L. Long-term safety of tobramycin inhalation powder in patients with cystic fibrosis: Phase IV (ETOILES) study. *Curr. Med. Res. Opin.* **2016**, *32*, 1789–1795. [CrossRef] [PubMed]
42. Geller, D.E.; Nasr, S.Z.; Piggott, S.; He, E.; Angyalosi, G.; Higgins, M. Tobramycin inhalation powder in cystic fibrosis patients: Response by age group. *Respir. Care* **2014**, *59*, 388–398. [CrossRef] [PubMed]
43. Geller, D.E.; Konstan, M.W.; Smith, J.; Noonberg, S.B.; Conrad, C. Novel tobramycin inhalation powder in cystic fibrosis subjects: Pharmacokinetics and safety. *Pediatr. Pulmonol.* **2007**, *42*, 307–313. [CrossRef] [PubMed]
44. Konstan, M.W.; Flume, P.A.; Kappler, M.; Chiron, R.; Higgins, M.; Brockhaus, F.; Zhang, J.; Angyalosi, G.; He, E.; Geller, D.E. Safety, efficacy and convenience of tobramycin inhalation powder in cystic fibrosis patients: The EAGER trial. *J. Cyst. Fibros.* **2011**, *10*, 54–61. [CrossRef] [PubMed]
45. Konstan, M.W.; Flume, P.A.; Galeva, I.; Wan, R.; Debonnett, L.M.; Maykut, R.J.; Angyalosi, G. One-year safety and efficacy of tobramycin powder for inhalation in patients with cystic fibrosis. *Pediatr. Pulmonol.* **2016**, *51*, 372–378. [CrossRef] [PubMed]
46. Galeva, I.; Konstan, M.W.; Higgins, M.; Angyalosi, G.; Brockhaus, F.; Piggott, S.; Thomas, K.; Chuchalin, A.G. Tobramycin inhalation powder manufactured by improved process in cystic fibrosis: The randomized EDIT trial. *Curr. Med. Res. Opin.* **2013**, *29*, 947–956. [CrossRef] [PubMed]
47. McCoy, K.S.; Quittner, A.L.; Oermann, C.M.; Gibson, R.L.; Retsch-Bogart, G.Z.; Montomery, A.B. Inhaled aztreonam lysine for chronic airway Pseudomonas aeruginosa in cystic fibrosis. *Am. J. Respir. Crit. Care Med.* **2008**, *178*, 921–928. [CrossRef] [PubMed]
48. Retsch-Bogart, G.Z.; Quittner, A.L.; Gibson, R.L.; Oermann, C.M.; McCoy, K.S.; Montgomery, A.B.; Cooper, P.J. Efficacy and safety of inhaled aztreonam lysine for airway Pseudomonas in cystic fibrosis. *Chest J.* **2009**, *135*, 1223–1232. [CrossRef] [PubMed]
49. Oermann, C.M.; Retsch-Bogart, G.Z.; Quittner, A.L.; Gibson, R.L.; McCoy, K.S.; Montgomery, A.B.; Cooper, P.J. An 18-month study of the safety and efficacy of repeated courses of inhaled aztreonam lysine in cystic fibrosis. *Pediatr. Pulmonol.* **2010**, *45*, 1121–1134. [CrossRef] [PubMed]
50. Oermann, C.M.; McCoy, K.S.; Retsch-Bogart, G.Z.; Gibson, R.L.; McKevitt, M.; Montgomery, A.B. Pseudomonas aeruginosa antibiotic susceptibility during long-term use of aztreonam for inhalation solution (AZLI). *J. Antimicrob. Chemother.* **2011**, *66*, 2398–2404. [CrossRef] [PubMed]

51. Assael, B.M.; Pressler, T.; Bilton, D.; Fayon, M.; Fischer, R.; Chiron, R.; La Rosa, M.; Knoop, C.; McElvaney, N.; Lewis, S.A.; et al. Inhaled aztreonam lysine vs. inhaled tobramycin in cystic fibrosis: A comparative efficacy trial. *J. Cyst. Fibros.* **2013**, *12*, 130–140. [CrossRef] [PubMed]
52. Tullis, D.E.; Burns, J.L.; Retsch-Bogart, G.Z.; Bresnik, M.; Henig, N.R.; Lewis, S.A.; Lipuma, J.J. Inhaled aztreonam for chronic Burkholderia infection in cystic fibrosis: A placebo-controlled trial. *J. Cyst. Fibros.* **2014**, *13*, 296–305. [CrossRef] [PubMed]
53. Retsch-Bogart, G.Z.; Burns, J.L.; Otto, K.L.; Liou, T.G.; McCoy, K.; Oermann, C.; Gibson, R.L. A phase 2 study of aztreonam lysine for inhalation to treat patients with cystic fibrosis and Pseudomonas aeruginosa infection. *Pediatr. Pulmonol.* **2008**, *43*, 47–58. [CrossRef] [PubMed]
54. Koyama, Y.; Kurosawa, A.; Tsuchiya, A.; Takakuta, K. A new antibiotic, colistin, produced by spore-forming soil bacteria. *J. Antibiot. Tokyo* **1950**, *3*, 457.
55. Jensen, T.; Pedersen, S.S.; Garne, S.; Heilmann, C.; Høiby, N.; Koch, C. Colistin inhalation therapy in cystic fibrosis patients with chronic *Pseudomonas aeruginosa* lung infection. *J. Antimicrob. Chemother.* **1987**, *19*, 831–838. [CrossRef] [PubMed]
56. Hodson, M.E.; Gallagher, C.G.; Govan, J.R. A randomised clinical trial of nebulised tobramycin or colistin in cystic fibrosis. *Eur. Resp. J.* **2002**, *20*, 658–664. [CrossRef]
57. Schuster, A.; Haliburn, C.; Döring, G.; Goldman, M.H. Safety, efficacy and convenience of colistimethate sodium dry powder for inhalation (Colobreathe DPI) in patients with cystic fibrosis: A randomised study. *Thorax* **2013**, 344–350. [CrossRef] [PubMed]
58. Dodd, M.E.; Abbott, J.; Maddison, J.; Moorcroft, A.J.; Webb, A.K. Effect of tonicity of nebulised colistin on chest tightness and pulmonary function in adults with cystic fibrosis. *Thorax* **1997**, *52*, 656–658. [CrossRef] [PubMed]
59. Cunningham, S.; Prasad, A.; Collyer, L.; Carr, S.; Lynn, I.B.; Wallis, C. Bronchoconstriction following nebulised colistin in cystic fibrosis. *Arch. Dis. Child.* **2001**, *84*, 432–433. [CrossRef] [PubMed]
60. Alothman, G.A.; Ho, B.; Alsaadi, M.M.; Ho, S.L.; O'Drowsky, L.; Louca, E.; Coates, A.L. Bronchial constriction and inhaled colistin in cystic fibrosis. *Chest J.* **2005**, *127*, 522–599. [CrossRef] [PubMed]
61. McCoy, K.S. Compounded colistimethate as possible cause of fatal acute respiratory distress syndrome. *N. Engl. J. Med.* **2007**, *357*, 2310–2311. [CrossRef] [PubMed]
62. Geller, D.E.; Flume, P.A.; Staab, D.; Fischer, R.; Loutit, J.S.; Conrad, D.J. Levofloxacin inhalation solution (MP-376) in patients with cystic fibrosis with *Pseudomonas aeruginosa*. *Am. J. Respir. Crit. Care Med.* **2011**, *183*, 1510–1516. [CrossRef] [PubMed]
63. Stuart Elborn, J.S.; Geller, D.E.; Conrad, D.; Aaron, S.D.; Smyth, A.R.; Fischer, R. A phase 3, open-label, randomized trial to evaluate the safety and efficacy of levofloxacin inhalation solution (APT-1026) verses tobramycin inhalation solution in stable cystic fibrosis patients. *J. Cyst. Fibros.* **2015**, *14*, 507–514. [CrossRef] [PubMed]
64. Flume, P.A.; VanDevanter, D.R.; Morgan, E.E.; Dudley, M.N.; Loutit, J.S.; Bell, S.C.; Kerem, E.; Fischer, R.; Smyth, A.R.; Aaron, S.D.; et al. A phase 3, multi-center, multinational, randomized, double-blind, placebo-controlled study to evaluate the efficacy and safety of levofloxacin inhalation solution (APT-1026) in stable cystic fibrosis patients. *J. Cyst. Fibros.* **2016**, *15*, 495–502. [CrossRef] [PubMed]
65. Stass, H.; Nagelschmitz, J.; Willmann, S.; Delesen, H.; Gupta, A.; Baumann, S. Inhalation of a dry powder ciprofloxacin formulation in healthy subjects: A phase I study. *Clin. Drug Investig.* **2013**, *33*, 419–427. [CrossRef] [PubMed]
66. Stass, H.; Nagelschmitz, J.; Kappeler, D.; Sommerer, K.; Kietzig, C.; Weimann, B. Ciprofloxacin Dry Powder for Inhalation in Patients with Non-Cystic Fibrosis Bronchiectasis or Chronic Obstructive Pulmonary Disease, and in Healthy Volunteers. *J. Aerosol. Med. Pulm. Drug Deliv.* **2017**, *30*, 53–63. [CrossRef] [PubMed]
67. Bruinenberg, P.; Blanchard, J.D.; Cipolla, D.C.; Dayton, F.; Mudumba, S.; Gonda, I. Inhaled liposomal ciprofloxacin: Once a day management of respiratory infections. *Respir. Drug Deliv.* **2010**, *1*, 73–81.
68. Justo, J.A.; Danziger, L.H.; Gotfried, M.H. Efficacy of inhaled ciprofloxacin in the management of non-cystic fibrosis bronchiectasis. *Ther. Adv. Respir. Dis.* **2013**, *7*, 272–287. [CrossRef] [PubMed]
69. Stass, H.; Weimann, B.; Nagelschmitz, J.; Rolinck-Werninghaus, C.; Staab, D. Tolerability and pharmacokinetic properties of ciprofloxacin dry powder for inhalation in patients with cystic fibrosis: A phase I, randomized, dose-escalation study. *Clin. Ther.* **2013**, *35*, 1571–1581. [CrossRef] [PubMed]
70. Stass, H.; Delesen, H.; Nagelschmitz, J.; Staab, D. Safety and pharmacokinetics of ciprofloxacin dry powder for inhalation in cystic fibrosis: A phase I, randomized, single-dose, dose-escalation study. *J. Aerosol. Med. Pulm. Drug Deliv.* **2015**, *28*, 106–115. [CrossRef] [PubMed]

71. Dorkin, H.L.; Staab, D.; Operschall, E.; Alder, J.; Criollo, M. Ciprofloxacin DPI: A randomised, placebo-controlled, phase IIb efficacy and safety study on cystic fibrosis. *BMJ Open Respir. Res.* **2015**, *2*, e000100. [CrossRef] [PubMed]
72. Barker, A.F. Bronchiectasis. *N. Engl. J. Med.* **2002**, *346*, 1383–1393. [CrossRef] [PubMed]
73. Seitz, A.E.; Olivier, K.N.; Adjemian, J.; Holland, S.M.; Prevots, R. Trends in bronchiectasis among medicare beneficiaries in the United States, 2000 to 2007. *Chest J.* **2012**, *142*, 432–439. [CrossRef] [PubMed]
74. Kang, E.Y.; Miller, R.R.; Müller, N.L. Bronchiectasis: Comparison of preoperative thin-section CT and pathologic findings in resected specimens. *Radiology* **1995**, *195*, 649–654. [CrossRef] [PubMed]
75. Grenier, P.; Maurice, F.; Musset, D.; Menu, Y.; Nahum, H. Bronchiectasis: Assessment by thin-section CT. *Radiology* **1986**, *161*, 95–99. [CrossRef] [PubMed]
76. Weycker, D.; Edelsberg, J.; Oster, G.; Tino, G. Prevalence and economic burden of bronchiectasis. *Clin. Pulm. Med.* **2005**, *12*, 205–209. [CrossRef]
77. Quint, J.K.; Millett, E.R.; Joshi, M.; Navaratnam, V.; Thomas, S.L.; Hurst, J.R.; Smeeth, L.; Brown, J.S. Changes in the incidence, prevalence and mortality of bronchiectasis in the UK from 2004 to 2013: A population-based cohort study. *Eur. Respir. J.* **2016**, *47*, 186–193. [CrossRef] [PubMed]
78. Seitz, A.E.; Olivier, K.N.; Steiner, C.A.; Montes de Oca, R.; Holland, S.M.; Prevots, D.R. Trends and burden of bronchiectasis-associated hospitalizations in the United States, 1993–2006. *Chest J.* **2010**, *138*, 944–949. [CrossRef] [PubMed]
79. King, P.T.; Holdsworth, S.R.; Freezer, N.J.; Villanueva, E.; Holmes, P.W. Microbiologic follow-up study in adult bronchiectasis. *Respir. Med.* **2007**, *101*, 1633–1638. [CrossRef] [PubMed]
80. Angrill, J.; Agustí, C.; de Celis, R.; Rañó, A.; Gonzalez, J.; Solé, T.; Xaubet, A.; Rodriguez-Roisin, R.; Torres, A. Bacterial colonisation in patients with bronchiectasis: Microbiological pattern and risk factors. *Thorax* **2002**, *57*, 15–19. [CrossRef] [PubMed]
81. Rogers, G.B.; Zain, N.M.; Bruce, K.D.; Burr, L.D.; Chen, A.C.; Rivett, D.W.; McGuckin, M.A.; Serisier, D.J. A novel microbiota stratification system predicts future exacerbations in bronchiectasis. *Ann. Am. Thorac. Soc.* **2014**, *11*, 496–503. [CrossRef] [PubMed]
82. Tunney, M.M.; Einarsson, G.G.; Wei, L.; Drain, M.; Klem, E.R.; Cardwell, C.; Ennis, M.; Boucher, R.C.; Wolfgang, M.C.; Elborn, J.S. Lung microbiota and bacterial abundance in patients with bronchiectasis when clinically stable and during exacerbation. *Am. J. Respir. Crit. Care Med.* **2013**, *187*, 1118–1126. [CrossRef] [PubMed]
83. Dickson, R.P.; Martinez, F.J.; Huffnagle, G.B. The role of the microbiome in exacerbations of chronic lung diseases. *Lancet* **2014**, *384*, 691–702. [CrossRef]
84. Aksamit, T.R.; O'Donnell, A.E.; Barker, A.; Olivier, K.N.; Winthrop, K.L.; Daniels, M.L.; Johnson, M.; Eden, E.; Griffith, D.; Knowles, M.; et al. Adult Bronchiectasis Patients: A First Look at the United States Bronchiectasis Research Registry. *Chest J.* **2017**, *151*, 982–992. [CrossRef] [PubMed]
85. Goeminne, P.C.; Scheers, H.; Decraene, A.; Seys, S.; Dupont, L.J. Risk factors for morbidity and death in non-cystic fibrosis bronchiectasis: A retrospective cross-sectional analysis of CT diagnosed bronchiectatic patients. *Respir. Res.* **2012**, *13*, 21. [CrossRef] [PubMed]
86. Guan, W.J.; Gao, Y.H.; Xu, G.; Lin, Z.Y.; Tang, Y.; Li, H.M.; Lin, Z.M.; Zheng, J.P.; Chen, R.C.; Zhong, N.S. Characterization of lung function impairment in adults with bronchiectasis. *PLoS ONE* **2014**, *9*, e113373. [CrossRef] [PubMed]
87. Martínez-García, M.A.; Soler-Cataluña, J.J.; Perpiñá-Tordera, M.; Román-Sánchez, P.; Soriano, J. Factors associated with lung function decline in adult patients with stable non-cystic fibrosis bronchiectasis. *Chest J.* **2007**, *132*, 1565–1572. [CrossRef] [PubMed]
88. McDonnell, M.J.; Jary, H.R.; Perry, A.; MacFarlane, J.G.; Hester, K.L.; Small, T.; Molyneux, C.; Perry, J.D.; Walton, K.E.; De Soyza, A. Non cystic fibrosis bronchiectasis: A longitudinal retrospective observational cohort study of Pseudomonas persistence and resistance. *Respir. Med.* **2015**, *109*, 716–726. [CrossRef] [PubMed]
89. Wilson, C.B.; Jones, P.W.; O'Leary, C.J.; Hansell, D.M.; Cole, P.J.; Wilson, R. Effect of sputum bacteriology on the quality of life of patients with bronchiectasis. *Eur. Respir. J.* **1997**, *10*, 1754–1760. [CrossRef] [PubMed]
90. Chalmers, J.D.; Goeminne, P.; Aliberti, S.; McDonnell, M.J.; Lonni, S.; Davidson, J.; Poppelwell, L.; Salih, W.; Pesci, A.; Dupont, L.J.; et al. The bronchiectasis severity index. An international derivation and validation study. *Am. J. Respir. Crit. Care Med.* **2014**, *189*, 576–585. [CrossRef] [PubMed]

91. Loebinger, M.R.; Wells, A.U.; Hansell, D.M.; Chinyanganya, N.; Devaraj, A.; Meister, M.; Wilson, R. Mortality in bronchiectasis: A long-term study assessing the factors influencing survival. *Eur. Respir. J.* **2009**, *34*, 843–849. [CrossRef] [PubMed]
92. Aliberti, S.; Lonni, S.; Dore, S.; McDonnell, M.J.; Goeminne, P.C.; Dimakou, K.; Fardon, T.C.; Rutherford, R.; Pesci, A.; Restrepo, M.I.; et al. Clinical phenotypes in adult patients with bronchiectasis. *Eur. Respir. J.* **2016**, *47*, 1113–1122. [CrossRef] [PubMed]
93. Williams, B.J.; Dehnbostel, J.; Blackwell, T.S. *Pseudomonas aeruginosa*: Host defence in lung diseases. *Respirology* **2010**, *15*, 1037–1056. [CrossRef] [PubMed]
94. Gellatly, S.L.; Hancock, R.E. *Pseudomonas aeruginosa*: New insights into pathogenesis and host defenses. *Pathog. Dis.* **2013**, *67*, 159–173. [CrossRef] [PubMed]
95. Barker, A.F.; Couch, L.; Fiel, S.B.; Gotfried, M.H.; Ilowite, J.; Meyer, K.C.; O'Donnell, A.; Sahn, S.A.; Smith, L.J.; Stewart, J.O.; et al. Tobramycin solution for inhalation reduces sputum *Pseudomonas aeruginosa* density in bronchiectasis. *Am. J. Respir. Crit. Care Med.* **2000**, *162*, 481–485. [CrossRef] [PubMed]
96. Scheinberg, P.; Shore, E. A pilot study of the safety and efficacy of tobramycin solution for inhalation in patients with severe bronchiectasis. *Chest J.* **2005**, *127*, 1420–1426. [CrossRef]
97. Drobnic, M.E.; Suñé, P.; Montoro, J.B.; Ferrer, A.; Orriols, R. Inhaled tobramycin in non-cystic fibrosis patients with bronchiectasis and chronic bronchial infection with Pseudomonas aeruginosa. *Ann. Pharmacother.* **2005**, *39*, 39–44. [CrossRef] [PubMed]
98. Bilton, D.; Henig, N.; Morrissey, B.; Gotfried, M. Addition of inhaled tobramycin to ciprofloxacin for acute exacerbations of Pseudomonas aeruginosa infection in adult bronchiectasis. *Chest J.* **2006**, *130*, 1503–1510. [CrossRef] [PubMed]
99. Hoppentocht, M.; Akkerman, O.W.; Hagedoorn, P.; Alffenaar, J.W.; van der Werf, T.S.; Kerstjens, H.A.; Frijlink, H.W.; de Boer, A.H. Tolerability and Pharmacokinetic Evaluation of Inhaled Dry Powder Tobramycin Free Base in Non-Cystic Fibrosis Bronchiectasis Patients. *PLoS ONE* **2016**, *11*, e0149768. [CrossRef] [PubMed]
100. Wilson, R.; Welte, T.; Polverino, E.; De Soyza, A.; Greville, H.; O'Donnell, A.; Alder, J.; Reimnitz, P.; Hampel, B. Ciprofloxacin dry powder for inhalation in non-cystic fibrosis bronchiectasis: A phase II randomised study. *Eur. Respir. J.* **2013**, *41*, 1107–1115. [CrossRef] [PubMed]
101. Bilton, D.; De Soyza, A.; Hayward, C.; Bruinenberg, P. Effect Of a 28-Day Course Of Two Different Doses Of Once A Day Liposomal Ciprofloxacin For Inhalation On Sputum Pseudomonas Aeruginosa Density In Non-CF Bronchiectasis. *Am. J. Respir. Crit. Care Med.* **2010**, *181*, A3191.
102. Bilton, D.; Serisier, D.; De Soyza, A.; Wolfe, R.; Bruinenberg, P. Multicenter, randomized, double-blind, placebo-controlled study (ORBIT 1) to evaluate the efficacy, safety, and tolerability of once daily ciprofloxacin for inhalation in the management of Pseudomonas aeruginosa infections in patients with non-cystic fibrosis bronchiectasis. *Eur. Respir. J.* **2011**, *38*, 1925.
103. Serisier, D.J.; Bilton, D.; De Soyza, A.; Thompson, P.J.; Kolbe, J.; Greville, H.W.; Cipolla, D.; Bruinenberg, P.; Gonda, I. Inhaled, dual release liposomal ciprofloxacin in non-cystic fibrosis bronchiectasis (ORBIT-2): A randomised, double-blind, placebo-controlled trial. *Thorax* **2013**, *68*, 812–817. [CrossRef] [PubMed]
104. Haworth, C.; Wanner, A.; Foehlich, J.; O'Neal, T.; Davis, A.; Gonda, I.; O'Donell, A. Inhaled liposomal ciprofloxacin in patient with bronchiectasis and chronic pseudomonas aeruginosa infection: Results from two parallel phase III trials (ORBIT-3 and -4). *Am. J. Respir. Crit. Care Med.* **2017**, in press.
105. Chono, S.; Tanino, T.; Seki, T.; Morimoto, K. Efficient drug delivery to alveolar macrophages and lung epithelial lining fluid following pulmonary administration of liposomal ciprofloxacin in rats with pneumonia and estimation of its antibacterial effects. *Drug Dev. Ind. Pharm.* **2008**, *34*, 1090–1096. [CrossRef] [PubMed]
106. Murray, M.P.; Govan, J.R.; Doherty, C.J.; Simpson, A.J.; Wilkinson, T.S.; Chalmers, J.D.; Greening, A.P.; Haslett, C.; Hill, A.T. A randomized controlled trial of nebulized gentamicin in non-cystic fibrosis bronchiectasis. *Am. J. Respir. Crit. Care Med.* **2011**, *183*, 491–499. [CrossRef] [PubMed]
107. Barker, A.F.; O'Donnell, A.E.; Flume, P.; Thompson, P.J.; Ruzi, J.D.; de Gracia, J.; Boersma, W.G.; De Soyza, A.; Shao, L.; et al. Aztreonam for inhalation solution in patients with non-cystic fibrosis bronchiectasis (AIR-BX1 and AIR-BX2): Two randomised double-blind, placebo-controlled phase 3 trials. *Lancet Respir. Med.* **2014**, *2*, 738–749. [CrossRef]
108. Haworth, C.S.; Foweraker, J.E.; Wilkinson, P.; Kenyon, R.F.; Bilton, D. Inhaled colistin in patients with bronchiectasis and chronic *Pseudomonas aeruginosa* infection. *Am. J. Respir. Crit. Care Med.* **2014**, *189*, 975–982. [CrossRef] [PubMed]

109. Denyer, J.; Dyche, T. The Adaptive Aerosol Delivery (AAD) technology: Past, present, and future. *J. Aerosol. Med. Pulm. Drug Deliv.* **2010**, *23* (Suppl. S1), S1–S10. [CrossRef] [PubMed]
110. Tabernero Huguet, E.; Gil Alaña, P.; Alkiza Basañez, R.; Hernández Gil, A.; Garros Garay, J.; Artola Igarza, J.L. Inhaled colistin in elderly patients with non-cystic fibrosis bronchiectasis and chronic *Pseudomonas aeruginosa* bronchial infection. *Rev. Esp. Geriatr. Gerontol.* **2015**, *50*, 111–115. [CrossRef] [PubMed]
111. O'Brien, R.J.; Geiter, L.J.; Snider, D.E., Jr. The epidemiology of nontuberculous mycobacterial diseases in the United States. Results from a national survey. *Am. Rev. Respir. Dis.* **1987**, *135*, 1007–1014. [PubMed]
112. Griffith, D.E.; Aksamit, T.R. Understanding nontuberculous mycobacterial lung disease: It's been a long time coming. *F1000 Res.* **2016**, *5*, 2797. [CrossRef] [PubMed]
113. Skolnik, K.; Kirkpatrick, G.; Quon, B.S. Nontuberculous Mycobacteria in Cystic Fibrosis. *Curr. Treat. Options Infect. Dis.* **2016**, *8*, 259–274. [CrossRef] [PubMed]
114. Park, I.K.; Olivier, K.N. Nontuberculous mycobacteria in cystic fibrosis and non-cystic fibrosis bronchiectasis. *Semin. Respir. Crit. Care Med.* **2015**, *36*, 217–224. [CrossRef] [PubMed]
115. Catherinot, E.; Roux, A.L.; Vibet, M.A.; Bellis, G.; Lemonnier, L.; Le Roux, E.; Bernède-Bauduin, C.; Le Bourgeois, M.; Herrmann, J.L.; Guillemot, D.; et al. Inhaled therapies, azithromycin and *Mycobacterium abscessus* in cystic fibrosis patients. *Eur. Respir. J.* **2013**, *41*, 1101–1106. [CrossRef] [PubMed]
116. Olivier, K.N.; Shaw, P.A.; Glaser, T.S.; Bhattacharyya, D.; Fleshner, M.; Brewer, C.C.; Zalewski, C.K.; Folio, L.R.; Siegelman, J.R.; Shallom, S.; et al. Inhaled amikacin for treatment of refractory pulmonary nontuberculous mycobacterial disease. *Ann. Am. Thorac. Soc.* **2014**, *11*, 30–35. [CrossRef] [PubMed]
117. Rose, S.J.; Neville, M.E.; Gupta, R.; Bermudez, L.E. Delivery of aerosolized liposomal amikacin as a novel approach for the treatment of nontuberculous mycobacteria in an experimental model of pulmonary infection. *PLoS ONE* **2014**, *9*, e108703. [CrossRef] [PubMed]
118. Olivier, K.N.; Griffith, D.E.; Eagle, G.; McGinnis, J.P.; Micioni, L.; Liu, K.; Daley, C.L.; Winthrop, K.L.; Ruoss, S.; Addrizzo-Harris, D.J.; et al. Randomized Trial of Liposomal Amikacin for Inhalation in Nontuberculous Mycobacterial Lung Disease. *Am. J. Respir. Crit. Care Med.* **2017**, *195*, 814–823. [CrossRef] [PubMed]
119. Bermudez, L.E.; Blanchard, J.D.; Hauck, L.; Gonda, I. Treatment of *Mycobacterium avium* subsp hominissuis (MAH) lung infection with liposome-encapsulated ciprofloxacin resulted in significant decrease in bacterial load in the lung. *Am. J. Respir. Crit. Care Med.* **2015**, *191*, A6293.
120. Bermudez, L.E.; Blanchard, J.; Babrak, L.; Gonda, I. Liposome-ciprofloxacin inhibits *Mycobacterium avium* subs hominissuis (MAH) microaggregate formation in a dose and time dependent manner. *Am. J. Respir. Crit. Care Med.* **2016**, *193*, A3734.
121. Blanchard, J.; Danelishvili, L.; Gonda, I.; Bermudez, L. Liposomal ciprofloxacin preparation is active against *Mycobacterium avium* subsp hominissuis and *Mycobacterium abscessus* in macrophages and in biofilm. *Am. J. Respir. Crit. Care Med.* **2014**, *189*, A6677.
122. Jennings, M.T.; Boyle, M.P.; Weaver, D.; Callahan, K.A.; Dasenbrook, E.C. Eradication strategy for persistent methicillin-resistant Staphylococcus aureus infection in individuals with cystic fibrosis—The PMEP trial: Study protocol for a randomized controlled trial. *Trials* **2014**, *15*, 223. [CrossRef] [PubMed]
123. Nick, J.A.; Moskowitz, S.M.; Chmiel, J.F.; Forssén, A.V.; Kim, S.H.; Saavedra, M.T.; Saiman, L.; Taylor-Cousar, J.L.; Nichols, D.P. Azithromycin may antagonize inhaled tobramycin when targeting *Pseudomonas aeruginosa* in cystic fibrosis. *Ann. Am. Thorac. Soc.* **2014**, *11*, 342–350. [CrossRef] [PubMed]
124. Nichols, D.P.; Happoldt, C.L.; Bratcher, P.E.; Caceres, S.M.; Chmiel, J.F.; Malcolm, K.C.; Saavedra, M.T.; Saiman, L.; Taylor-Cousar, J.L.; Nick, J.A. Impact of azithromycin on the clinical and antimicrobial effectiveness of tobramycin in the treatment of cystic fibrosis. *J. Cyst. Fibros.* **2016**, *16*, 358–366. [CrossRef] [PubMed]
125. Gao, Y.H.; Guan, W.J.; Xu, G.; Tang, Y.; Gao, Y.; Lin, Z.Y.; Lin, Z.M.; Zhong, N.S.; Chen, R.C. Macrolide therapy in adults and children with non-cystic fibrosis bronchiectasis: A systematic review and meta-analysis. *PLoS ONE* **2014**, *9*, e90047. [CrossRef] [PubMed]
126. Fan, L.C.; Lu, H.W.; Wei, P.; Ji, X.B.; Liang, S.; Xu, J.F. Effects of long-term use of macrolides in patients with non-cystic fibrosis bronchiectasis: A meta-analysis of randomized controlled trials. *BMC Infect. Dis.* **2015**, *15*, 160. [CrossRef] [PubMed]
127. Chen, H.; Woods, A.; Forbes, B.; Jones, S. Controlled drug release from lung-targeted nanocarriers via chemically mediated shell permeabilisation. *Int. J. Pharm.* **2016**, *511*, 1033–1041. [CrossRef] [PubMed]

128. Pai, R.V.; Jain, R.R.; Bannalikar, A.S.; Menon, M.D. Development and Evaluation of Chitosan Microparticles Based Dry Powder Inhalation Formulations of Rifampicin and Rifabutin. *J. Aerosol. Med. Pulm. Drug Deliv.* **2016**, *29*, 179–195. [CrossRef] [PubMed]
129. Gaspar, M.C.; Grégoire, N.; Sousa, J.J.; Pais, A.A.; Lamarche, I.; Gobin, P.; Olivier, J.C.; Marchand, S.; Couet, W. Pulmonary pharmacokinetics of levofloxacin in rats after aerosolization of immediate-release chitosan or sustained-release PLGA microspheres. *Eur. J. Pharm. Sci.* **2016**, *93*, 184–191. [CrossRef] [PubMed]
130. Rogers, G.B.; van der Gast, C.J.; Cuthbertson, L.; Thomson, S.K.; Bruce, K.D.; Martin, M.L.; Serisier, D.J. Clinical measures of disease in adult non-CF bronchiectasis correlate with airway microbiota composition. *Thorax* **2013**, *68*, 731–737. [CrossRef] [PubMed]

15

Immunological Roles of Elevated Plasma Levels of Matricellular Proteins in Japanese Patients with Pulmonary Tuberculosis

Beata Shiratori [1,†,‡], Jingge Zhao [1,†], Masao Okumura [2], Haorile Chagan-Yasutan [1], Hideki Yanai [3], Kazue Mizuno [3], Takashi Yoshiyama [2], Tadashi Idei [3], Yugo Ashino [1], Chie Nakajima [4], Yasuhiko Suzuki [4] and Toshio Hattori [5,*]

1 Division of Disaster-Related Infectious Diseases, International Research Institute of Disaster Science, Tohoku University, 2-1 Seiryo-machi, Aoba-ku, Sendai, Miyagi 980-8575, Japan; beatabucekova@gmail.com (B.S.); zhaojingge1987@gmail.com (J.Z.); haorile@gmail.com (H.C.-Y.); ya82@yahoo.co.jp (Y.A.)

2 Department of Respiratory Medicine, Fukujuji Hospital, Japan Anti-Tuberculosis Association, 3-1-24 Matsuyama, Kiyose, Tokyo 204-8533, Japan; okumuram@fukujuji.org (M.O.); yoshiyamat@fukujuji.org (T.Y.)

3 Department of Clinical Laboratory, Fukujuji Hospital, Japan Anti-Tuberculosis Association, 3-1-2 4 Matsuyama, Kiyose, Tokyo 204-8533, Japan; yanaih@fukujuji.org (H.Y.); hiralin99@yahoo.co.jp (K.M.); ideit@fukujuji.org (T.I.)

4 Division of Global Epidemiology, Research Center for Zoonosis Control, Hokkaido University, North 20, West 10, Kita-ku, Sapporo, Hokkaido 001-0020, Japan; cnakajim@czc.hokudai.ac.jp (C.N.); suzuki@czc.hokudai.ac.jp (Y.S.)

5 Department of Health Science and Social Welfare, Kibi International University, 8 Igamachi, Takahashi 716-8508, Japan

* Correspondence: hattorit@kiui.ac.jp;

† These authors contributed equally to this work.

‡ Current address: KKR Tohoku Kosai Hospital, Kokubun-cho 2-3-11, Aoba-ku, Sendai-shi, Miyagi 980-0803, Japan.

Academic Editor: Francesco B. Blasi

Abstract: Elevated matricellular proteins (MCPs), including osteopontin (OPN) and galectin-9 (Gal-9), were observed in the plasma of patients with Manila-type tuberculosis (TB) previously. Here, we quantified plasma OPN, Gal-9, and soluble CD44 (sCD44) by enzyme-linked immunosorbent assay (ELISA), and another 29 cytokines by Luminex assay in 36 patients with pulmonary TB, six subjects with latent tuberculosis (LTBI), and 19 healthy controls (HCs) from Japan for a better understanding of the roles of MCPs in TB. All TB subjects showed positive results of enzyme-linked immunospot assays (ELISPOTs). Spoligotyping showed that 20 out of 36 *Mycobacterium tuberculosis* (MTB) strains belong to the Beijing type. The levels of OPN, Gal-9, and sCD44 were higher in TB (positivity of 61.1%, 66.7%, and 63.9%, respectively) than in the HCs. Positive correlations between OPN and Gal-9, between OPN and sCD44, and negative correlation between OPN and ESAT-6-ELISPOT response, between chest X-ray severity score of cavitary TB and ESAT-6-ELISPOT response were observed. Instead of OPN, Gal-9, and sCD44, cytokines G-CSF, GM-CSF, IFN-α, IFN-γ, IL-12p70, and IL-1RA levels were higher in Beijing MTB-infected patients. These findings suggest immunoregulatory, rather than inflammatory, effect of MCPs and can advance the understanding of the roles of MCPs in the context of TB pathology.

Keywords: tuberculosis; osteopontin; galectin-9; CD44; Beijing genotype MTB

1. Introduction

In 2000, Bornstein et al. proposed that there is a family of secreted extracellular matrix (ECM) proteins termed "matricellular" proteins to highlight their influence on cell-matrix interactions [1]. Based on this definition, several proteins have now been identified as matricellular proteins (MCPs), including connective-tissue growth factors, galectins [2] and osteopontin (OPN) [3]. MCPs participate in wound repair, inflammation, and cancer progression by binding to their receptor [3]. The multitasking aspects of MCPs are derived from the different structural proteins, cell-surface receptors, proteases, and cytokines with which these proteins come into contact in the local environment of various tissues.

Among infectious diseases, *Mycobacterium tuberculosis* (MTB) infection remains a global public threat due to its ability to evade the host immune system by various mechanisms, including inhibition of phagolysosome fusion within phagocytes or induction of anti-inflammatory cytokine secretion [4]. Abnormal turnover of MCPs in the development of granulomas and cavities are the typical pulmonary manifestations of TB [5], in which chronic inflammation is activated, leading to tissue damage and subsequent tissue remodeling [6]. MCPs are expressed at low levels in normal adult tissues but are promptly up-regulated during tissue repair and remodeling processes [7]. In a previous study, we observed the expression of OPN and Gal-9 in TB granuloma [8]. We also confirmed the high level of plasma OPN in subjects with Manila genotype MTB from the Philippines [9] and in TB patients from Indonesia [8]. The intact form of OPN, also reported as full-length OPN (FL-OPN), is involved in the complex pathways of coagulation and fibrinolysis, where multiple sites of FL-OPN serve as a thrombin-cleaved target. During this process, the OPN fragments are produced. Among those fragments, proteolytic cleavage of FL-OPN by thrombin (between Arg168 and Ser169) generates a functional fragment of N-terminal thrombin-cleaved OPN (trOPN), which contains a cryptic binding site for integrins $\alpha 9\beta 1$ and $\alpha 4\beta 1$ that enhances the attachment of trOPN to integrins. Elevation of trOPN levels has been reported in the recovery phase of dengue virus infection [10].

Galectin-9 (Gal-9), a β-galactoside-binding MCP that induces apoptosis, chemoattraction, and necrosis, stimulates bactericidal activity in mouse TB models by binding to its receptor, T-cell immunoglobulin and mucin domain-containing molecule-3 (Tim3) [11,12]. Tim3-expressing T cells accumulate during chronic TB infection, produce less IL-2 and TNF but more IL-10, and are functionally exhausted. Such T-cell exhaustion impairs immunity and is detrimental to the outcome of MTB infection [13]. On the other hand, Gal-9 is reported to stimulate regulatory T cells and is produced by them in an autocrine manner, indicating that they have immunoregulatory functions [14]. Gal-9 and Tim-3 expression in $CD4^+$ and $CD8^+$ T cells increases during TB infection in humans compared to healthy individuals [15]. As a result, the recovery of T-cell function against MTB is associated with the blockage of TIM3 [16]. The associations of Gal-9 with the severity of the diseases were also found in dengue virus [17] and malaria infection [18], suggesting that manipulation of Gal-9 signals has an immunotherapeutic potential and may represent an alternative approach to improving immune responses to infections and/or vaccines [19]. Based on these findings, Gal-9 is proposed to be a soluble molecule responsible for an immune checkpoint [20].

CD44, a polymorphic transmembrane glycoprotein encoded by a single gene located on chromosome 11, one of OPN receptors, is involved in signaling and in regulating immune responses, and contributes to clinical manifestations [21]. Increased OPN and CD44 expression was reported in adult T-cell leukemia cells [22]. Meanwhile, CD44 glycosylation directly controls binding affinity of Gal-9 for fibrin and for immobilized fibrinogen and, therefore, participates in a wide variety of cell-cell or cell-matrix interactions, including tumor invasion and metastases [23]. CD44, along with CD25, is used to track early T-cell development in the thymus, and CD44 expression is an indicative marker for effector-memory T cells. Both functions involve a mechanism of CD44-regulated apoptosis resistance in T-cell subpopulations, namely T_h1 cells [24]. On the other hand, the sCD44 level in TB patients has not been examined.

Interferon γ (IFN-γ)-producing TB antigen-specific $CD4^+$ effector T cells and memory T cells can be monitored by an enzyme-linked immunospot assay (ELISPOT) [25], in which galectin-9–CD44 interaction enhances stability and function of adaptive regulatory T cells (Tregs), promoting Foxp3 expression and, therefore, suppressing effector T cell responses during infection [26]. Spoligotyping methods have been applied to identify the Beijing genotype of MTB that has been demonstrated as an independent risk factor of treatment failure [27]. In this study, results of various current diagnostic methods and clinical findings were also analyzed in view of the function of MCPs. Our results showed an important immunological role of elevated OPN, Gal-9, and sCD44 levels in MTB infection.

2. Results

2.1. Clinical Findings

The study includes 36 patients with active pulmonary TB, six LTBI patients, and 19 HCs. All HCs tested negative for T-SPOT.TB, and all TB patients tested positive for T-SPOT.TB. Laboratory data on the TB patients are summarized in Table 1. The majority of TB patients had low values of hemoglobin and hematocrit. Analysis of differential blood cell counts in TB patients showed frequent neutrophilia and lymphocytopenia. Plasma C-reactive protein (CRP) levels were above the reference range in 32 (88.8%) TB patients. Among the 36 patients with active pulmonary TB, 20 and 16 were infected with Beijing and non-Beijing type MTB, respectively. Moreover, 16 non-Beijing MTB isolates were found to be Latin American-Mediterranean-9 strain (one patient) and T2 strain (one patient); EAI2_Manila strain (two patients) and T3-OSA strain (two patients); a new type of strain (five patients) and T1 strain (five patients).

Table 1. Characteristics of HC, LTBI, and TB individuals.

Parameter	Ref.	HC (n = 19)	LTBI (n = 6)	TB (n = 36)	p Value
Antropometric data					
Age: year; median (range)		34 (19–67)	63 (36–71)	59.5 (19–86)	0.007
Gender: male; n (%)		12 (63)	5 (83)	28 (78)	0.43
Laboratory findings: median (range)					
RBC ($10^6/\mu$L)	Male 4.5–5.5; Female 4.0–5.0	na	4.65 (4.35–5.12)	4.44 (2.72–5.57)	0.443
Hemoglobin (g/dL)	14–18	na	14.6 (14.2–15.3)	13.1 (8.9–17.5)	0.064
Hematocrit (%)	40–48	na	43.6 (40.9–46.0)	39.65 (25.5–51.9)	0.059
WBC ($10^3/\mu$L)	4.5–11	na	7.64 (5.34–9.96)	7.33 (3.84–16.22)	0.945
Neutrophil (%)	38–80	na	57.35(51.9–75.7)	75.2 (57.0–89.6)	0.014
Lymphocyte (%)	15–40	na	33.1 (18.2–39.6)	14.1 (2.8–34.8)	0.007
Monocyte (%)	4–7	na	6 (4.9–7.7)	6.9 (3.4–11.2)	0.035
Eosinophil (%)	0–8	na	1.1 (0.4–4.1)	1.4 (0–11.4)	0.902
Platelet ($10^3/\mu$L)	140–390	na	267 (203–280)	305 (125–564)	0.228
CRP (mg/dL)	0–0.3	na	0.055 (0.04–0.07)	6 (0.04–21.5)	0.002
Genotype (Beijing strain MTB %)	73.0, year 2010, Japan	na	na	55.6	na
ALT (Units)	4–37	na	20.5 (11–29)	15 (8–103)	na
Creatinine (mg/dL)	0.5–1.5	na	0.74 (0.42–11)	0.71 (0.57–0.86)	na

Age differences among the groups were analyzed by the *Kruskal-Wallis* test, gender differences by the *Chi-square* test, and laboratory findings by the *Mann-Whitney* test; $p < 0.05$ means a significant difference; na: not applicable.

2.2. Luminex and ELISA

Luminex assay was applied to determine the levels of pro-inflammatory markers that are important in cell signaling and promote systemic inflammation. The results showed high levels of IFN-γ, IL-8, IP-10, and TNF-α in the TB group compared to HCs (Table 2). Plasma levels of other 25 biomarkers were below the measurable levels or did not show differences among the groups. Plasma OPN, Gal-9, and sCD44 were significantly higher in TB patients than in HCs. Plasma Gal-9 and sCD44 concentrations were higher in patients with LTBI than in HCs. In contrast, despite low levels of OPN in both HCs and LTBI, there was no significant difference between patients with TB and patients with LTBI (Figure 1A–C). Unlike OPN, the FL-OPN and trOPN levels in the TB group did not differ from those in the HCs (Table 2). Spearman's correlation analysis revealed a significant correlation between OPN and Gal-9, and between sCD44 and OPN, but not between Gal-9 and sCD44 in TB patients (Figure 2D–F). In TB patients, the levels of both OPN and sCD44 were associated with lymphocytopenia and the levels of CRP, IL-8, IP-10, and OPN significantly correlated with neutrophils, whereas sCD44 correlated with white blood cell counts and TNF-α, but such a correlation was not observed in HCs. In spite of the significant correlation between OPN and FL-OPN in the TB patients, OPN did not correlate with trOPN (Figure 3A,B). Although Gal-9 did not show a correlation with either OPN or sCD44 (Table 3), there was a correlation of Gal-9 with alanine aminotransferase (ALT) and creatinine. Plasma OPN, Gal-9, and sCD44 did not discriminate between patients with Beijing and non-Beijing MTB (Figure 1G–I).

Table 2. Biomarker levels measured by Luminex assay and ELISA in HCs and TB patients.

Biomarker	HC	TB	*p* Value
IFNγ (pg/mL)	4.46 (0.42–19.38)	8.13 (2.12–41)	0.0065
IL-8 (pg/mL)	1.585 (0.38–7.52)	7.26 (0.6–31.07)	<0.0001
IP-10 (pg/mL)	235.8 (132.2–472.8)	864.6 (219.3–3051)	<0.0001
TNFα (pg/mL)	3.88 (2.83–8.34)	10.11 (2.19–24.83)	<0.0001
OPN (ng/mL)	19.63 (9.31–111.64)	28.62 (10.59–170)	0.012
Gal-9 (ng/mL)	14.0 (0–120)	171.5 (0–470)	0.0002
sCD44 (ng/mL)	118.57 (91.02–141.41)	159.66 (98.89–346.2)	<0.0001
FL-OPN (nmol/mL)	5.20 (2.83–14.45)	1.75 (0.52–43.91)	>0.05
rtOPN (pmol/mL)	0 (0–26.73)	0.87 (0–347.95)	>0.05

Of the 29 cytokine/chemokine indicators examined in each group, 15 indicators (IL-1α, IL-1β, IL-2, IL-3, IL-4, IL-5, IL-6, IL-7, IL-10, IL-12p40, IL-13, IL-15, IL-17A, MIP-1α, and TNF-β) were excluded from statistical analyses because their median levels were below the detection level. EGF, VEGF, MCP-1, MIP-1β, eotaxin, G-CSF, GM-CSF, IFN-α2, IL-12p70, and IL-1RA did not differ among the groups. OPN, Gal-9, and sCD44 differed between groups. FL-OPN and trOPN did not differ among the groups.

Table 3. Correlations of OPN, Gal-9, and sCD44 with other laboratory parameters and biomarkers in TB patients.

Measurements	OPN	sCD44	Gal-9
	r (*P*)	r (*P*)	r (*P*)
WBC ($10^3/\mu$L)	Ns	0.388 (0.019)	Ns
Neutrophil (%)	0.517 (<0.0001)	Ns	Ns
Lymphocyte (%)	−0.569 (<0.0001)	−0.558 (<0.0001)	Ns
CRP (mg/dL)	0.757 (<0.0001)	0.534 (0.001)	Ns
IL-8 (pg/mL)	0.474 (0.013)	0.524 (0.005)	Ns
IP-10 (pg/mL)	0.420 (0.029)	0.542 (0.003)	Ns
TNFα	Ns	0.446 (0.020)	Ns
ALT	Ns	Ns	0.375 (0.024)
Cre	Ns	Ns	0.377 (0.023)

Ns: not significant.

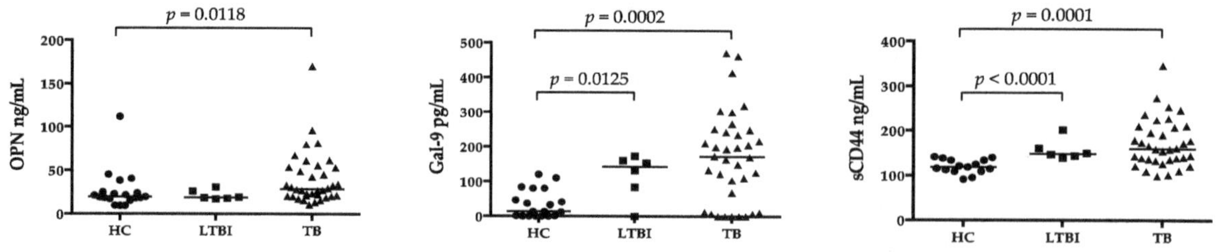

(A) (B) (C)

Figure 1. *Cont.*

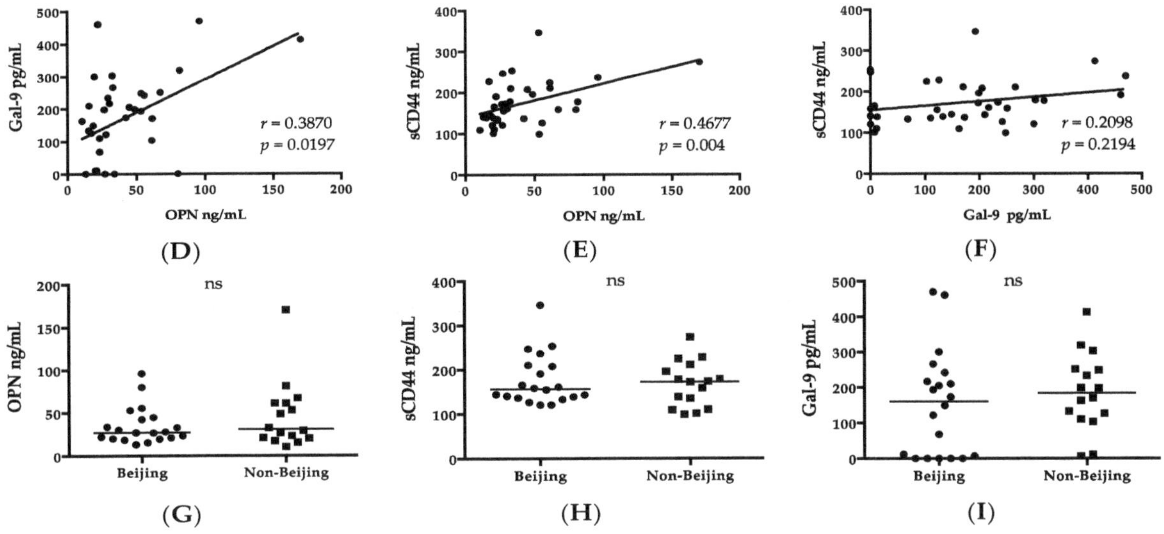

Figure 1. OPN, Gal-9 and sCD44 in groups under study. Comparison of plasma levels of OPN (**A**); Gal-9 (**B**); and sCD44 (**C**) among HC, LTBI, and TB patients. Correlations among OPN, Gal-9, and sCD44 in TB patients (**D–F**); comparison of OPN (**G**); Gal-9 (**H**); and sCD44 (**I**) between Beijing and non-Beijing genotype.

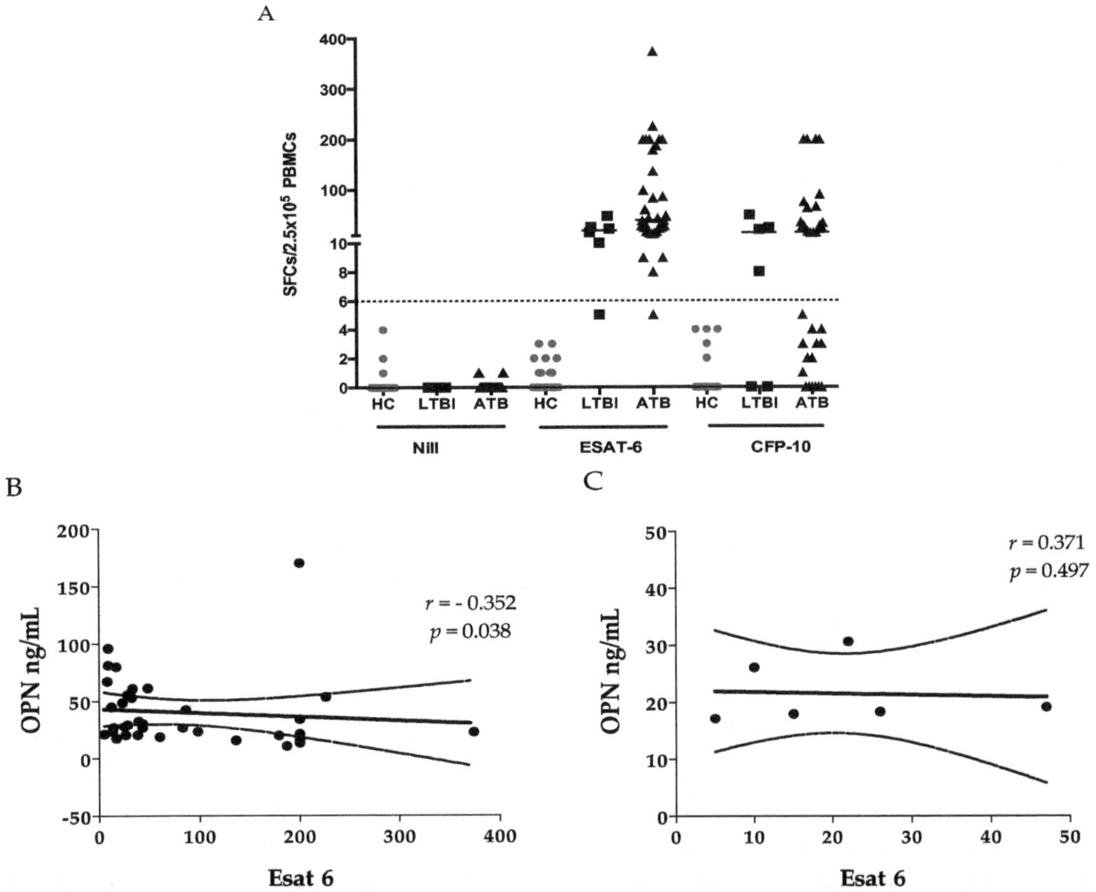

Figure 2. ELISPOTs reaction and OPN levels. ELISPOT assays are plotted as the number of specific PBMCs against the indicated stimulus (**A**); a negative correlation was observed between the ELISPOT for ESAT-6 and OPN in TB (**B**); and this correlation was not seen in the LTBI group (**C**).

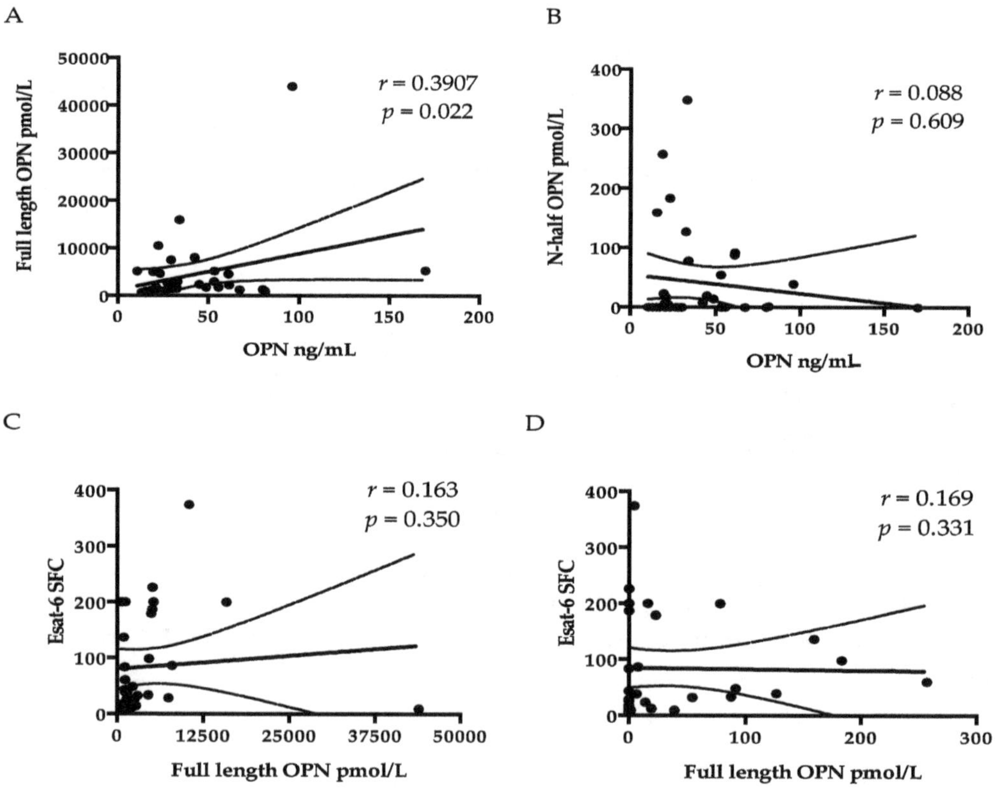

Figure 3. OPN, full-length OPN, n-half OPN, and ESAT-6 SFC count in TB patients. A comparison of plasma levels of OPN with full-length OPN (**A**) and with n-half OPN (**B**); and a comparison of ESAT-6 ELISPOT SFC counts with full-length OPN (**C**) and with n-half OPN (**D**).

2.3. ELISPOTS

All HCs tested negative for ESAT-6 or CFP-10 because the SFC (cutoff = 6) was lower than the cutoff; none of them showed total SFC $\geq$ 8 in ESAT-6 and CFP-10 assays. In the TB group, one sample was negative for ESAT-6 (SFC = 5) and CFP-10 (SFC = 3); the total SFC was no less than 8, and the result was considered positive. In the LTBI group, one sample with negative Esat-6 (SFC = 5) and CFP-10 (SFC = 0) was considered indeterminate because total SFC was less than 8. Therefore, the sensitivity of ELISPOTs for TB and LTBI was 100% and 83.3%, respectively (Figure 1A). There was a negative correlation between ESAT-6 SFC and OPN levels (Figure 1B) in TB but not in LTBI (Figure 1C). Nonetheless, ESAT-6 did not correlate with either FL-OPN or trOPN (Figure 3C,D), nor was a correlation detected between OPN levels and CFP10. Moreover, none of 19 markers tested by Luminex showed any correlation with either ESAT-6 or CFP-10 responses.

2.4. Sensitivity and Specificity

ROC analysis revealed that OPN, Gal-9, sCD44, IP-10, and anti-TBGL IgG could discriminate active TB (ATB) from HC, in spite of varied discriminatory power indicated by an AUC comparison. IP-10 (92.6% sensitivity and 93.3% specificity) was more effective than OPN ($p < 0.001$) and anti-TBGL IgG ($p < 0.05$). sCD44 (63.9% sensitivity and 100% specificity) was more effective than OPN (Table 4). Of note, in spite of greater discriminatory power of IP-10 and sCD44, there was no significant difference between these two tests (Figure 4B), nor was a difference found between OPN and anti-TBGL assays (Figure 4A). No valid discrimination was found between ATB and LTBI in terms of the MCPs due to small number of LTBI subjects (Figure 4C).

Table 4. Sensitivity and specificity.

Analytes	Youden Index	Cutoff	Sensitivity (%)	Specificity (%)	AUC	Comparison		
OPN	0.4006	25.1	61.1	79	0.706	*a*	*b*	
Gal-9	0.6667	120	66.7	100	0.798			
sCD44	0.6389	141.4	63.9	100	0.846	*a*		
IP-10	0.8593	400.3	92.6	93.3	0.965		*b*	*a*
Anti-TBGL IgG	0.5058	1.6	61.1	89.4	0.762			*a*

A cutoff was calculated based on TB and HC data from the Youden index. The discriminatory power of each test was evaluated by the area under curve (AUC) comparison. ***a***, ***b***, a significant difference between the AUCs of the indicated tests; ***a***, $p < 0.05$, ***b***, $p < 0.001$.

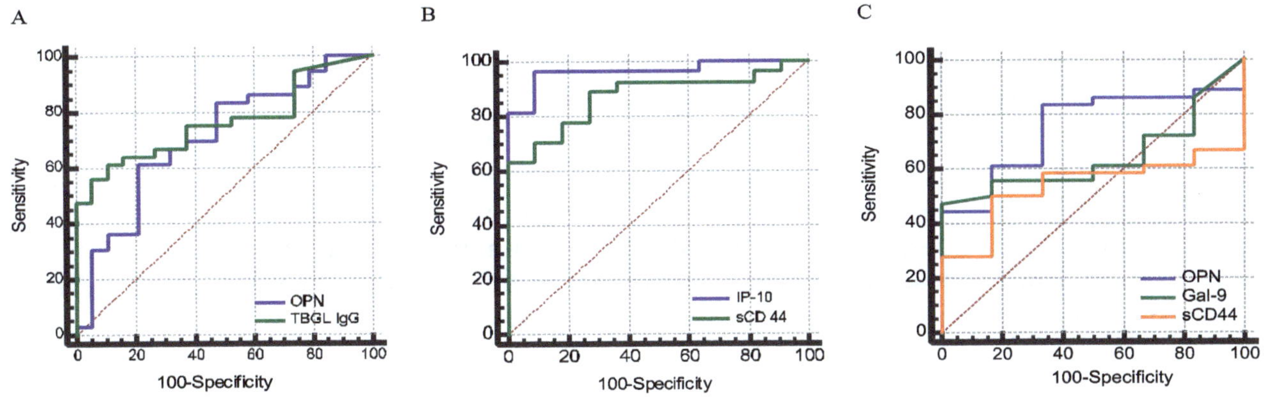

Figure 4. Sensitivity and specificity analysis for OPN, anti-TBGL IgG, IP-10, and sCD44. Comparison between ATB and HCs (**A**,**B**), no significant difference between the areas under curve (AUC) of OPN and anti-TBGL IgG, IP-10, or sCD44, $p > 0.05$. Strong discriminatory power of IP-10 and sCD44; $p < 0.0001$ for both (**A**). Comparison between ATB and LTBI, no significant discriminatory power of OPN, Gal-9, and sCD44 in LTBI and ATB ($p > 0.05$) due to the inadequacy of LTBI subjects (**C**). No significant difference between the AUC of OPN and Gal-9, between Gal-9 and sCD44, but difference between OPN and sCD44 ($p = 0.014$) (**C**).

2.5. Clinical Biomarkers, Chest X-rays, and Genotype

OPN and sCD44 showed positive correlations with inflammatory markers and a negative correlation with lymphocyte counts ($p < 0.001$). On the contrary, Gal-9 levels did not show any correlation with inflammatory and hematological markers, but correlated positively with ALT and creatinine (Table 3). Analysis of patients' chest radiographs showed cavity formation in 12 (33.3%) patients. Patients with lung cavities had significantly lower levels of hemoglobin and hematocrit and a higher differential number of monocytes and higher CRP, anti-TBGL IgG, and IP-10 levels (Table 5). In contrast, the levels of OPN, sCD44, and Gal-9 were not significantly higher in cavity-positive ATB subjects.

Table 5. Comparison of laboratory findings between TB patients with and without cavity lung formation.

Parameter	Normal Value (Range)	Cavity (−) (n = 24)	Cavity (+) (n = 12)	p Value
Hemoglobin (g/dL)	14–18	13.8 (8.9–17.5)	12.4 (9.9–14.7)	0.0454
Hematocrit (%)	40–48	42 (25.5–51.9)	37.5 (28.4–41.4)	0.0208
Monocyte (%)	4–7	6.2 (3.4–10)	8.3 (4.9–10.2)	0.0054
CRP (mg/dL)	0–0.3	3.27 (0.04–21.5)	8.67 (0.08–17.97)	0.0478
IP-10 (pg/mL)	132.2–472.8	751.5 (219.3–2735)	1570 (369.7–3051)	0.0408
Anti-TBGL IgG (U/mL)	<2	13.3 (0.1–62.6)	1.11 (0–72.6)	0.0123
CXR Score	0	92.46 (82.4–100)	131.84 (104.34–140)	0.0001

The CXR score correlated with a higher proportion or higher number of monocytes and IL-12p70. The CXR score in cavity-positive and cavity-negative TB patients was analyzed further. In the former subgroup, ESAT-6 SFC showed an inverse correlation with CXR (Table 6). In the latter subgroup, IL-12p70 correlated with CXR (Table 6). No significant differences in plasma OPN, Gal-9, or sCD44 were observed between subjects with Beijing and non-Beijing MTB (Figure 1G–I). Nonetheless, higher G-CSF, GM-CSF, IFN-α, IFN-γ, IL-12p70, and IL-1RA concentrations were detected in Beijing MTB subjects (Table 7). Among these six makers, levels of IFN-α, IFN-γ, and IL-1RA were higher in Beijing MTB subjects compared to the HCs (Table 7, *Kruskal-Wallis* test, $p < 0.05$).

Table 6. CXR score and biomarkers in TB patients.

Parameter	CXR Scorer (p)	CXR Scorer (p)	
		Cavity (+)	Cavity (−)
Monocytes (%)	0.502 (0.003)	Ns	Ns
OPN	Ns	Ns	Ns
sCD44	Ns	Ns	Ns
IP-10	0.452 (0.027)	Ns	Ns
Gal-9	Ns	Ns	Ns
IL-12p70	0.517 (0.01)	Ns	0.574 (0.032)
ESAT-6 SFC	Ns	−0.6185 (0.0425)	Ns

Ns: no significant.

Table 7. Laboratory and biomarker values in patients infected by Beijing or non-Beijing strains of *Mycobacterium tuberculosis* (MTB).

Parameter	HC	Beijing Type (n = 20)	Non-Beijing Type (n = 16)	p Value
Laboratory findings				
RBC ($10^6/\mu L$)	na.	4.28 (2.72–5.16)	4.64 (3.86–5.57)	0.0465
Total protein (g/dL)	na.	7.05 (5.41–8.03)	7.69 (6.54–8.14)	0.0323
Biomarker (pg/mL)				
G-CSF	48.48 (12.19–90.49)	56.94 (21.69–106.36)	38.12 (14.06–73.07)	0.0388
GM-CSF	4.24 (0.44–18.98)	12.29 (0.83–48.8)	5.84 (0.44–14.6)	0.0300
IFNα	11.07 (0–56.49)	32.87 (1.67–60.81) [a]	7.53 (0–40.97)	0.0034
IFNγ	4.46 (0.42–19.38)	16.02 (3.09–41) [a]	4.71 (2.12–17.84)	0.0141
IL-12p70	2.74 (1.35–15.06)	8.22 (1.85–29.77)	2.62 (0.03–7.13)	0.0007
IL-1RA	17.79 (0–81.26)	51.96 (8.56–217.37) [a]	14.02 (0–78.44)	0.0095
IP-10	235.78 (132.2–472.75)	877.12 (219.29–2814.69) [a]	864.57 (369.67–3051.48) [b]	>0.05
Cavity n (%)	0	8 (40)	4 (25)	>0.05
CXR score	0	102.23 (82.4–140)	109.74 (82.77–140)	>0.05

Differences among the groups in terms of laboratory biomarkers were analyzed by the *Kruskal-Wallis* test; $p < 0.05$ indicates a significant difference between Beijing and non-Beijing MTB groups; [a] indicates a significant difference between groups Beijing MTB and HC, $p < 0.05$; [b] indicates a significant difference between groups non-Beijing MTB and HC; $p < 0.05$. na., no applicable.

3. Discussion

It is known that cells producing IFN-γ after stimulation with ESAT-6 and CFP-10 are $CD4^+$ effector memory cells in both HIV-infected [28] and uninfected subjects [29]. A very low proportion of MTB-specific effector T cells is found in the blood compared with the infected tissue, indicating the differences in the cellular immune response and regulatory mechanisms between focal sites and systemic levels [30]. OPN is a multifunctional phosphorylated glycoprotein that is synthesized by a variety of immune and non-immune cells, and it participates in the balance between the T_h1 and T_h2 responses and in granulomatous reactions [31,32]. A negative correlation was observed between OPN and ESAT-6 ELISPOTs (Figure 1B), in addition to the negative correlation of OPN with lymphocyte counts (Table 3), which could be explained by increased migration of lymphocytes toward the lesion in response to OPN signaling [33]. OPN-induced T-cell migration may initiate suppression of hyperinflammation [33] and prevent the contact between peripheral lymphocytes and MTB bacilli, to the extent of compartmentalization of MTB bacteria and lower risk of dissemination [34,35]. Since OPN showed a correlation with sCD44, one of the memory T-cell markers [36], it may also reflect the activation of memory T cells in the lesion. Of note, we did not observe a correlation between OPN and a CFP-10 cellular response, in support of the discrepancies between results of ESAT-6 and CFP-10 assays [37]. Nevertheless, the component of secreted OPN responsible for summoning T-cell immigration is still unknown. Therefore, we tested the correlation among ESAT-6 SFC, FL-OPN, and trOPN, which did not show a statistical association with one another. It is more than obvious that the FL-OPN level exceeds the trOPN level, in addition to a correlation between OPN and FL-OPN, suggesting that FL-OPN is responsible as one of components of OPN. Another culprit may be MMP-cleaved OPN [32]. Nevertheless, these components were not demonstrated in this study.

OPN levels are higher in patients with extensive TB/HIV coinfection than in patients with a single disease of TB or HIV [38]. HIV has been proposed to infect memory T cells preferentially, and efficient transfer of the R5 virus to effector memory T cells has also been observed [39,40]. We have reported the increased amount of OPN in an AIDS-TB case, though this patient showed lymphadenopathy and did not have granuloma of the lungs [41]. Probably, OPN was synthesized in activated lymph nodes and immune cells in this patient, and we have reported that macrophages are the main producer in the lymph nodes of adult T-cell leukemia patients [21]. In this particular case of AIDS/TB, OPN did not decrease after antiretroviral therapy despite the fall of the viral load [41], and OPN was retained as a component of the immune reconstitution (IRIS) that takes place during antiretroviral therapy [42]. These data suggest that OPN could be synthesized in response to both TB and HIV infection and serve as a marker of complex disease activity such as IRIS.

Gal-9 appeared to reflect disease severity as reported for other diseases, such as malaria and dengue, because of its association with ALT and creatinine [17,18] (Table 3). The levels of ALT and creatinine are indicators of systemic severity of TB infection [43]. The association of these molecules with Gal-9 in TB cases supports the idea that Gal-9 could either influence the outcome of MTB infection or indicate the state of disease [44]. Like many immunological pathways, the Gal-9 pathway functions via binding of Gal-9 to its receptor TIM3 prior to the initiation of the MCP-mediated signaling, before regulation of intracellular antimicrobial processes and of long-term immunological memory, as well as physiological homeostasis [45]. In vitro TIM3 blockade—in co-culture experiments with MTB-infected macrophages from TB patients with or without HIV co-infection—promotes bacterial killing and enhances IL-1β secretion by infected cells, as well as the IFN-γ release by T cells [12]. Therefore, the interaction of Gal-9 and TIM3 serves as an immune checkpoint rather than leading to inflammation [20]. Regimens incorporating therapeutics targeting such immune checkpoints are urgently needed to improve the clinical management of multidrug-resistant TB (MDR-TB) when the TB drug options are diminished for patients with MDR-TB infection [46]. Drugs enhancing T-cell activity, depleting Treg cells, and inhibiting the immune checkpoint have been reported, in agreement with the potential of targeting of the Gal-9–TIM3 interaction.

In this study, for the first time, we reported a high plasma concentration of sCD44 in ATB compared to HCs, in the sense of discriminatory power comparable to that of IP-10 (Figure 4B, $p > 0.05$). The discriminatory power of sCD44 is higher than that of OPN. Nonetheless, like OPN and Gal-9, sCD44 is related to immune regulation. Without the recruitment of other non-MTB inflammatory diseases in this study, it is implausible to make a conclusion about the reliability of these markers for TB diagnosis. IP-10, a chemokine secreted from cells stimulated with interferon and lipopolysaccharides, is a chemoattractant for activated T cells [47]. IP-10 concentrations correlated with the plasma OPN level (Table 3). A similar finding has also been reported, except that decreased IP-10 and OPN levels were reported as markers of negative conversion in sputum smears. Nevertheless, only IP-10 correlates with CRP and inflammation [48]. In our study, significantly higher levels of plasma IP-10 in cavitary TB patients (Table 5), and the correlation between IP-10 and CXR score (Table 6) are in agreement with IP-10's role as an inflammation inducer. In addition to an inflammatory marker of TB [49], serum IP-10 also increased in chronic hepatitis C [50] and autoimmune diseases [51].

Beijing genotype MTB has been the most prevalent in East Asia [52] because of its virulence and resistance to drugs and BCG vaccination. Treatment failure and relapse have also been found to be associated with Beijing genotype MTB [53]. On the other hand, other researchers, and our group, have reported that the rates of MDR-MTB among Beijing and non-Beijing family strains are not statistically significantly different in Beijing MTB-predominant regions [27,54]. Highly intense inflammation of Beijing genotype MTB infection may be detected by assaying inflammatory cytokines. Nevertheless, we did not detect differences in IP-10, sCD44, OPN, or Gal-9 concentrations between Beijing and non-Beijing TB infections; plasma concentrations of other cytokines, including G-CSF, GM-CSF, IFN-α, IFN-γ, IL-12p70, and IL-1RA, were found to be higher in Beijing MTB-infected subjects than in non-Beijing MTB-infected subjects. An increased level of IL-12p70 was found to be associated with a high CXR sore, in support of the more severe lung damage in Beijing MTB infection compared to non-Beijing MTB infection [55]. G-CSF and GM-CSF also play a role in the regulation of macrophages and dendritic cells to facilitate granuloma in the development of a cavity [56]. Therefore, a high percentage of patients with a cavity were observed in the Beijing MTB group (40%) compared to the non-Beijing MTB group (25%) in this study. Unlike those cytokines, MCPs are involved in not only inflammation, but also immune regulation, and their concentrations were not affected by the genotype of MTB in this study.

4. Materials and Methods

4.1. Study Subjects

The study was conducted at Double-Barred Hospital, Tokyo, Japan, and Tohoku University, Sendai, Japan, between May 2014 and 2015. The study protocol was approved by the Ethics Committee of Fukujuji Hospital, Japan Anti-Tuberculosis Association and Graduate School of Medicine (NO. 2014-1-122, January 2014), Tohoku University. Written informed consent was obtained from all the enrolled subjects. All of the procedures were conducted in accordance with the Declaration of Helsinki.

Patients with culture-confirmed TB diagnosis according to WHO guidelines [57] were included in the active TB group ($n = 36$); none of these patients had taken anti-TB medication. Healthy control subjects (HCs; $n = 19$) had no TB-related symptoms, and exhibited negative T-SPOT.TB (Oxford Immunotec, Oxford, UK) results. Subjects who showed positive T-SPOT.TB results or were positive in Interferon-γ release assays (IGRAs) and without TB clinical manifestations were categorized as patients with latent tuberculosis (LTBI; $n = 6$). Exclusion criteria were as follows: impossibility to obtain informed consent, cancer, and human immunodeficiency virus infection.

Each subject donated a 7-mL heparinized and 7-mL EDTA-treated peripheral-blood sample. The EDTA-blood samples were centrifuged within 30 min of collection, and plasma was stored at −80 °C until further analyses. Heparinized blood samples were sent from Double-Barred Cross Hospital and delivered to Tohoku University by a courier service within 24 h. All laboratory data were obtained from patients' medical records and at the point of sample collection.

The TB patients were categorized into cavity-positive or cavity-negative in accordance with the presence or absence of cavities on chest X-ray images. A scoring method was used on the basis of the affected lung area and the presence of a cavity in order to conduct the comparison of TB lung lesion severity. The score was calculated as the percentage of lung affected plus 40 if cavitation was present [58].

4.2. Spoligotyping

To differentiate Beijing and non-Beijing genotypes of MTB, spoligotypes of clinical MTB isolates were determined as described previously [19]. Acid-fast bacilli (AFB) smear staining and Ogawa medium culture were conducted to confirm the MTB infection. To identify the most prevalent genotype, DNA samples were isolated from the colonies in culture. One colony was picked and resuspended in 0.5 mL of Tris-EDTA. The mixture was subjected to a 95 °C boil-and-cool cycle for decontamination before processing for spoligotyping. Briefly, the DR region was amplified with a primer pair, and the polymerase chain reaction (PCR) products were hybridized to a set of 43 spacer-specific oligonucleotide probes, which were covalently bound to membranes. The spoligo-international type was determined by comparing spoligotypes with the international spoligotyping database [20].

4.3. ELISPOTs

Peripheral blood mononuclear cells (PBMCs) were isolated from heparinized blood samples over Ficoll-Paque Plus (GE Healthcare Bio-Sciences AB, Uppsala, Sweden) and resuspended in the AIM V medium (Gibco, Grand Island, NE, USA) at the concentration of 2.5×10^5 per 100 µL. *M. tuberculosis* infection was determined using T-SPOT.TB (Oxford Immunotec, Oxford, UK), according to the manufacturer's recommendation. A test result was considered reliable if the spot-forming cell

(SFC) number in the positive-control well was >20, and in the negative control well was <10. Positive results were scored as positive if the SFC number of either ESAT-6 or CFP-10 well was >6. If the total number of SFCs of ESAT-6 and CFP-10 was ≤ 8, the test result was considered indeterminate. Spots were counted with an automated Immunospot Analyzer, CTL (Cellular Technologies, Cleveland, OH, USA).

4.4. ELISA

Plasma concentrations of OPN were determined using the Human Osteopontin DuoSet ELISA Development System Kit (R and D Systems, Minneapolis, MN, USA) [21]. In this ELISA kit, the proprietary capture monoclonal antibody and the detection polyclonal antibodies were both raised against recombinant human OPN (NS0-derived, amino acids Ile17-Asn300). To determine the full-length OPN and trOPN, two separate ELISA kits (IBL, Gunma, Japan) were used. In the FL-OPN kit, a polyclonal rabbit antibody (O-17) specific to the N terminus of OPN (Ile17-Gln31, accession # NP_000573.1) was used as a capture antibody, and a mouse monoclonal antibody (10A16) raised against synthetic peptides corresponding to the internal sequence of human OPN (Lys166-Glu187) served as a detector antibody. Therefore, this kit does not allow us to detect trOPN. Meanwhile, the trOPN ELISA assay was performed using an anti-trOPN monoclonal antibody (34E3) as the capture antibody, and the O-17 antibody as the detection antibody. This capture antibody specifically reacts to the epitope Ser162–Arg168 exposed by thrombin and does not react with matrix metalloproteinase 3 or 7 (MMP-3 or -7)-cleaved N-terminal trOPN [10,59]. Gal-9 was quantified using a human Gal-9 ELISA kit (Galpharma Co., Ltd., Takamatsu, Japan), as described previously [17]. The concentration of soluble CD44 was measured by means of the Human CD44 ELISA kit (Abcam, Cambridge, MA, USA), as described previously [21]. Samples, reagents, and buffers were prepared according to the manufacturers' manuals.

4.5. Luminex Assays

Twenty-nine cytokine and chemokine species, including epidermal growth factor (EGF), eotaxin, granulocyte macrophage-colony stimulating factor (GM-CSF), G-CSF, interferon-alpha2 (IFN-α), IFN-γ, interleukin 1 alpha (IL-1α), IL-1β, IL-1 receptor antagonist (IL-1RA), IL-2, IL-3, IL-4, IL-5, IL-6, IL-7, IL-8, IL-10, IL-12p40, IL-12p70, IL-13, IL-15, IL-17a, IFN-γ-inducible protein-10 (IP-10), monocyte chemotactic protein 1 (MCP-1), macrophage-inducible protein 1α (MIP-1α), MIP-1β, tumor necrosis factor α (TNF-α), TNF-β, and vascular endothelial growth factor (VEGF), in plasma were measured using a commercially available kit (Milliplex Human Cytokine and Chemokine multiplex assay kit, Merck Millipore, Billerica, MA, USA) by Luminex methods, as reported previously [17]. The assay was performed according to manufacturer's instructions and the concentrations of cytokines/chemokines were calculated by comparing the assay readings with a five-parameter logistic standard curve on a Bioplex-200 instrument (Bio-Rad, Hercules, CA, USA). All of the results were expressed in pg/mL.

4.6. Data Analyses

Data are expressed as the median and range. Significance of differences for more than two groups was tested by the Kruskal–Wallis analysis. Significance of differences between two groups was tested by the Mann-Whitney *U* analysis. Correlations were determined using Spearman's nonparametric test. These analyses were carried out in the GraphPad Prism 6 software (GraphPad, San Diego, CA, USA). Furthermore, receiver operating characteristic (ROC) curves were constructed to study the diagnostic utility of OPN, Gal-9, sCD44, and IP-10. The area under curve (AUC) and cutoff analyses were conducted by means of the MedCalc statistical software Version 16.8.4 (Ostend, Belgium). A difference was assumed to be significant at $p < 0.05$.

5. Conclusions

In conclusion, this study showed that the levels of OPN, Gal-9, sCD44, and IP-10 could help to understand the immune network of MCPs in TB, in addition to their diagnostic value in MTB infections, especially in the presence of a lung cavity. Higher plasma concentration of OPN in association with a low-ESAT-6-ELISPOT-response could help to understand the immunopathogenesis of TB. A high level of sCD44 and Gal-9 in MTB infection could also predict MTB-related inflammation and clinical severity.

Acknowledgments: We acknowledge Toshiro Niki from Department of Immunology, Kagawa University, Takamatsu, for his comments on the biological function of Gal-9, and Yuka Sasaki from Double-Barred Cross Hospital, for her assessment on clinical severity of TB patients. This research is supported by the Research Program on Emerging and Re-emerging Infectious Diseases from Japan Agency for Medical Research and development, AMED, Grant Number 16fk0108302h0003. In addition, this study was partially supported by a grant from the Ministry of Education, Culture, Sports, Science and Technology of Japan for the Joint Research Program of the Research Center for Zoonosis Control at Hokkaido University and a special research grant from the International Research Institute of Disaster Science of Tohoku University.

Author Contributions: Toshio Hattori conceived and designed the projects; Masao Okumura, Hideki Yanai, Kazue Mizuno, Takashi Yoshiyama, Tadashi Idei collected samples and performed clinical data analysis; Yugo Ashino and Jingge Zhao performed chest X-ray assessment; Haorile Chagan-Yasutan performed Luminex assays; Beata Shiratori performed ELISPOTs assay; Beata Shiratori and Jingge Zhao performed ELISA assays; Chie Nakajima and Yasuhiko Suzuki performed spoligotyping. All the authors analyzed the data, discussed the results and contributed to the proof-editing of the manuscripts; and Jingge Zhao wrote the manuscript.

References

1. Bornstein, P.; Sage, E.H. Matricellular proteins: Extracellular modulators of cell function. *Curr. Opin. Cell Biol.* **2002**, *14*, 608–616. [CrossRef]
2. Elola, M.T.; Wolfenstein-Todel, C.; Troncoso, M.F.; Vasta, G.R.; Rabinovich, G.A. Galectins: Matricellular glycan-binding proteins linking cell adhesion, migration, and survival. *Cell. Mol. Life Sci. CMLS* **2007**, *64*, 1679–1700. [CrossRef] [PubMed]
3. Murphy-Ullrich, J.E.; Sage, E.H. Revisiting the matricellular concept. *Matrix Biol. J. Int. Soc. Matrix Biol.* **2014**, *37*, 1–14. [CrossRef] [PubMed]
4. Deretic, V.; Singh, S.; Master, S.; Harris, J.; Roberts, E.; Kyei, G.; Davis, A.; de Haro, S.; Naylor, J.; Lee, H.H.; et al. *Mycobacterium tuberculosis* inhibition of phagolysosome biogenesis and autophagy as a host defence mechanism. *Cell. Microbiol.* **2006**, *8*, 719–727. [CrossRef] [PubMed]
5. Elkington, P.T.; Emerson, J.E.; Lopez-Pascua, L.D.; O'Kane, C.M.; Horncastle, D.E.; Boyle, J.J.; Friedland, J.S. *Mycobacterium tuberculosis* up-regulates matrix metalloproteinase-1 secretion from human airway epithelial cells via a p38 MAPK switch. *J. Immunol.* **2005**, *175*, 5333–5340. [CrossRef] [PubMed]
6. Dheda, K.; Booth, H.; Huggett, J.F.; Johnson, M.A.; Zumla, A.; Rook, G.A. Lung remodeling in pulmonary tuberculosis. *J. Infect. Dis.* **2005**, *192*, 1201–1209. [CrossRef] [PubMed]
7. Cox, T.R.; Erler, J.T. Remodeling and homeostasis of the extracellular matrix: Implications for fibrotic diseases and cancer. *Dis. Models Mech.* **2011**, *4*, 165–178. [CrossRef] [PubMed]
8. Hasibuan, F.M.; Shiratori, B.; Senoputra, M.A.; Chagan-Yasutan, H.; Koesoemadinata, R.C.; Apriani, L.; Takahashi, Y.; Niki, T.; Alisjahbana, B.; Hattori, T. Evaluation of matricellular proteins in systemic and local immune response to *Mycobacterium tuberculosis* infection. *Microbiol. Immunol.* **2015**, *59*, 623–632. [CrossRef] [PubMed]
9. Shiratori, B.; Leano, S.; Nakajima, C.; Chagan-Yasutan, H.; Niki, T.; Ashino, Y.; Suzuki, Y.; Telan, E.; Hattori, T. Elevated OPN, IP-10, and neutrophilia in loop-mediated isothermal amplification confirmed tuberculosis patients. *Mediat. Inflamm.* **2014**, *2014*, 513263. [CrossRef] [PubMed]
10. Chagan-Yasutan, H.; Lacuesta, T.L.; Ndhlovu, L.C.; Oguma, S.; Leano, P.S.A.; Telan, E.F.O.; Kubo, T.; Morita, K.; Uede, T.; Dimaano, E.M.; et al. Elevated levels of full-length and thrombin-cleaved osteopontin during acute dengue virus infection are associated with coagulation abnormalities. *Thromb. Res.* **2014**, *134*, 449–454. [CrossRef] [PubMed]

11. Jayaraman, P.; Sada-Ovalle, I.; Beladi, S.; Anderson, A.C.; Dardalhon, V.; Hotta, C.; Kuchroo, V.K.; Behar, S.M. Tim3 binding to galectin-9 stimulates antimicrobial immunity. *J. Exp. Med.* **2010**, *207*, 2343–2354. [CrossRef] [PubMed]
12. Sada-Ovalle, I.; Chavez-Galan, L.; Torre-Bouscoulet, L.; Nava-Gamino, L.; Barrera, L.; Jayaraman, P.; Torres-Rojas, M.; Salazar-Lezama, M.A.; Behar, S.M. The Tim3–galectin 9 pathway induces antibacterial activity in human macrophages infected with *Mycobacterium tuberculosis*. *J. Immunol.* **2012**, *189*, 5896–5902. [CrossRef] [PubMed]
13. Jayaraman, P.; Jacques, M.K.; Zhu, C.; Steblenko, K.M.; Stowell, B.L.; Madi, A.; Anderson, A.C.; Kuchroo, V.K.; Behar, S.M. Tim3 mediates T cell exhaustion during *Mycobacterium tuberculosis* infection. *PLoS Pathog.* **2016**, *12*, e1005490. [CrossRef] [PubMed]
14. Oomizu, S.; Arikawa, T.; Niki, T.; Kadowaki, T.; Ueno, M.; Nishi, N.; Yamauchi, A.; Hattori, T.; Masaki, T.; Hirashima, M. Cell surface galectin-9 expressing th cells regulate Th17 and Foxp3+ treg development by galectin-9 secretion. *PLoS ONE* **2012**, *7*, e48574. [CrossRef] [PubMed]
15. Qiu, Y.; Chen, J.; Liao, H.; Zhang, Y.; Wang, H.; Li, S.; Luo, Y.; Fang, D.; Li, G.; Zhou, B.; et al. Tim-3-expressing $CD4^+$ and $CD8^+$ T cells in human tuberculosis (TB) exhibit polarized effector memory phenotypes and stronger anti-TB effector functions. *PLoS Pathog.* **2012**, *8*, e1002984. [CrossRef] [PubMed]
16. Sada-Ovalle, I.; Ocana-Guzman, R.; Perez-Patrigeon, S.; Chavez-Galan, L.; Sierra-Madero, J.; Torre-Bouscoulet, L.; Addo, M.M. Tim-3 blocking rescue macrophage and T cell function against *Mycobacterium tuberculosis* infection in HIV^+ patients. *J. Int. AIDS Soc.* **2015**, *18*, 20078. [CrossRef] [PubMed]
17. Chagan-Yasutan, H.; Ndhlovu, L.C.; Lacuesta, T.L.; Kubo, T.; Leano, P.S.; Niki, T.; Oguma, S.; Morita, K.; Chew, G.M.; Barbour, J.D.; et al. Galectin-9 plasma levels reflect adverse hematological and immunological features in acute dengue virus infection. *J. Clin. Virol.* **2013**, *58*, 635–640. [CrossRef] [PubMed]
18. Dembele, B.P.; Chagan-Yasutan, H.; Niki, T.; Ashino, Y.; Tangpukdee, N.; Shinichi, E.; Krudsood, S.; Kano, S.; Hattori, T. Plasma levels of galectin-9 reflect disease severity in malaria infection. *Malar. J.* **2016**, *15*, 403. [CrossRef] [PubMed]
19. Merani, S.; Chen, W.; Elahi, S. The bitter side of sweet: The role of galectin-9 in immunopathogenesis of viral infections. *Rev. Med. Virol.* **2015**, *25*, 175–186. [CrossRef] [PubMed]
20. Anderson, A.C.; Joller, N.; Kuchroo, V.K. Lag-3, Tim-3, and Tigit: Co-inhibitory receptors with specialized functions in immune regulation. *Immunity* **2016**, *44*, 989–1004. [CrossRef] [PubMed]
21. Chagan-Yasutan, H.; Tsukasaki, K.; Takahashi, Y.; Oguma, S.; Harigae, H.; Ishii, N.; Zhang, J.; Fukumoto, M.; Hattori, T. Involvement of osteopontin and its signaling molecule CD44 in clinicopathological features of adult T cell leukemia. *Leuk. Res.* **2011**, *35*, 1484–1490. [CrossRef] [PubMed]
22. Zhang, J.; Yamada, O.; Kida, S.; Matsushita, Y.; Yamaoka, S.; Chagan-Yasutan, H.; Hattori, T. Identification of CD44 as a downstream target of noncanonical NF-kappab pathway activated by human T-cell leukemia virus type 1-encoded tax protein. *Virology* **2011**, *413*, 244–252. [CrossRef] [PubMed]
23. Alves, C.S.; Yakovlev, S.; Medved, L.; Konstantopoulos, K. Biomolecular characterization of CD44-fibrin(ogen) binding: Distinct molecular requirements mediate binding of standard and variant isoforms of CD44 to immobilized fibrin (ogen). *J. Biol. Chem.* **2009**, *284*, 1177–1189. [CrossRef] [PubMed]
24. Baaten, B.J.; Li, C.R.; Deiro, M.F.; Lin, M.M.; Linton, P.J.; Bradley, L.M. CD44 regulates survival and memory development in T_h1 cells. *Immunity* **2010**, *32*, 104–115. [CrossRef] [PubMed]
25. Goletti, D.; Butera, O.; Bizzoni, F.; Casetti, R.; Girardi, E.; Poccia, F. Region of difference 1 antigen-specific $CD4^+$ memory T cells correlate with a favorable outcome of tuberculosis. *J. Infect. Dis.* **2006**, *194*, 984–992. [CrossRef] [PubMed]
26. Wu, C.; Thalhamer, T.; Franca, R.F.; Xiao, S.; Wang, C.; Hotta, C.; Zhu, C.; Hirashima, M.; Anderson, A.C.; Kuchroo, V.K. Galectin-9–CD44 interaction enhances stability and function of adaptive regulatory T cells. *Immunity* **2014**, *41*, 270–282. [CrossRef] [PubMed]
27. Wang, J.; Liu, Y.; Zhang, C.L.; Ji, B.Y.; Zhang, L.Z.; Shao, Y.Z.; Jiang, S.L.; Suzuki, Y.; Nakajima, C.; Fan, C.L.; et al. Genotypes and characteristics of clustering and drug susceptibility of *Mycobacterium tuberculosis* isolates collected in Heilongjiang province, China. *J. Clin. Microbiol.* **2011**, *49*, 1354–1362. [CrossRef] [PubMed]
28. Chiacchio, T.; Petruccioli, E.; Vanini, V.; Cuzzi, G.; Pinnetti, C.; Sampaolesi, A.; Antinori, A.; Girardi, E.; Goletti, D. Polyfunctional T-cells and effector memory phenotype are associated with active TB in HIV-infected patients. *J. Infect.* **2014**, *69*, 533–545. [CrossRef] [PubMed]

29. Petruccioli, E.; Petrone, L.; Vanini, V.; Sampaolesi, A.; Gualano, G.; Girardi, E.; Palmieri, F.; Goletti, D. IFNγ/TNFα specific-cells and effector memory phenotype associate with active tuberculosis. *J. Infect.* **2013**, *66*, 475–486. [CrossRef] [PubMed]
30. Brighenti, S.; Andersson, J. Local immune responses in human tuberculosis: Learning from the site of infection. *J. Infect. Dis.* **2012**, *205*, S316–S324. [CrossRef] [PubMed]
31. Koguchi, Y.; Kawakami, K.; Uezu, K.; Fukushima, K.; Kon, S.; Maeda, M.; Nakamoto, A.; Owan, I.; Kuba, M.; Kudeken, N.; et al. High plasma osteopontin level and its relationship with interleukin-12-mediated type 1 T helper cell response in tuberculosis. *Am. J. Respir. Crit. Care Med.* **2003**, *167*, 1355–1359. [CrossRef] [PubMed]
32. Uede, T. Osteopontin, intrinsic tissue regulator of intractable inflammatory diseases. *Pathol. Int.* **2011**, *61*, 265–280. [CrossRef] [PubMed]
33. Inoue, M.; Shinohara, M.L. Cutting edge: Role of osteopontin and integrin α V in T cell-mediated anti-inflammatory responses in endotoxemia. *J. Immunol.* **2015**, *194*, 5595–5598. [CrossRef] [PubMed]
34. Nau, G.J.; Chupp, G.L.; Emile, J.F.; Jouanguy, E.; Berman, J.S.; Casanova, J.L.; Young, R.A. Osteopontin expression correlates with clinical outcome in patients with mycobacterial infection. *Am. J. Pathol.* **2000**, *157*, 37–42. [CrossRef]
35. Nau, G.J.; Guilfoile, P.; Chupp, G.L.; Berman, J.S.; Kim, S.J.; Kornfeld, H.; Young, R.A. A chemoattractant cytokine associated with granulomas in tuberculosis and silicosis. *Proc. Natl. Acad. Sci. USA* **1997**, *94*, 6414–6419. [CrossRef] [PubMed]
36. Krishnan, L.; Gurnani, K.; Dicaire, C.J.; van Faassen, H.; Zafer, A.; Kirschning, C.J.; Sad, S.; Sprott, G.D. Rapid clonal expansion and prolonged maintenance of memory $CD8^+$ T cells of the effector ($CD44^{high}$ $CD62l^{low}$) and central ($CD44^{high}$ $CD62l^{high}$) phenotype by an archaeosome adjuvant independent of TLR2. *J. Immunol.* **2007**, *178*, 2396–2406. [CrossRef] [PubMed]
37. Gey van Pittius, N.C.; Warren, R.M.; van Helden, P.D. ESAT-6 and CFP-10: What is the diagnosis? *Infect. Immunity* **2002**, *70*, 6509–6510. [CrossRef]
38. Ridruechai, C.; Sakurada, S.; Yanai, H.; Yamada, N.; Kantipong, P.; Piyaworawong, S.; Dhepakson, P.; Khusmith, S.; Keicho, N. Association between circulating full-length osteopontin and IFN-γ with disease status of tuberculosis and response to successful treatment. *Southeast Asian J. Trop. Med. Public Health* **2011**, *42*, 876–889. [PubMed]
39. Schnittman, S.M.; Lane, H.C.; Greenhouse, J.; Justement, J.S.; Baseler, M.; Fauci, A.S. Preferential infection of $CD4^+$ memory T cells by human immunodeficiency virus type 1: Evidence for a role in the selective T-cell functional defects observed in infected individuals. *Proc. Natl. Acad. Sci. USA* **1990**, *87*, 6058–6062. [CrossRef] [PubMed]
40. Groot, F.; van Capel, T.M.; Schuitemaker, J.; Berkhout, B.; de Jong, E.C. Differential susceptibility of naive, central memory and effector memory T cells to dendritic cell-mediated HIV-1 transmission. *Retrovirology* **2006**, *3*, 52. [CrossRef] [PubMed]
41. Chagan-Yasutan, H.; Saitoh, H.; Ashino, Y.; Arikawa, T.; Hirashima, M.; Li, S.; Usuzawa, M.; Oguma, S.; EF, O.T.; Obi, C.L.; et al. Persistent elevation of plasma osteopontin levels in hiv patients despite highly active antiretroviral therapy. *Tohoku J. Exp. Med.* **2009**, *218*, 285–292. [CrossRef] [PubMed]
42. Li, Q.; Lifson, J.D.; Duan, L.; Schacker, T.W.; Reilly, C.; Carlis, J.; Estes, J.D.; Haase, A.T. Potential roles of follicular dendritic cell-associated osteopontin in lymphoid follicle pathology and repair and in B cell regulation in HIV-1 and SIV infection. *J. Infect. Dis.* **2005**, *192*, 1269–1276. [CrossRef] [PubMed]
43. Eastwood, J.B.; Corbishley, C.M.; Grange, J.M. Tuberculosis and the kidney. *J. Am. Soc. Nephrol. JASN* **2001**, *12*, 1307–1314. [PubMed]
44. Berry, M.P.; Graham, C.M.; McNab, F.W.; Xu, Z.; Bloch, S.A.; Oni, T.; Wilkinson, K.A.; Banchereau, R.; Skinner, J.; Wilkinson, R.J.; et al. An interferon-inducible neutrophil-driven blood transcriptional signature in human tuberculosis. *Nature* **2010**, *466*, 973–977. [CrossRef] [PubMed]
45. Kaufmann, S.H.; Lange, C.; Rao, M.; Balaji, K.N.; Lotze, M.; Schito, M.; Zumla, A.I.; Maeurer, M. Progress in tuberculosis vaccine development and host-directed therapies—A state of the art review. *Lancet Respir. Med.* **2014**, *2*, 301–320. [CrossRef]
46. Zumla, A.; Rao, M.; Dodoo, E.; Maeurer, M. Potential of immunomodulatory agents as adjunct host-directed therapies for multidrug-resistant tuberculosis. *BMC Med.* **2016**, *14*, 89. [CrossRef] [PubMed]

47. Dufour, J.H.; Dziejman, M.; Liu, M.T.; Leung, J.H.; Lane, T.E.; Luster, A.D. IFN-γ-inducible protein 10 (IP-10; CXCL10)-deficient mice reveal a role for IP-10 in effector T cell generation and trafficking. *J. Immunol.* **2002**, *168*, 3195–3204. [CrossRef] [PubMed]
48. Zhu, Y.A.; Jia, H.Y.; Chen, J.N.; Cui, G.Y.; Gao, H.; Wei, Y.F.; Lu, C.; Wang, L.; Uede, T.; Diao, H.Y. Decreased osteopontin expression as a reliable prognostic indicator of improvement in pulmonary tuberculosis: Impact of the level of interferon-γ-inducible protein 10. *Cell. Physiol. Biochem.* **2015**, *37*, 1983–1996. [CrossRef] [PubMed]
49. Petrone, L.; Cannas, A.; Vanini, V.; Cuzzi, G.; Aloi, F.; Nsubuga, M.; Sserunkuma, J.; Nazziwa, R.A.; Jugheli, L.; Lukindo, T.; et al. Blood and urine inducible protein 10 as potential markers of disease activity. *Int. J. Tuberc. Lung Dis.* **2016**, *20*, 1554–1561. [CrossRef] [PubMed]
50. Petrone, L.; Chiacchio, T.; Vanini, V.; Petruccioli, E.; Cuzzi, G.; di Giacomo, C.; Pucci, L.; Montalbano, M.; Lionetti, R.; Testa, A.; et al. High urine IP-10 levels associate with chronic HCV infection. *J. Infect.* **2014**, *68*, 591–600. [CrossRef] [PubMed]
51. Antonelli, A.; Ferrari, S.M.; Corrado, A.; di Domenicantonio, A.; Fallahi, P. Autoimmune thyroid disorders. *Autoimmun. Rev.* **2015**, *14*, 174–180. [CrossRef] [PubMed]
52. Bifani, P.J.; Mathema, B.; Kurepina, N.E.; Kreiswirth, B.N. Global dissemination of the *Mycobacterium tuberculosis* W-Beijing family strains. *Trends Microbiol.* **2002**, *10*, 45–52. [CrossRef]
53. Parwati, I.; van Crevel, R.; van Soolingen, D. Possible underlying mechanisms for successful emergence of the *Mycobacterium tuberculosis* Beijing genotype strains. *Lancet Infect. Dis.* **2010**, *10*, 103–111. [CrossRef]
54. Zhang, J.; Mi, L.; Wang, Y.; Liu, P.; Liang, H.; Huang, Y.; Lv, B.; Yuan, L. Genotypes and drug susceptibility of *Mycobacterium tuberculosis* isolates in Shihezi, Xinjiang province, China. *BMC Res. Notes* **2012**, *5*, 309. [CrossRef] [PubMed]
55. Kato-Maeda, M.; Shanley, C.A.; Ackart, D.; Jarlsberg, L.G.; Shang, S.; Obregon-Henao, A.; Harton, M.; Basaraba, R.J.; Henao-Tamayo, M.; Barrozo, J.C.; et al. Beijing sublineages of *Mycobacterium tuberculosis* differ in pathogenicity in the guinea pig. *Clin. Vaccine Immunol.* **2012**, *19*, 1227–1237. [CrossRef] [PubMed]
56. Szeliga, J.; Daniel, D.S.; Yang, C.H.; Sever-Chroneos, Z.; Jagannath, C.; Chroneos, Z.C. Granulocyte-macrophage colony stimulating factor-mediated innate responses in tuberculosis. *Tuberculosis* **2008**, *88*, 7–20. [CrossRef] [PubMed]
57. Who Guidelines on Tuberculosis. Available online: http://www.who.int/publications/guidelines/tuberculosis/en/ (accessed on 24 September 2016).
58. Ralph, A.P.; Ardian, M.; Wiguna, A.; Maguire, G.P.; Becker, N.G.; Drogumuller, G.; Wilks, M.J.; Waramori, G.; Tjitra, E.; Sandjaja; et al. A simple, valid, numerical score for grading chest X-ray severity in adult smear-positive pulmonary tuberculosis. *Thorax* **2010**, *65*, 863–869. [CrossRef] [PubMed]
59. Grassinger, J.; Haylock, D.N.; Storan, M.J.; Haines, G.O.; Williams, B.; Whitty, G.A.; Vinson, A.R.; Be, C.L.; Li, S.H.; Sorensen, E.S.; et al. Thrombin-cleaved osteopontin regulates hemopoietic stem and progenitor cell functions through interactions with $\alpha_9\beta_1$ and $\alpha_4\beta_1$ integrins. *Blood* **2009**, *114*, 49–59. [CrossRef] [PubMed]

16

A Different Microbiome Gene Repertoire in the Airways of Cystic Fibrosis Patients with Severe Lung Disease

Giovanni Bacci [1], Alessio Mengoni [1], Ersilia Fiscarelli [2], Nicola Segata [3], Giovanni Taccetti [4], Daniela Dolce [4], Patrizia Paganin [5], Patrizia Morelli [6], Vanessa Tuccio [2], Alessandra De Alessandri [6], Vincenzina Lucidi [2] and Annamaria Bevivino [5,*]

1 Department of Biology, University of Florence, Florence 50019, Italy; giovanni.bacci@unifi.it (G.B.); alessio.mengoni@unifi.it (A.M.)
2 Cystic Fibrosis Microbiology and Cystic Fibrosis Center, "Bambino Gesù" Children's Hospital and Research Institute, Rome 00165, Italy; ersilia.fiscarelli@opbg.net (E.F.); vanessa.tuccio@opbg.net (V.T.); vincenzina.lucidi@opbg.net (V.L.)
3 Centre for Integrative Biology, University of Trento, Trento 38123, Italy; nicola.segata@unitn.it
4 Department of Pediatric Medicine, Cystic Fibrosis Center, Anna Meyer Children's University Hospital, Florence 50139, Italy; giovanni.taccetti@meyer.it (G.T.); daniela.dolce@meyer.it (D.D.)
5 Territorial and Production Systems Sustainability Department, ENEA, Italian National Agency for New Technologies, Energy and Sustainable Economic Development, Casaccia Research Center, Rome 00123, Italy; patrypaganin@yahoo.it
6 Cystic Fibrosis Center, IRCCS G. Gaslini Institute, Genoa 16146, Italy; patriziamorelli@gaslini.org (P.M.); aledeales@gmail.com (A.D.A.)
* Correspondence: annamaria.bevivino@enea.it

Abstract: In recent years, next-generation sequencing (NGS) was employed to decipher the structure and composition of the microbiota of the airways in cystic fibrosis (CF) patients. However, little is still known about the overall gene functions harbored by the resident microbial populations and which specific genes are associated with various stages of CF lung disease. In the present study, we aimed to identify the microbial gene repertoire of CF microbiota in twelve patients with severe and normal/mild lung disease by performing sputum shotgun metagenome sequencing. The abundance of metabolic pathways encoded by microbes inhabiting CF airways was reconstructed from the metagenome. We identified a set of metabolic pathways differently distributed in patients with different pulmonary function; namely, pathways related to bacterial chemotaxis and flagellar assembly, as well as genes encoding efflux-mediated antibiotic resistance mechanisms and virulence-related genes. The results indicated that the microbiome of CF patients with low pulmonary function is enriched in virulence-related genes and in genes encoding efflux-mediated antibiotic resistance mechanisms. Overall, the microbiome of severely affected adults with CF seems to encode different mechanisms for the facilitation of microbial colonization and persistence in the lung, consistent with the characteristics of multidrug-resistant microbial communities that are commonly observed in patients with severe lung disease.

Keywords: cystic fibrosis; lung disease; lung microbiome; shotgun metagenomics; bioinformatics; metabolic pathways; virulence genes

---

1. Introduction

Subjects affected by cystic fibrosis (CF) experience a progressive loss of pulmonary functions accompanied by an increased burden of chronic infections. The respiratory microbial composition is particularly relevant for patients with CF. In fact, bacterial lung infections reduce life expectancy in patients with CF (the median predicted survival age is equal to 41.6, as reported in the Cystic Fibrosis Foundation Patient Registry [1]), and represent the primary cause of morbidity and mortality in CF patients [2]. In the last decade, the emergence of high-throughput sequencing approaches, coupled with the development of new bioinformatics pipelines designed to cope with metagenomics data, has revolutionized the study of complex bacterial communities such as the airway microbiota of CF patients, thereby improving our understanding of this largely unknown "microbial black-box". This understanding of how a bacterial community changes over time and over the course of CF disease progression has revealed a different bacterial community structure upon pulmonary exacerbations (such as a reduced bacterial diversity and an increasingly conserved community composition) coupled with a decline in pulmonary health, antibiotic treatment, and patient age [3–11]. No overall changes in total bacterial density with exacerbation was observed [12], suggesting that shifts in the relative abundance of bacterial community members, rather than changes in total bacterial density, are more likely to be associated with alterations in clinical state [12].

In previous studies [13,14], we provided new insights into the features of the bacterial communities of patients with CF, improving our current knowledge about the airway microbiota composition and polymicrobial interactions in patients following a severe decline in lung function and with different lung disease statuses (normal/mild vs. moderate vs. severe). Although the description of taxonomic groups colonizing the airways of CF patients has helped in the understanding of how bacterial species change during disease progression, the overall gene content harbored by these communities remains largely unknown. Since metabolic and functional features of a microbial species are the dominant factors determining its ability to survive in a given environment (e.g., CF patients' lungs) [15], untargeted metagenomic approaches may provide deep insights into the microbial CF lung metagenome, permitting the identification of gene sets involved in functional pathways associated with a worsening clinical condition [16].

In the present study, we performed a deep metagenomic investigation to probe the lung microbiome of twelve CF patients with mild (Forced expiratory volume in one second (FEV_1) > 70%) and severe (FEV_1 < 40%) lung disease. We aimed to investigate whether patients with different disease severities may indeed have a different representation of "keystone genes" in their lung microbiota. To the best of our knowledge, only a few works have already inspected the CF microbiome through shotgun metagenomes, and most of them are case reports on a limited number of patients [17,18] or on specific metabolic functions [19]. Moving away from taxonomic inventories towards a better understanding of CF microbiome genes opens a new avenue for the identification of the microbial gene repertoire associated with CF lung disease.

2. Results

2.1. Clinical Characteristics of Enrolled Patients and Culture-Based Diagnostic Microbiology

The clinical status of the individual subjects is reported in Table 1. The study cohort includes twelve patients (aged 18–46 years; median = 28) with CF who were in stable clinical conditions, without any pulmonary exacerbation and not undergoing antibiotic therapy (*i.v.* or oral) in the previous four weeks before specimen collection. The normal/mild (FEV_1 > 70% predicted) and severe (FEV_1 < 40% predicted) groups also differed in the extent of repeated antibiotic exposure and in their mean age being equal to (mean $\pm$ standard error) 25.33 $\pm$ 2.216 and 33.83 $\pm$ 3.146 years in the normal/mild and the severe group, respectively (two-tailed *t*-test; p value = 0.0313). In addition, the severe group tended to receive more uniform antimicrobial agents by the inhalation of aerosolised antibiotics during maintenance therapy, such as aerolized colistimethate and azithromycin, with respect to the normal/mild group (Table 1). Traditional culture-based diagnostic microbiology revealed the presence of *Pseudomonas aeruginosa* and *Staphylococcus aureus*, being the dominant bacterial species in patients with severe and mild respiratory function, respectively (Table S1). Other minor taxa were *Achromobacter xylosoxidans*, *Rothia mucilaginosa*, *Veillonella parvula*, *Stenotrophomonas maltophilia*, *Gemella sanguinis* and *Escherichia coli*.

Table 1. Demographic and clinical characteristics of patients with normal/mild (Forced expiratory volume in one second (FEV_1) > 70%) and severe (FEV_1 < 40%) lung disease status enrolled in the study.

Study ID	Age	Gender	CFTR Genotype	BMI	Average Annual FEV_1% Value	Lung Disease Status	Number of Exacerbations in the Last 5 Years	Maintenance Antimicrobial Therapy [1]
BS29	25	F	F508del/L1077P	23.1	72	normal/mild	20 (2–7)	AT
BS47	33	M	F508del/N1303K	23.8	94	normal/mild	5 (1–2)	AA, AC
MS1	30	F	G1244 E/G1244 E	22.9	83	normal/mild	5 (0–4)	AC
GNR19	18	M	F508del/F508del	21.4	80	normal/mild	9 (1–3)	None
GNR5	24	M	F508del/12491G>A	22.7	72	normal/mild	9 (0–3)	None
BNR22	22	F	F508del/G85E	22.1	81	normal/mild	23 (2–7)	AT, AZ
BS19	36	M	F508del/W1282X	24.9	37	severe	18 (3–4)	AC, AZ
BS51	36	M	F508del/2789+5G>A	21	38	severe	16 (2–6)	AC, AZ
BS85	34	M	F508del/1259insA	18.8	21	severe	15 (2–5)	AC, AZ
BNR15	46	F	F508del/F508del	19.7	37	severe	16 (2–4)	AC, AZ
BNR20	25	M	F508del/F508del	23.3	36	severe	36 (4–11)	AA, AC
BNR49	26	M	N1303K/G85E	19.9	29	severe	10 (1–3)	AC

[1] AT, aerosolized tobramycin; AA, aerosolized aztreonam; AC, aerosolized colistimethate; AA, aerosolized aztreonam; AZ, azithromycin.

2.2. Metabolic Community Structure between Patient Groups

Sequencing yielded > 15 M paired-end sequences for each sample, with 1–5% of them being of putative microbial origin (the remaining being human DNA). This confirmed that human contamination still represents a considerable drawback in the metagenomic analysis of human sputum samples, as already reported in other metagenomics studies [20,21]. From 12 samples, a total of 5.4 M microbial sequences (mean ± standard error per sample, 453,824 ± 41,349) were included in the analysis (Table S2). The HMP Unified Metabolic Analysis Network (HUMAnN) analysis revealed 47 pathways which were differently distributed across all samples (Figure S1). The principal component analysis (PCA) analysis on metabolic and regulatory data (Figure 1) explained almost 80% of the total variance reporting a distinct sample distribution for normal/mild and severe patient groups.

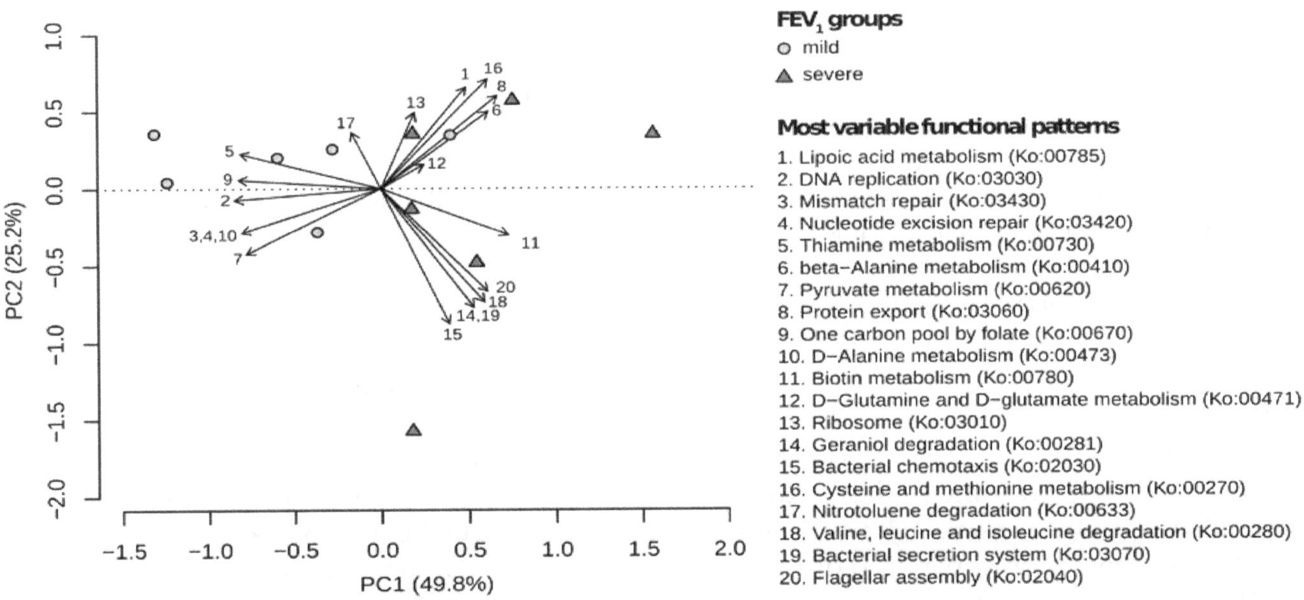

Figure 1. Principal component analysis (PCA) based on the top twenty metabolic patterns. Each number corresponds to a pathway reported in the figure legend, whereas each point corresponds to a different patient. Point shape reflects patient groups.

In particular, the separation of normal/mild samples from severe samples was largely driven by 6 pathways: biotin metabolism (Ko:00780), geraniol degradation (Ko:00281), bacterial chemotaxis (Ko:02030), valine leucine and isoleucine degradation (Ko:00280), the bacterial secretion system (Ko:03070), and flagellar assembly (Ko:02040). The Kruskal–Wallis one-way analysis of variance confirmed this result with five out of six previously identified pathways displaying higher values in the severe group patients compared to the normal/mild ones (Figure 2). Overall, 31 pathways were equally distributed between the two groups considered (Figures S2 and S3), whereas 16 pathways were differentially distributed in the two groups, being found mainly in patients with normal/mild (5 pathways) and severe disease (11 pathways), respectively (Figure 2).

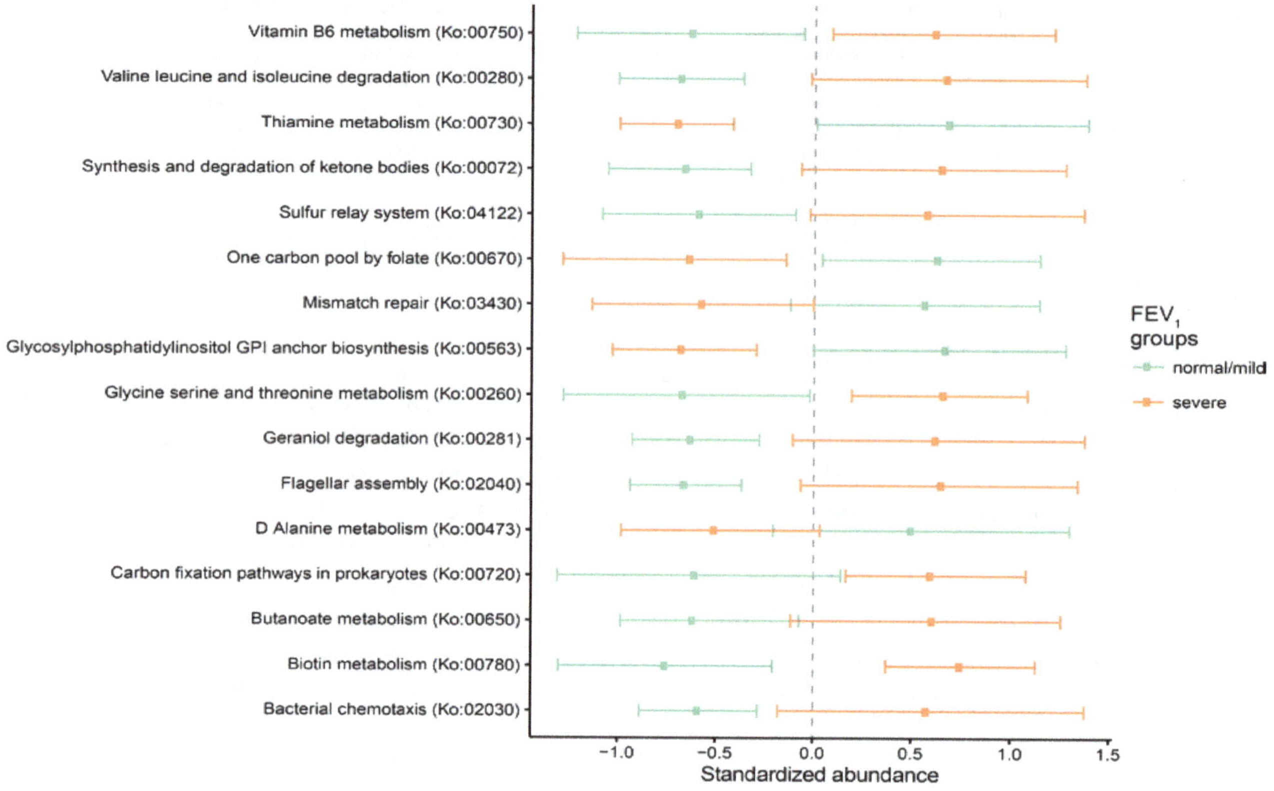

Figure 2. Differences in metabolic and regulatory pathways detected with HMP Unified Metabolic Analysis Network HUMAnN. Colors indicate statistically significant differences (p-value < 0.05) after Kruskal–Wallis one-way analysis of variance. Values indicate mean and one standard deviation (bars). Standardized abundances (x axis) were calculated as: $[x - m(x)]/sd(x)$, where "SD" is the standard deviation and "m" is the mean value.

2.3. *Metagenomic Functional Differences Suggest Distinct Ecological Roles within the Cystic Fibrosis Microbiome*

In order to establish a set of gene putatively available in CF lung communities, metagenomic reads were assembled into contigs. We were able to assemble an average of 1655 contigs (s.e. 526) per sample (N50 values ranging from 645 to 1655) (Figure S4 and Table S2). The gene-calling step predicted a mean of 5014 open reading frames (ORFs) with a standard error of 1266. The functional potential harbored by microbiomes was inferred, predicting gene functions by homology using the evolutionary genealogy of genes: non-supervised orthologous groups (eggNOG) database (Figure 3).

Both patient groups showed a massive presence of transporter proteins, with the severe group reporting higher values than the normal/mild group. The Transporter Classification Database (TCDB) analysis highlighted the possible presence of antibiotic resistance proteins indicating an imbalanced distribution of the multidrug resistance efflux pumps of the ATP-binding cassette (ABC) and resistance–nodulation–cell division (RND) super-families between the two groups of patients. In particular, patients with severe disease showed a high presence of both ABC and RND super-families members (Figure S5), thus suggesting the presence of efflux-mediated antibiotic resistance mechanisms. Virulence protein counts were normalized using the total number of ORFs predicted in each sample. Virulence (and virulence-related) factors displaying a significant difference between groups (two-tailed Student's t-test p-value ≤ 0.05, alpha = 0.05) are shown in Figure 4 (individual values for each patient are reported in Figures S6 and S7).

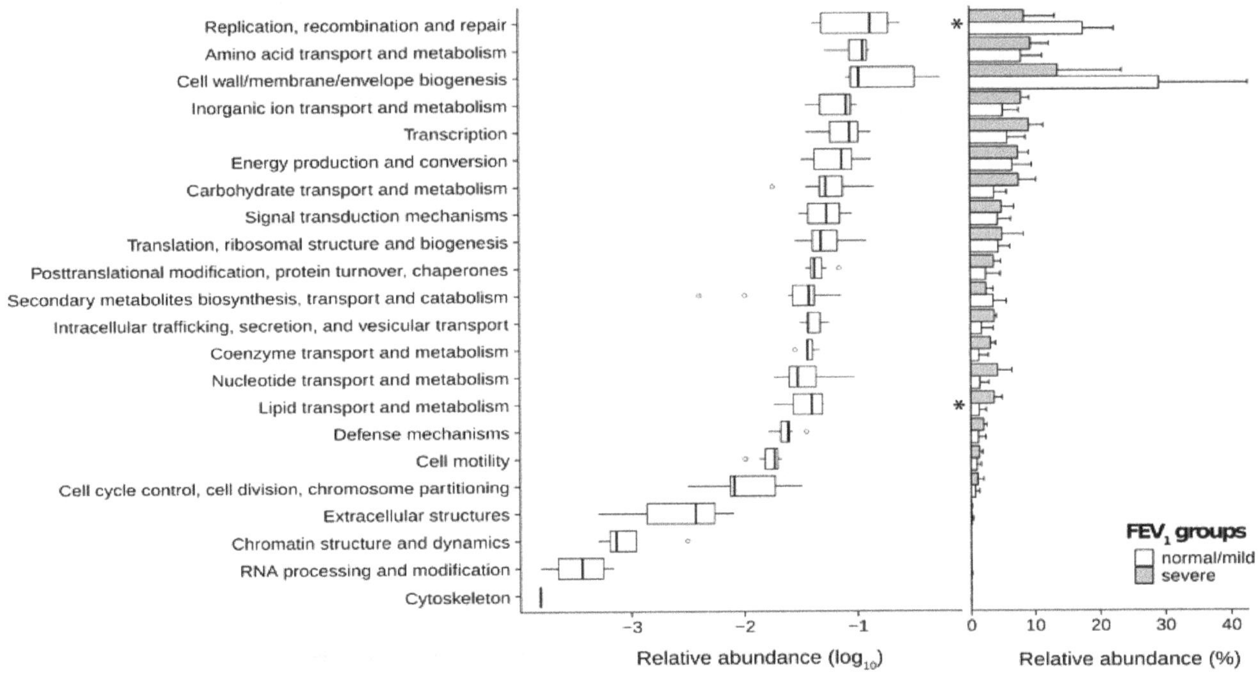

Figure 3. Distribution of functional categories obtained with an evolutionary genealogy of genes: non-supervised orthologous groups (eggnog) analysis. Box plots for each eggNOG category found for both groups of patients are reported in the left panel, whereas relative abundances for each group are reported in the right panel (bars represent the average value and error bars indicate the standard error for each measure). Significant differences between normal/mild and severe groups are flagged with an asterisk. Boxes denote the interquartile range (IQR) between the 25th and the 75th percentile (first and third quartiles), whereas the inner line represents the median. Whiskers represent the lowest and highest values within 1.5 times IQR from the first and third quartiles. Outliers are reported using white circles.

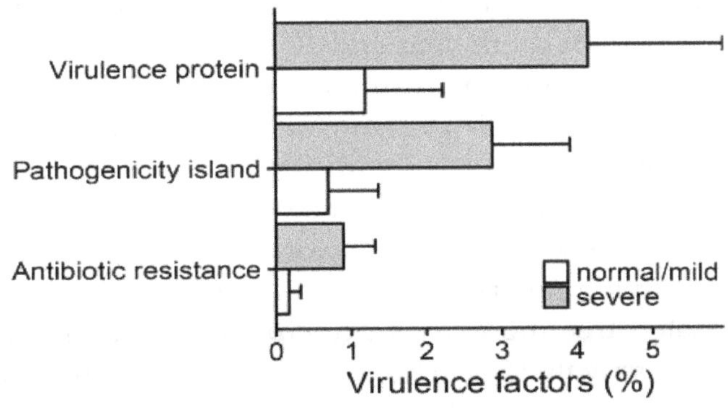

Figure 4. Virulence factor distribution across patient groups. Only factors displaying a significant (Student's t-test p-value ≤ 0.05) diverging distribution are reported. The bars represent the average value for each category whereas the error bars indicate the standard error.

A larger presence of virulence factors was found in patients with severe disease, with antibiotic resistance as the third most abundant category. The Resfams analysis [22] suggests that the microbes in CF airways encode a diverse set of antibiotic resistance mechanisms; among them, the multidrug resistance efflux pumps are the most represented (Figure 5). Overall, 17 out of 18 antibiotic resistance categories showed higher values in patients with severe disease, with 8 of them reporting significant differences. As expected, efflux mediated systems were the most abundant categories, all reporting higher values for severe patients than for normal/mild ones (Figure 5 and Figure S8). Our results are supported by culture-based analysis, which reveals the presence of multi-drug resistant bacteria in the severe group (Table S1).

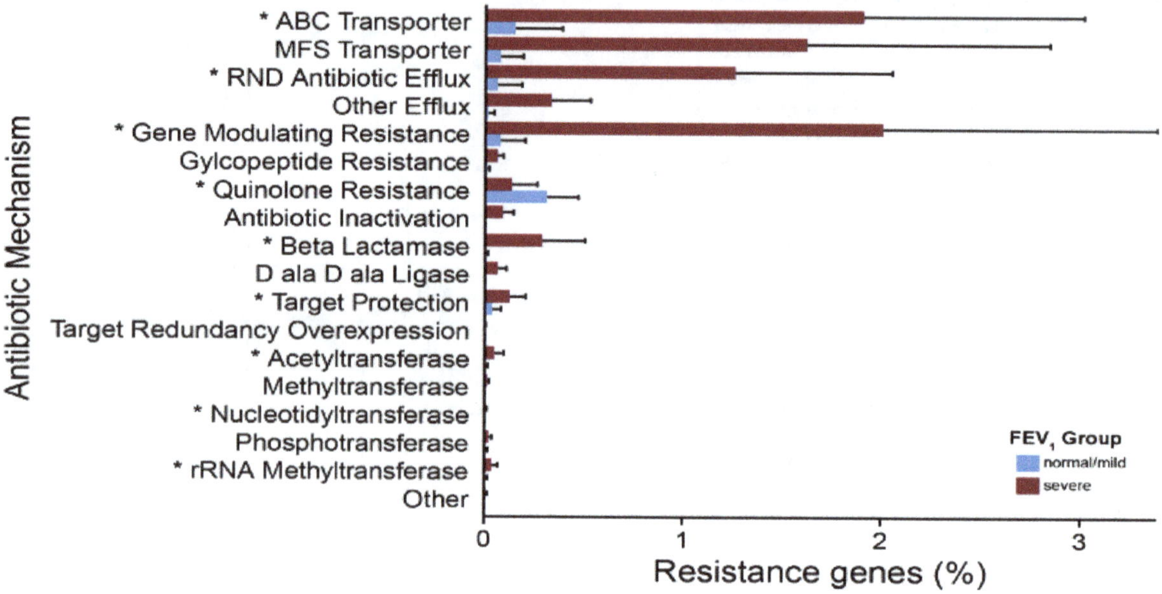

Figure 5. Antibiotic resistance gene differentiate patient groups. Bar charts report the percentage values of antibiotic resistance gene detected. Significant differences are reported with one asterisk (p-value < 0.05). P values were obtained through a Student's t-test on the number of genes detected. Bars were drawn by computing the average percentage value of each resistance category whereas error bars are reported using standard errors.

2.4. Relationship between Functional Potential and Taxonomic Microbial Composition

To further characterize the airway microbiome of CF patients, the correlation between the taxonomic and functional structure of the microbial community was examined. The dissimilarity of the taxonomic community was significantly correlated with the functional community dissimilarity (Mantel test with Pearson correlation coefficient and 1000 permutations; p-values < 0.05), implying a relation between the species distribution patterns and the functional distribution of the whole airway community. Otherwise, the metabolic pathway distribution (Kyoto Encyclopedia of Genes and Genomes (KEGG) analysis) was poorly correlated with other features, reporting significant correlations only with antibiotic resistance gene distribution and taxonomic structure (Table S3).

To further identify the driving forces for the taxonomic distribution, the relative influence of functional genes, metabolic pathway distribution, virulence factors, and antibiotic resistance genes were rendered by using boosted tree models on principal components derived from each feature. Principal components with an eigenvalue > 1 in total accounted for more than 85% of the total variance and were therefore chosen for training boosted regression trees (Table S4). In boosted tree models, measures of relative influence quantify the importance of a given predictor; the variables that have a weak effect on prediction therefore have, by extension, scarcely an influence on the variable that the model tries to predict [23]. Therefore, factors that have a minimal relative influence in predicting the abundance of a given taxon are poorly connected with the distribution of that taxon. Although the use of orthogonal composite variables (as reported in the method section) reduced type I errors, the contribution of each original variable cannot be inferred directly. To partially overcome this limitation, the most dominant variables contributing to each component (top-50% eigenvalues of K, E, A, and V) were reported in Table S4.

Based on the results reported in this study, the metabolic pathway distribution inferred with KEGG (K) was the major factor able to predict the microbial taxonomic structure, whereas the gene distribution obtained with eggNOG (E) had little influence on the whole community, affecting only the distribution of a limited number of species (Figure 6).

Surprisingly, antibiotic resistance genes (A) were related to three bacterial species only: *Achromobacter xylosoxidans*, *Fusobacterium periodonticum*, and an unclassified member of the *Bordetella* genus. *A. xylosoxidans* strains, intrinsically resistant to many classes of antimicrobial agents, have been associated with CF [24,25], as well as *F. periodonticum*, which has been reported to increase its presence during exacerbation [26]. Conversely, virulence factors (V) (mainly comprising genes previously identified in pathogenicity islands, virulence proteins, and antibiotic resistance genes Figures S7 and 4) were not related to any particular species reporting the lowest values of relative influence.

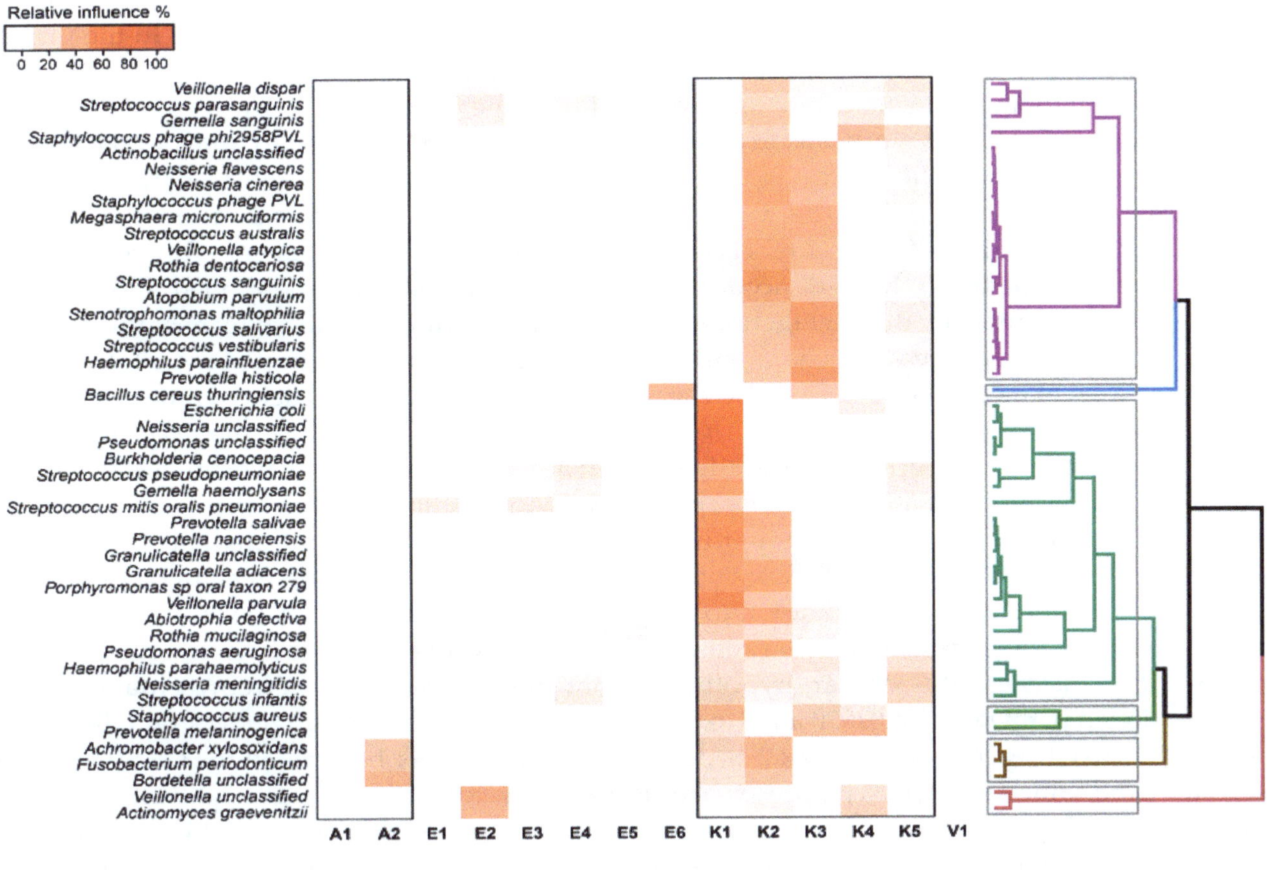

Figure 6. Relative influence of Kyoto Encyclopedia of Genes and Genomes (KEGG) pathways (K1 to K5), gene frequencies (evolutionary genealogy of genes: non-supervised orthologous groups (eggnog) database, E1 to E6), antibiotic resistance genes (Resfam database A1 and A2), and virulence factors (microbial database of protein toxins, virulence factors and antibiotic resistance genes for bio-defense applications (MvirDB), V1) for taxonomic structure of microbial lung community evaluated through "booster regression trees" models. The relative influence of different principal component to each bacterial species detected was clustered with the unweighted pair-group method with arithmetic mean (UPGMA) method based on Pearson's correlation and a tree was reported on the right side of the plot. Boxes report the main group of taxa detected through a cluster analysis.

3. Discussion

In an endeavor to better understand the complexity of CF microbiomes in patients with high/low pulmonary function, we performed a metagenomics investigation of the bacterial communities in the airways of patients with CF focusing on the identification of a set of functional features associated with different lung disease statuses in the present study.

Sputum specimens, which represent by far the most widely used sample to access the airway microbiota of CF disease [27–30], were collected from twelve patients with CF. As recently indicated by Dickson and colleagues [31], although use of sputum can introduce an additional risk of upper airway contamination, the presence of oropharyngeal microbiota does not obscure the meaningful microbial signal in sputum which is correlated with established indices of lung health. To date, in CF metagenomics, published studies have focused on the sputum derived from CF patients [17,32–34]. The shotgun metagenomics approach, which provides the gene catalogue of the microbial community, allows an insight into some functional features to be gained (e.g., the presence of metabolic pathways and potential antibiotic resistance genes), in addition to accurate species-level taxonomic assignments.

In the first metagenomic study performed by Willner and colleagues [33], the airways of diseased and non-diseased individuals showed a potentially different microbial community metabolism (inferred from the recovered gene catalogue of the microbiome), suggesting that the community metabolism is dynamic and variable among patients differing in their health status. In the present work, the abundances of metabolic pathways encoded by microbes inhabiting CF airways of patients with high/low pulmonary function were reconstructed from the metagenome. The metabolic pathway distribution described in this work was in accordance with the one described in other studies [19,32], with pathways related to amino acid catabolism, nucleotide metabolism, and stress responses reporting high values in both normal/mild and severe patients. Several pathways were uniformly distributed among patients, regardless of their clinical condition, reflecting a large set of core functions typical of host-associated microbes. Indeed, according to the previous studies mentioned above [19,32], there was little variation in the metagenome pathway distribution, with sixteen pathways only reporting different abundance values between the two groups of patients inspected here. Interestingly, we identified a set of metabolic pathways correlated with the worsening of patients' clinical conditions; in particular, two pathways, the *bacterial chemotaxis pathway* (Ko:02030) and the *flagellar assembly pathway* (Ko:02040), were reported as clinically relevant according to previous works [35–39]. Indeed, one pathway was associated with *Pseudomonas aeruginosa* lung infection (bacterial chemotaxis pathway), whereas the second (flagellar assembly pathway) was classified as a potent mediator of virulence in Gram-negative bacteria such as *P. aeruginosa* strains. Moreover, the *motB* gene (a component of the flagellar assembly pathway) is known to aid bacterial chemotaxis and flagellar assembly; also, its product (a membrane protein, flagellar motor protein) was recognized as a potential novel vaccine target in *Vibrio cholerae* [40]. We can hypothesize that the difference in the representation of the above-mentioned pathways (Ko:02030 and Ko:02040) could rely on both *P. aeruginosa* strain differences (between the two disease groups) as well as on the presence of other bacteria in the CF microbiome which carry the same gene sets. The presence of *P. aeruginosa* and other Gram-negative strains that could be responsible for the appearance of these pathways were also revealed by cultivation methods analysis, as reported in Figure S9. However, the limited number of patients analyzed in our study does not allow for definitive, statistically-based conclusion on this issue.

In addition to microbial genes involved in metabolic metabolism, genes involved in antibiotic resistance are also powerful indicators of the microbial community's adaptation to the CF lung [17]. Indeed, the top-50% KEGG pathways (reported in Table S4) were mainly involved in the metabolism of amino acids and nucleotides and may be linked to bacterial proliferation and adaptation in the lungs. An increased presence of genes involved in both nucleotide and amino acid metabolism may, in fact, indicate a huge presence of both types of molecules which, in turn, may come from neutrophil extracellular traps, bacterial biofilms and the action of human and bacterial proteases [32,41–44]. Moreover, a large number of genes classified with eggNOG belonged to the transporter families. Their further analysis by using the Transporter Classification Database (TCDB) permitted us to identify a massive presence of families connected with antibiotic resistance mechanisms, especially in patients with severe lung disease. The presence of genes related to antibiotic resistance mechanisms was confirmed by the Hidden Markov model (HMM) (Resfams), which accurately predicts new resistance functions from sequence alone [22]. The efflux-mediated system, which represents the widespread drug resistance mechanism common to many microorganisms, was the most represented gene function. Interestingly, the presence of *P. aeruginosa* and *Staphylococcus aureus* was not related to the differential abundance of antibiotic resistance genes and virulence factors. Indeed, virulence and resistance genes have been found to be spread throughout the whole CF bacterial community and are poorly related to the presence of single taxa, suggesting that the emergence of these mechanisms should be attributed to a particular clinical condition (normal/mild or severe lung disease) of CF patients. In fact, significant differences in the percentage of total Antibiotic Resistance (AR) functions encoded in microbial genomes between normal/mild and severe groups were found. Overall, there was a significant AR mechanism enrichment in patients with severe lung disease due to several years of exposure to antimicrobial drugs. It is well known that several antimicrobial agents and complex regimens are used for prophylaxis, eradication, treatment of exacerbations, and chronic suppressive therapy [45,46], paving the way for the emergence and spreading of AR mechanisms throughout the lung microbial community. In particular, oral, intravenous, and inhaled antibiotic courses are often frequent and prolonged, especially with increasing age and declining pulmonary status [47] as those characterizing the patients with severe lung disease. As underlined by Zhao and colleagues [28], an antibiotic administered closer to the time of sampling would be expected to have a greater impact on the microbial community than that same antibiotic would have when administered at a longer interval from the sampling time. Even if, on the date of sampling and in the 30 days before sample collection, antibiotic administration through an IV route was not given to our patients, we can hypothesize that patients with severe lung disease, having an average higher age than those from the normal/mild group, experienced several years of exposure to antimicrobial drugs, leading to periodic selection for an AR microbiota and resulting in a higher frequency and diversity of AR genes in their lung microbiota. The depth and diversity of AR genes uncovered by metagenomic studies in CF patients with different disease statuses brings to light the need for new strategies to combat antibiotic-resistant pathogens [48]. As reported by King and colleagues [49], the metagenomic profiles of human microbiota are becoming increasingly characterized, and growing data suggests that imbalances of the microbiota could lead to a disease status [50].

4. Materials and Methods

4.1. Ethics Statement

The study was approved by the Ethics Committees of Children's Hospital and Research Institute Bambino Gesù (Rome, Italy), Cystic Fibrosis Center, Anna Meyer Children's University Hospital (Florence, Italy) and G. Gaslini Institute (University of Genoa, Genoa, Italy) (Prot. N. 681 CM of 2 November 2012; Prot. N. 85 of 27 February 2014; Prot. N. FCC 2012 Partner 4-IGG of 18 September 2012). Informed written consent was given by all adult subjects before enrollment in the study. All sputum specimens were produced voluntarily. All procedures were performed in agreement with the "Guidelines of the European Convention on Human Rights and Biomedicine for Research in Children" and the Ethics Committee of the three CF Centers involved. All measures were obtained and processed ensuring patient data protection and confidentiality.

4.2. Patients

Twelve patients with CF (aged 18–46 years), older than six years, were enrolled in the study between September 2012 and April 2013. The cohort consisted of clinically stable patients without any pulmonary exacerbation and who were not undergoing antibiotic therapy (*i.v.* or oral) in the previous four weeks before specimen collection [51,52]. Patients were treated according to the current standards of care [53] with at least four microbiological controls per year [54]. At each visit, clinical data collection and microbiological status (colonizing pathogens with available cultivation protocols) were performed according to the European CF Society standards of care [55]. Forced expiratory volume in one second as a percentage of predicted (%FEV_1) is a key outcome of the monitoring of lung function in CF [56]. All enrolled patients had an absence of an acute pulmonary exacerbation. Patients were classified into two groups, "normal/mild" ($FEV_1 > 70\%$) and "severe" ($FEV_1 < 40\%$), by estimating their average annual FEV_1 value on the basis of multiple spirometric measurements over the two years before their enrollment. FEV_1 values were measured according to the American Thoracic Society (ATS) and the European Respiratory Society (ERS) standards [57,58]. The lower limit of age for subjects with "normal/mild" disease was 15 years old, while that of subjects with severe disease was 25 years old. The study was approved by the Ethics Committees of Children's Hospital and Research Institute Bambino Gesù (Rome, Italy), Cystic Fibrosis Center, Anna Meyer Children's University Hospital (Florence, Italy) and G. Gaslini Institute (University of Genoa, Genoa, Italy), as stated in the ethical statement. The demographic and clinical characteristics of patients are reported in Table 1. The number of exacerbations (as defined by a cluster of symptoms and signs as previously indicated [51,52]) was determined in the five years before the enrollment.

4.3. Sample Processing

The microbiome analysis was performed on sputum samples. Upon expectoration, CF sputum samples were immediately treated for 15 min with Sputolysin (Calbiochem, La Jolla, CA, USA) in accordance with the manufacturer's instructions and split into aliquots for culture and molecular analyses. Aliquots for culturable analysis were immediately examined, and the remaining aliquots were frozen and stored at −80 °C for subsequent DNA extraction and metagenomic analysis. Bacterial detection and identification were performed as previously reported [13]. The microbiological status of the individual subjects is reported in Table S2.

4.4. DNA Extraction Procedures and Sequencing

About 400 μl aliquots of frozen sputum were subjected to genomic DNA extraction using acetyl trimethylammonium bromide (CTAB) protocol, according to the procedure previously reported [59]. Sample aliquots were spun at 10,000× g to pellet cellular material. After the removal of the supernatant, cell pellets were re-suspended in 567 μL of autoclaved and 0.2 filtered TE pH 8 and incubated for 1 h at 37 °C with 30 μL 10% sodium dodecyl sulfate (SDS) and 3 μL 20 mg/mL Proteinase K (Sigma-Aldrich, St. Louis, MO, USA). Samples were then incubated for 10 min with 100 μL of 5 M NaCl prepared with sterile water and 80 μL of CTAB/NaCl solution (4.1 g NaCl, 10 g CTAB in 100 mL sterile water). Following incubation, extracts were purified using phenol chloroform extraction, and DNA was recovered by isopropanol precipitation. Pelleted DNA was washed twice with cold 70% ethanol, allowed to air dry, and re-suspended in 30 μL of sterile water. Quantity and integrity of DNA extracted were assessed by Qubit 2.0 fluorometer (Invitrogen, Life technologies) and gel electrophoresis, respectively. Library preparation and DNA sequencing were performed following the standard pipelines for Illumina HiSeq 2000, PE100 sequencing (Beijing Genomics Institute, BGI, Shenzhen, Guangdong, China), as described in Supplementary Information S1. Raw sequence data reported in this study have been deposited in the National Center for Biotechnology Information (NCBI) "Sequence Read Archive" (SRA) under the project accession PRJNA316056.

4.5. Bioinformatic Analyses

Sequence quality was ensured by trimming reads using StreamingTrim 1.0 [60], with a quality cutoff of 20. Bowtie2 [61] was used to screen out human-derived sequences from metagenomic data with the latest version of the human genome available in the NCBI database (GRCh38) as reference. Sequences displaying a concordant alignment (a mate pair that aligns with the expected relative mate orientation and with the expected range of distances between mates) against the human genomes were then removed from all subsequent analyses. Metabolic and regulatory patterns were estimated using HUMAnN [62] and considered only those pathways with a coverage value $\geq$ 80%, whereas the taxonomic microbial community composition was assessed using MetaPhlAn2 [63]. Reads were assembled into contigs using the SPAdes microbial assembler [64] with automatic k-mer length selection. To establish an airway microbiome gene catalog [65], we first removed contigs smaller than 500bp and then used MetaGeneMark [66] to predict open reading frames (ORFs). Translated protein sequences obtained from assembled contigs were classified using Hmmer [67] with the eggNOG [68] database trained on bacterial sequences (bactNOG). Each protein was classified according to its best hit with an e-value lower than 0.001 as suggested in [69]. Proteins classified as transporters were further inspected using Basic Local Alignment Search Tool (BLAST) against the Transporter Classification Database (TCDB) [70] to obtain a more detailed classification. Similarly, the MvirDB [71] database was used to inspect the distribution of virulence factors among our samples. We classified each sequence based on its BLAST best hit with an e-value lower than 1×10^{-20} in order to minimize the number of alignments that could be found by chance. Proteins that did not match any reference sequence were excluded from the analysis. Finally, predicted proteins were screened for antibiotic resistance activity based on the workflow described in [22] and validated for the Resfams database.

4.6. Statistical Analyses

All statistical analyses were implemented in R (R Core Team (2015), version 3.2.3, R Foundation for Statistical Computing, Vienna, Austria) with the help of various packages. The distribution of metabolic pathways was assessed using the principal component analysis (PCA) on normalized data using the "rda" function of the vegan package version 2.3.2 [72]. The 20 metabolic pathways that varied greatly between normal/mild and severe groups were selected through the similarity of the percentages analysis ("simper" function) and used for PCA analysis (vegan 2.3.2). The Kruskal–Wallis one-way analysis of variance was used to test whether the metabolic and regulatory pathways of different patient groups originated from distinct distributions using the "Kruskal" function of the agricolae package (version 1.2.3). The distribution of ortholog genes, virulence factors, and antibiotic resistance mechanisms was normalized by the total number of open reading frames (ORFs) detected for each sample, and the differences between normal/mild and severe groups were assessed using the two-tailed Student's *t*-test for each category ("t.test" function). The correlation between two dissimilarity matrices, obtained from metagenomics data such as the metabolic pathway or gene distribution, was assessed by using the Mantel test (vegan 2.3.2) as reported in other studies [73,74]. Basically, each table was transformed into a dissimilarity matrix using the "Bray–Curtis" dissimilarity index. By doing so, all dissimilarity matrices were reduced to the same rank, making it possible to use the Mantel test to inspect the correlation between them. The influence of gene patterns, metabolic modules distribution, virulence factors, and antibiotic-resistance genes on the taxonomic microbial composition was evaluated using "boosted regression tree" models [23] with 5000 trees, 10-fold cross-validation, and three-way interactions (gbm package version 2.1.1). Testing multiple individual variables assumed to be correlated with each other may inflate type I errors due to the high number of comparisons made [75]. To reduce the number of comparisons, and therefore to minimize the number of false positive correlations [75], orthogonal composite variables were derived from principal component analysis (PCA) for each factor explored, retaining only those components with an eigenvalue > 1. The derived variables were used for training boosted regression trees, minimizing the number of comparisons and, thus, reducing potential type I errors. A hierarchical cluster analysis was performed based on the average linkage method with "Pearson's distance" metrics ("hclust" function). All graphical representations of data were performed using the ggplot2 package version 2.0.0 [76]. To minimize the type I errors in multiple comparisons, p-values where adjusted using a false discovery rate (FDR).

5. Conclusions

Our results highlight that different pulmonary conditions in patients with CF co-occur with a different microbiome gene repertoire. In particular, an imbalanced distribution of virulence factors along with AR genes and metabolic pathways has been found. Understanding the role of the CF airway microbiome and detecting microbiome genes associated with lower lung function are key challenges for the delivery of new potential biomarkers for the management of bacterial infection in CF patients and the improvement of health care treatment. Our study was limited to twelve subjects; therefore, a larger scale study is needed to more completely characterize the spectrum of microbiome changes associated with the decreasing of pulmonary function. Longitudinal metagenomic analysis, which we plan to evaluate in ongoing studies, may help in understanding imbalances down to the single gene level, possibly helping to find new therapeutic strategies for targeting personalized disease phenotypes.

Acknowledgments: This study was supported by Italian Grants funded by the Italian Cystic Fibrosis Research Foundation (FFC) (http://www.fibrosicisticaricerca.it/) to Annamaria Bevivino (Research Project number FFC#14/2015 (with the contribution of "Delegazione FFC di Latina", "Latteria Montello Nonno Nanni", and "Gruppo di Sostegno FFC Valle Scrivia Alessandria"), and partially supported by MIUR "Futuro in Ricerca" RBFR13EWWI_001 to Nicola Segata. Giovanni Bacci was supported by a postdoctoral fellowship by Italian Cystic Fibrosis Research Foundation. The funders had no role in study design, data collection and analysis, decision to publish, or preparation of the manuscript. The authors greatly acknowledge the Italian Cystic Fibrosis Research Foundation (FCC) for its support and administrative tasks, and Ricciotti Gabriella and Campana Silvia for their technical support.

Author Contributions: Annamaria Bevivino conceived and designed the experiments, supervised analyses, interpreted data, and drafted the manuscript. Alessio Mengoni supervised analyses, interpreted data, and drafted the manuscript. Giovanni Bacci carried out bioinformatic analyses, statistically evaluated the results and wrote the manuscript. Vincenzina Lucidi, Ersilia Fiscarelli, Giovanni Taccetti, Alessandra De Alessandri, Vanessa Tuccio, Patrizia Morelli and Daniela Dolce collected and processed the clinical specimens, and provided clinical expertise for the discussion of the results. Patrizia Paganin performed DNA extraction. Nicola Segata provided bioinformatics expertise and critically revised the manuscript. All authors read, reviewed, and approved the final version to be published.

References

1. Cystic Fibrosis Foundation. *Patient Registry Annual Data Report 2015*; Cystic Fibrosis Foundation: Bethesda, MD, USA, 2016.
2. Gibson, R.L.; Burns, J.L.; Ramsey, B.W. Pathophysiology and Management of Pulmonary Infections in Cystic Fibrosis. *Am. J. Respir. Crit. Care Med.* **2003**, *168*, 918–951. [CrossRef] [PubMed]
3. Lipuma, J.J. The changing microbial epidemiology in cystic fibrosis. *Clin. Microbiol. Rev.* **2010**, *23*, 299–323. [CrossRef] [PubMed]
4. Carmody, L.A.; Zhao, J.; Schloss, P.D.; Petrosino, J.F.; Murray, S.; Young, V.B.; Li, J.Z.; LiPuma, J.J. Changes in cystic fibrosis airway microbiota at pulmonary exacerbation. *Ann. Am. Thorac. Soc.* **2013**, *10*, 179–187. [CrossRef] [PubMed]
5. Coburn, B.; Wang, P.W.; Diaz Caballero, J.; Clark, S.T.; Brahma, V.; Donaldson, S.; Zhang, Y.; Surendra, A.; Gong, Y.; Elizabeth Tullis, D.; et al. Lung microbiota across age and disease stage in cystic fibrosis. *Sci. Rep.* **2015**, *5*, 10241. [CrossRef] [PubMed]
6. Hogan, D.A.; Willger, S.D.; Dolben, E.L.; Hampton, T.H.; Stanton, B.A.; Morrison, H.G.; Sogin, M.L.; Czum, J.; Ashare, A. Analysis of lung microbiota in bronchoalveolar lavage, protected brush and sputum samples from subjects with mild-to-moderate cystic fibrosis lung disease. *PLoS ONE* **2016**, *11*, e0149998. [CrossRef] [PubMed]
7. Rogers, G.B.; Shaw, D.; Marsh, R.L.; Carroll, M.P.; Serisier, D.J.; Bruce, K.D. Respiratory microbiota: addressing clinical questions, informing clinical practice. *Thorax* **2015**, *70*, 74–81. [CrossRef] [PubMed]

8. Cuthbertson, L.; Rogers, G.B.; Walker, A.W.; Oliver, A.; Green, L.E.; Daniels, T.W.V.; Carroll, M.P.; Parkhill, J.; Bruce, K.D.; van der Gast, C.J. Respiratory microbiota resistance and resilience to pulmonary exacerbation and subsequent antimicrobial intervention. *ISME J.* **2015**, *10*, 1081–1091. [CrossRef] [PubMed]
9. Maughan, H.; Wang, P.W.; Diaz Caballero, J.; Fung, P.; Gong, Y.; Donaldson, S.L.; Yuan, L.; Keshavjee, S.; Zhang, Y.; Yau, Y.C.W.; et al. Analysis of the cystic fibrosis lung microbiota via serial Illumina sequencing of bacterial 16S rRNA hypervariable regions. *PLoS ONE* **2012**, *7*, e45791. [CrossRef] [PubMed]
10. Huang, Y.J.; LiPuma, J.J. The Microbiome in Cystic Fibrosis. *Clin. Chest Med.* **2016**, *37*, 59–67. [CrossRef] [PubMed]
11. Surette, M.G. The cystic fibrosis lung microbiome. *Ann. Am. Thorac. Soc.* **2014**, *11*, 61–65. [CrossRef] [PubMed]
12. Carmody, L.A.; Zhao, J.; Kalikin, L.M.; LeBar, W.; Simon, R.H.; Venkataraman, A.; Schmidt, T.M.; Abdo, Z.; Schloss, P.D.; LiPuma, J.J. The daily dynamics of cystic fibrosis airway microbiota during clinical stability and at exacerbation. *Microbiome* **2015**, *3*, 12. [CrossRef] [PubMed]
13. Paganin, P.; Fiscarelli, E.V.; Tuccio, V.; Chiancianesi, M.; Bacci, G.; Morelli, P.; Dolce, D.; Dalmastri, C.; de Alessandri, A.; Lucidi, V.; et al. Changes in cystic fibrosis airway microbial community associated with a severe decline in lung function. *PLoS ONE* **2015**, *10*, e0124348. [CrossRef] [PubMed]
14. Bacci, G.; Paganin, P.; Lopez, L.; Vanni, C.; Dalmastri, C.; Cantale, C.; Daddiego, L.; Perrotta, G.; Dolce, D.; Morelli, P.; et al. Pyrosequencing unveils cystic fibrosis lung microbiome differences associated with a severe lung function decline. *PLoS ONE* **2016**, *11*, e0156807. [CrossRef]
15. Narayanamurthy, V.; Sweetnam, J.M.; Denner, D.R.; Chen, L.W.; Naureckas, E.T.; Laxman, B.; White, S.R. The metabolic footprint of the airway bacterial community in cystic fibrosis. *Microbiome* **2017**, *5*, 67. [CrossRef] [PubMed]
16. Sharon, G.; Garg, N.; Debelius, J.; Knight, R.; Dorrestein, P.C.; Mazmanian, S.K. Specialized metabolites from the microbiome in health and disease. *Cell Metab.* **2014**, *20*, 719–730. [CrossRef] [PubMed]
17. Lim, Y.W.; Evangelista, J.S.; Schmieder, R.; Bailey, B.; Haynes, M.; Furlan, M.; Maughan, H.; Edwards, R.; Rohwer, F.; Conrad, D. Clinical insights from metagenomic analysis of sputum samples from patients with cystic fibrosis. *J. Clin. Microbiol.* **2014**, *52*, 425–437. [CrossRef] [PubMed]
18. Willner, D.; Haynes, M.R.; Furlan, M.; Hanson, N.; Kirby, B.; Lim, Y.W.; Rainey, P.B.; Schmieder, R.; Youle, M.; Conrad, D.; et al. Case studies of the spatial heterogeneity of DNA viruses in the cystic fibrosis lung. *Am. J. Respir. Cell Mol. Biol.* **2012**, *46*, 127–131. [CrossRef] [PubMed]
19. Whiteson, K.L.; Meinardi, S.; Lim, Y.W.; Schmieder, R.; Maughan, H.; Quinn, R.; Blake, D.R.; Conrad, D.; Rohwer, F. Breath gas metabolites and bacterial metagenomes from cystic fibrosis airways indicate active pH neutral 2,3-butanedione fermentation. *ISME J.* **2014**, *8*, 1247–1258. [CrossRef] [PubMed]
20. Losada, P.M.; Chouvarine, P.; Dorda, M.; Hedtfeld, S.; Mielke, S.; Schulz, A.; Wiehlmann, L.; Tümmler, B. The cystic fibrosis lower airways microbial metagenome. *ERJ Open Res.* **2016**, *2*, 00096-2015. [CrossRef]
21. Dhooghe, B.; Noël, S.; Huaux, F.; Leal, T.; Diaz Caballero, J.; Clark, S.T.; Coburn, B.; Zhang, Y.; Wang, P.W.; Donaldson, S.L.; et al. Sputum DNA sequencing in cystic fibrosis: Non-invasive access to the lung microbiome and to pathogen details. *J. Cyst. Fibros.* **2014**, *5*, 20. [CrossRef]
22. Gibson, M.K.; Forsberg, K.J.; Dantas, G. Improved annotation of antibiotic resistance determinants reveals microbial resistomes cluster by ecology. *ISME J.* **2014**, *9*, 1–10. [CrossRef] [PubMed]
23. Elith, J.; Leathwick, J.R.; Hastie, T. A working guide to boosted regression trees. *J. Anim. Ecol.* **2008**, *77*, 802–813. [CrossRef] [PubMed]
24. Lambiase, A.; Catania, M.R.; Del Pezzo, M.; Rossano, F.; Terlizzi, V.; Sepe, A.; Raia, V. *Achromobacter xylosoxidans* respiratory tract infection in cystic fibrosis patients. *Eur. J. Clin. Microbiol. Infect. Dis.* **2011**, *30*, 973–980. [CrossRef] [PubMed]
25. De Baets, F.; Schelstraete, P.; van Daele, S.; Haerynck, F.; Vaneechoutte, M. *Achromobacter xylosoxidans* in cystic fibrosis: Prevalence and clinical relevance. *J. Cyst. Fibros.* **2007**, *6*, 75–78. [CrossRef] [PubMed]
26. Worlitzsch, D.; Rintelen, C.; Böhm, K.; Wollschläger, B.; Merkel, N.; Borneff-Lipp, M.; Döring, G. Antibiotic-resistant obligate anaerobes during exacerbations of cystic fibrosis patients. *Clin. Microbiol. Infect.* **2009**, *15*, 454–460. [CrossRef] [PubMed]
27. Cox, M.J.; Allgaier, M.; Taylor, B.; Baek, M.S.; Huang, Y.J.; Daly, R.A.; Karaoz, U.; Andersen, G.L.; Brown, R.; Fujimura, K.E.; et al. Airway microbiota and pathogen abundance in age-stratified cystic fibrosis patients. *PLoS ONE* **2010**, *5*, e11044. [CrossRef] [PubMed]

28. Zhao, J.; Murray, S.; Lipuma, J.J. Modeling the impact of antibiotic exposure on human microbiota. *Sci. Rep.* **2014**, *4*, 4345. [CrossRef] [PubMed]
29. Zhao, J.; Schloss, P.D.; Kalikin, L.M.; Carmody, L.A.; Foster, B.K.; Petrosino, J.F.; Cavalcoli, J.D.; VanDevanter, D.R.; Murray, S.; Li, J.Z.; et al. Decade-long bacterial community dynamics in cystic fibrosis airways. *Proc. Natl. Acad. Sci. USA* **2012**, *109*, 5809–5814. [CrossRef] [PubMed]
30. Rogers, G.B.; van der Gast, C.J.; Cuthbertson, L.; Thomson, S.K.; Bruce, K.D.; Martin, M.L.; Serisier, D.J. Clinical measures of disease in adult non-CF bronchiectasis correlate with airway microbiota composition. *Thorax* **2013**, *68*, 731–737. [CrossRef] [PubMed]
31. Dickson, R.P.; Erb-Downward, J.R.; Martinez, F.J.; Huffnagle, G.B. The Microbiome and the respiratory tract. *Annu. Rev. Physiol.* **2016**, *78*, 481–504. [CrossRef] [PubMed]
32. Quinn, R.A.; Lim, Y.W.; Maughan, H.; Conrad, D.; Rohwer, F.; Whiteson, K.L. Biogeochemical forces shape the composition and physiology of polymicrobial communities in the cystic fibrosis lung. *MBio* **2014**, *5*. [CrossRef] [PubMed]
33. Willner, D.; Furlan, M.; Haynes, M.; Schmieder, R.; Angly, F.E.; Silva, J.; Tammadoni, S.; Nosrat, B.; Conrad, D.; Rohwer, F. Metagenomic analysis of respiratory tract DNA viral communities in cystic fibrosis and non-cystic fibrosis individuals. *PLoS ONE* **2009**, *4*, e7370. [CrossRef] [PubMed]
34. Lim, Y.W.; Schmieder, R.; Haynes, M.; Willner, D.; Furlan, M.; Youle, M.; Abbott, K.; Edwards, R.; Evangelista, J.; Conrad, D.; et al. Metagenomics and metatranscriptomics: Windows on CF-associated viral and microbial communities. *J. Cyst. Fibros.* **2013**, *12*, 154–164. [CrossRef] [PubMed]
35. Nelson, J.W.; Tredgett, M.W.; Sheehan, J.K.; Thornton, D.J.; Notman, D.; Govan, J.R. Mucinophilic and chemotactic properties of *Pseudomonas aeruginosa* in relation to pulmonary colonization in cystic fibrosis. *Infect. Immun.* **1990**, *58*, 1489–1495. [PubMed]
36. Feldman, M.; Bryan, R.; Rajan, S.; Scheffler, L.; Brunnert, S.; Tang, H.; Prince, A. Role of flagella in pathogenesis of *Pseudomonas aeruginosa* pulmonary infection. *Infect. Immun.* **1998**, *66*, 43–51. [PubMed]
37. Wolfgang, M.C.; Jyot, J.; Goodman, A.L.; Ramphal, R.; Lory, S. *Pseudomonas aeruginosa* regulates flagellin expression as part of a global response to airway fluid from cystic fibrosis patients. *Proc. Natl. Acad. Sci. USA* **2004**, *101*, 6664–6668. [CrossRef] [PubMed]
38. Luzar, M.A.; Thomassen, M.J.; Montie, T.C. Flagella and motility alterations in *Pseudomonas aeruginosa* strains from patients with cystic fibrosis: Relationship to patient clinical condition. *Infect. Immun.* **1985**, *50*, 577–582. [PubMed]
39. Deretic, V.; Govan, J.R.W.; Konyecsni, W.M.; Martin, D.W. Mucoid *Pseudomonas aeruginosa* in cystic fibrosis: Mutations in the *muc* loci affect transcription of the *algR* and *algD* genes in response to environmental stimuli. *Mol. Microbiol.* **1990**, *4*, 189–196. [CrossRef] [PubMed]
40. Chawley, P.; Samal, H.B.; Prava, J.; Suar, M.; Mahapatra, R.K. Comparative genomics study for identification of drug and vaccine targets in *Vibrio cholerae*: MurA ligase as a case study. *Genomics* **2014**, *103*, 83–93. [CrossRef] [PubMed]
41. Rubin, B.K. Mucus structure and properties in cystic fibrosis. *Paediatr. Respir. Rev.* **2007**, *8*, 4–7. [CrossRef] [PubMed]
42. Brinkmann, V.; Reichard, U.; Goosmann, C.; Fauler, B.; Uhlemann, Y.; Weiss, D.S.; Weinrauch, Y.; Zychlinsky, A. Neutrophil extracellular traps kill bacteria. *Science* **2004**, *303*, 1532–1535. [CrossRef] [PubMed]
43. Whitchurch, C.B.; Tolker-Nielsen, T.; Ragas, P.C.; Mattick, J.S. Extracellular DNA required for bacterial biofilm formation. *Science* **2002**, *295*, 1487. [CrossRef] [PubMed]
44. Voynow, J.A.; Fischer, B.M.; Zheng, S. Proteases and cystic fibrosis. *Int. J. Biochem. Cell Biol.* **2008**, *40*, 1238–1245. [CrossRef] [PubMed]
45. Doring, G.; Flume, P.; Heijerman, H.; Elborn, J.S.; Consensus Study Group. Treatment of lung infection in patients with cystic fibrosis: Current and future strategies. *J. Cyst. Fibros.* **2012**, *11*, 461–479. [CrossRef] [PubMed]
46. Doring, G.; Hoiby, N.; Consensus Study Group. Early intervention and prevention of lung disease in cystic fibrosis: A European consensus. *J. Cyst. Fibros.* **2004**, *3*, 67–91. [CrossRef] [PubMed]
47. Chavez, A.; Mian, A.; Scurlock, A.M.; Blackall, D.; Com, G. Antibiotic hypersensitivity in CF: Drug-induced life-threatening hemolytic anemia in a pediatric patient. *J. Cyst. Fibros.* **2010**, *9*, 433–438. [CrossRef] [PubMed]

48. Pehrsson, E.C.; Forsberg, K.J.; Gibson, M.K.; Ahmadi, S.; Dantas, G. Novel resistance functions uncovered using functional metagenomic investigations of resistance reservoirs. *Front. Microbiol.* **2013**, *4*. [CrossRef] [PubMed]
49. King, P.; Pham, L.K.; Waltz, S.; Sphar, D.; Yamamoto, R.T.; Conrad, D.; Taplitz, R.; Torriani, F.; Forsyth, R.A. Longitudinal metagenomic analysis of hospital air identifies clinically relevant microbes. *PLoS ONE* **2016**, *11*. [CrossRef]
50. Blaser, M.J. The microbiome revolution. *J. Clin. Investig.* **2014**, *124*, 4162–4165. [CrossRef] [PubMed]
51. Fuchs, H.J.; Borowitz, D.S.; Christiansen, D.H.; Morris, E.M.; Nash, M.L.; Ramsey, B.W.; Rosenstein, B.J.; Smith, A.L.; Wohl, M.E. Effect of aerosolized recombinant human DNase on exacerbations of respiratory symptoms and on pulmonary function in patients with cystic fibrosis. The Pulmozyme Study Group. *N. Engl. J. Med.* **1994**, *331*, 637–642. [CrossRef] [PubMed]
52. Ramsey, B.W.; Pepe, M.S.; Quan, J.M.; Otto, K.L.; Montgomery, A.B.; Williams-Warren, J.; Vasiljev-K, M.; Borowitz, D.; Bowman, C.M.; Marshall, B.C.; et al. Intermittent administration of inhaled tobramycin in patients with cystic fibrosis. Cystic Fibrosis Inhaled Tobramycin Study Group. *N. Engl. J. Med.* **1999**, *340*, 23–30. [CrossRef] [PubMed]
53. Kerem, E.; Conway, S.; Elborn, S.; Heijerman, H.; Committee, C. others Standards of care for patients with cystic fibrosis: A European consensus. *J. Cyst. Fibros.* **2005**, *4*, 7–26. [CrossRef] [PubMed]
54. Flume, P.A.; Mogayzel, P.J.; Robinson, K.A.; Goss, C.H.; Rosenblatt, R.L.; Kuhn, R.J.; Marshall, B.C.; Bujan, J.; Downs, A.; Finder, J.; et al. Cystic fibrosis pulmonary guidelines: Treatment of pulmonary exacerbations. *Am. J. Respir. Crit. Care Med.* **2009**, *180*, 802–808. [CrossRef] [PubMed]
55. Smyth, A.R.; Bell, S.C.; Bojcin, S.; Bryon, M.; Duff, A.; Flume, P.; Kashirskaya, N.; Munck, A.; Ratjen, F.; Schwarzenberg, S.J.; et al. European cystic fibrosis society standards of care: Best practice guidelines. *J. Cyst. Fibros.* **2014**, *13*, S23–S42. [CrossRef] [PubMed]
56. Taylor-Robinson, D.; Whitehead, M.; Diderichsen, F.; Olesen, H.V.; Pressler, T.; Smyth, R.L.; Diggle, P. Understanding the natural progression in %FEV_1 decline in patients with cystic fibrosis: A longitudinal study. *Thorax* **2012**, *67*, 860–866. [CrossRef] [PubMed]
57. Flume, P.A.; O'Sullivan, B.P.; Robinson, K.A.; Goss, C.H.; Mogayzel, P., Jr.; Willey-Courand, D.B.; Bujan, J.; Finder, J.; Lester, M. Cystic Fibrosis Pulmonary Guidelines: Chronic Medications for Maintenance of Lung Health. *Am. J. Respir. Crit. Care Med.* **2007**, *176*, 957–969. [CrossRef] [PubMed]
58. Miller, M.R.; Hankinson, J.; Brusasco, V.; Burgos, F.; Casaburi, R.; Coates, A.; Crapo, R.; Enright, P.; van der Grinten, C.P.M.; Gustafsson, P.; et al. Standardisation of spirometry. *Eur. Respir. J.* **2005**, *26*, 319–338. [CrossRef] [PubMed]
59. Willner, D.; Daly, J.; Whiley, D.; Grimwood, K.; Wainwright, C.E.; Hugenholtz, P. Comparison of DNA extraction methods for microbial community profiling with an application to pediatric bronchoalveolar lavage samples. *PLoS ONE* **2012**, *7*, e34605. [CrossRef] [PubMed]
60. Bacci, G.; Bazzicalupo, M.; Benedetti, A.; Mengoni, A. StreamingTrim 1.0: A Java software for dynamic trimming of 16S rRNA sequence data from metagenetic studies. *Mol. Ecol. Resour.* **2014**, *14*, 426–434. [CrossRef] [PubMed]
61. Langmead, B.; Salzberg, S.L. Fast gapped-read alignment with Bowtie 2. *Nat. Methods* **2012**, *9*, 357–359. [CrossRef] [PubMed]
62. Abubucker, S.; Segata, N.; Goll, J.; Schubert, A.M.; Izard, J.; Cantarel, B.L.; Rodriguez-Mueller, B.; Zucker, J.; Thiagarajan, M.; Henrissat, B.; et al. Metabolic reconstruction for metagenomic data and its application to the human microbiome. *PLoS Comput. Biol.* **2012**, *8*, e1002358. [CrossRef] [PubMed]
63. Truong, D.T.; Franzosa, E.A.; Tickle, T.L.; Scholz, M.; Weingart, G.; Pasolli, E.; Tett, A.; Huttenhower, C.; Segata, N. MetaPhlAn2 for enhanced metagenomic taxonomic profiling. *Nat. Methods* **2015**, *12*, 902–903. [CrossRef] [PubMed]
64. Bankevich, A.; Nurk, S.; Antipov, D.; Gurevich, A.A.; Dvorkin, M.; Kulikov, A.S.; Lesin, V.M.; Nikolenko, S.I.; Pham, S.; Prjibelski, A.D.; et al. SPAdes: A new genome assembly algorithm and its applications to single-cell sequencing. *J. Comput. Biol.* **2012**, *19*, 455–477. [CrossRef] [PubMed]
65. Qin, J.; Li, R.; Raes, J.; Arumugam, M.; Burgdorf, K.S.; Manichanh, C.; Nielsen, T.; Pons, N.; Levenez, F.; Yamada, T.; et al. A human gut microbial gene catalogue established by metagenomic sequencing. *Nature* **2010**, *464*, 59–65. [CrossRef] [PubMed]

66. Zhu, W.; Lomsadze, A.; Borodovsky, M. Ab initio gene identification in metagenomic sequences. *Nucleic Acids Res.* **2010**, *38*, e132. [CrossRef] [PubMed]
67. Eddy, S.R. Accelerated Profile HMM Searches. *PLoS Comput. Biol.* **2011**, *7*, e1002195. [CrossRef] [PubMed]
68. Powell, S.; Szklarczyk, D.; Trachana, K.; Roth, A.; Kuhn, M.; Muller, J.; Arnold, R.; Rattei, T.; Letunic, I.; Doerks, T.; et al. eggNOG v3.0: Orthologous groups covering 1133 organisms at 41 different taxonomic ranges. *Nucleic Acids Res.* **2012**, *40*, D284–D289. [CrossRef] [PubMed]
69. Pearson, W.R. An introduction to sequence similarity ("homology") searching. *Curr. Protoc. Bioinform.* **2013**. [CrossRef]
70. Saier, M.H.; Reddy, V.S.; Tamang, D.G.; Västermark, A. The transporter classification database. *Nucleic Acids Res.* **2014**, *42*, D251–D258. [CrossRef] [PubMed]
71. Zhou, C.E.; Smith, J.; Lam, M.; Zemla, A.; Dyer, M.D.; Slezak, T. MvirDB—A microbial database of protein toxins, virulence factors and antibiotic resistance genes for bio-defence applications. *Nucleic Acids Res.* **2007**, *35*, D391–D394. [CrossRef] [PubMed]
72. Oksanen, J.; Blanchet, F.; Kindt, R.; Legendre, P.; Minchin, P.; O'Hara, R.; Simpson, G.; Solymos, P.; Stevens, M.H.H.; Wagner, H. Vegan: Community ecology package. R package version 2.0–10. 2013. Available online: http://CRAN.R-project.org/package=vegan.
73. Kuang, J.; Huang, L.; He, Z.; Chen, L.; Hua, Z.; Jia, P.; Li, S.; Liu, J.; Li, J.; Zhou, J.; et al. Predicting taxonomic and functional structure of microbial communities in acid mine drainage. *ISME J.* **2016**, *10*, 1527–1539. [CrossRef] [PubMed]
74. Turnbaugh, P.J.; Hamady, M.; Yatsunenko, T.; Cantarel, B.L.; Duncan, A.; Ley, R.E.; Sogin, M.L.; Jones, W.J.; Roe, B.A.; Affourtit, J.P.; et al. A core gut microbiome in obese and lean twins. *Nature* **2009**, *457*, 480–484. [CrossRef] [PubMed]
75. John, R.; Dalling, J.W.; Harms, K.E.; Yavitt, J.B.; Stallard, R.F.; Mirabello, M.; Hubbell, S.P.; Valencia, R.; Navarrete, H.; Vallejo, M.; et al. Soil nutrients influence spatial distributions of tropical tree species. *Proc. Natl. Acad. Sci. USA* **2007**, *104*, 864–869. [CrossRef] [PubMed]
76. Wickham, H. *Ggplot2: Elegant Graphics for Data Analysis*; Springer: New York, NY, USA, 2009; ISBN 978-0-387-98140-6.

Permissions

All chapters in this book were first published by MDPI; hereby published with permission under the Creative Commons Attribution License or equivalent. Every chapter published in this book has been scrutinized by our experts. Their significance has been extensively debated. The topics covered herein carry significant findings which will fuel the growth of the discipline. They may even be implemented as practical applications or may be referred to as a beginning point for another development.

The contributors of this book come from diverse backgrounds, making this book a truly international effort. This book will bring forth new frontiers with its revolutionizing research information and detailed analysis of the nascent developments around the world.

We would like to thank all the contributing authors for lending their expertise to make the book truly unique. They have played a crucial role in the development of this book. Without their invaluable contributions this book wouldn't have been possible. They have made vital efforts to compile up to date information on the varied aspects of this subject to make this book a valuable addition to the collection of many professionals and students.

This book was conceptualized with the vision of imparting up-to-date information and advanced data in this field. To ensure the same, a matchless editorial board was set up. Every individual on the board went through rigorous rounds of assessment to prove their worth. After which they invested a large part of their time researching and compiling the most relevant data for our readers.

The editorial board has been involved in producing this book since its inception. They have spent rigorous hours researching and exploring the diverse topics which have resulted in the successful publishing of this book. They have passed on their knowledge of decades through this book. To expedite this challenging task, the publisher supported the team at every step. A small team of assistant editors was also appointed to further simplify the editing procedure and attain best results for the readers.

Apart from the editorial board, the designing team has also invested a significant amount of their time in understanding the subject and creating the most relevant covers. They scrutinized every image to scout for the most suitable representation of the subject and create an appropriate cover for the book.

The publishing team has been an ardent support to the editorial, designing and production team. Their endless efforts to recruit the best for this project, has resulted in the accomplishment of this book. They are a veteran in the field of academics and their pool of knowledge is as vast as their experience in printing. Their expertise and guidance has proved useful at every step. Their uncompromising quality standards have made this book an exceptional effort. Their encouragement from time to time has been an inspiration for everyone.

The publisher and the editorial board hope that this book will prove to be a valuable piece of knowledge for researchers, students, practitioners and scholars across the globe.

List of Contributors

Molly Easter and Seth Bollenbecker
Division of Pulmonary, Allergy and Critical Care Medicine, Department of Medicine, The University of Alabama at Birmingham, Birmingham, AL 35294, USA

Jarrod W. Barnes and Stefanie Krick
Division of Pulmonary, Allergy and Critical Care Medicine, Department of Medicine, The University of Alabama at Birmingham, Birmingham, AL 35294, USA
Gregory Fleming James Cystic Fibrosis Center, The University of Alabama at Birmingham, Birmingham, AL 35294, USA

Angela Cesaro, Eliana Dell'Olmo, Rocco Di Girolamo and Luca Tartaglione
Department of Chemical Sciences, University of Naples Federico II, Via Cintia 21, I-80126 Naples, Italy

Elio Pizzo
Department of Biology, University of Naples Federico II, Via Cintia 21, I-80126 Naples, Italy

Rosa Gaglione and Angela Arciello
Department of Chemical Sciences, University of Naples Federico II, Via Cintia 21, I-80126 Naples, Italy
Istituto Nazionale di Biostrutture e Biosistemi (INBB), I-00136 Rome, Italy

Anshu Agrawal
Division of Basic and Clinical Immunology, Department of Medicine, University of California Irvine, Irvine, CA 92697, USA

Aline Fastrès, Elodie Roels and Cécile Clercx
Department of Clinical Sciences, FARAH, Faculty of Veterinary Medicine, University of Liège, 4000 Liège, Belgium

Florence Felice, Catherine Moermans, Jean-Louis Corhay, Renaud Louis and Julien Guiot
Respiratory department, CHU Liège. Domaine universitaire du Sart Tilman, B35, 4000 Liège, Belgium

Fabrice Bureau
Laboratory of Cellular and Molecular Immunology, GIGA Research, University of Liège, 4000 Liège, Belgium

Jon M. Florence, Laela M. Booshehri and Anna K. Kurdowska
Department of Cellular and Molecular Biology, University of Texas Health Science Center, Tyler, TX 75708, USA

Agnieszka Krupa and Adrian L. Gajewski
Department of Cellular and Molecular Biology, University of Texas Health Science Center, Tyler, TX 75708, USA
Laboratory of Gastroimmunology, Department of Immunology and Infectious Biology, Faculty of Biology and Environmental Protection, University of Lodz, 90-237 Lodz, Poland

Luis Máiz and Rosa Nieto
Servicio de Neumología, Unidad de Bronquiectasias y Fibrosis Quística, Hospital Universitario Ramón y Cajal, 28034 Madrid, Spain

Rafael Cantón and Elia Gómez G. de la Pedrosa
Servicio de Microbiología, Hospital Universitario Ramón y Cajal and Instituto Ramón y Cajal de Investigación Sanitaria (IRYCIS), 28034 Madrid, Spain

Miguel Ángel Martinez-García
Servicio de Neumología, Hospital Universitario y Politécnico la Fe, 46016 Valencia, Spain

Sonya C. Carnell, Lee Borthwick and Anthony De Soyza
Institute of Cellular Medicine, Newcastle University, Newcastle NE2 4HH, UK

John D. Perry
Department of Microbiology, The Freeman Hospital, Newcastle NE7 7DN, UK

Daniela Vollmer, Jacob Biboy, Waldemar Vollmer and Anjam C. M. Khan
Centre for Bacterial Cell Biology, Institute for Cell and Molecular Biosciences, Newcastle University, Newcastle NE2 4HH, UK

Marcella Facchini
Infections & Cystic Fibrosis Unit, San Raffaele Scientific Institute, 20132 Milan, Italy

Alessandra Bragonzi
Division of Immunology, Transplantation and Infectious Diseases, IRCCS San Raffaele Scientific Institute, Milano 20132, Italy Infections & Cystic Fibrosis Unit, San Raffaele Scientific Institute, 20132 Milan, Italy

Alba Silipo
Department of Chemical Sciences, University of Naples Federico II, Via Cintia 4, 80026 Napoli, Italy

Annette C. Vergunst
VBMI, INSERM, Univ. Montpellier, 30908 Nimes, France

Jennifer E. Douglas
Perelman School of Medicine, University of Pennsylvania, Philadelphia, PA 19104, USA
Monell Chemical Senses Center, Philadelphia, PA 19104, USA

Noam A. Cohen
Monell Chemical Senses Center, Philadelphia, PA 19104, USA
Department of Otorhinolaryngology–Head and Neck Surgery, University of Pennsylvania Health System, Philadelphia, PA 19104, USA
Philadelphia Veterans Affairs Medical Center Surgical Services, Philadelphia, PA 19104, USA

Paola Faverio, Anna Stainer, Giulia Bonaiti, Stefano C. Zucchetti, Edoardo Simonetta, Almerico Marruchella and Alberto Pesci
Dipartimento Cardio-Toraco-Vascolare, University of Milan Bicocca, Respiratory Unit, San Gerardo Hospital, ASST di Monza, Via Pergolesi 33, 20900 Monza, Italy

Giuseppe Lapadula and Andrea Gori
Department of Internal Medicine, Division of Infectious Diseases, San Gerardo Hospital, ASST di Monza, Via Pergolesi 33, 20900 Monza, Italy

Francesco Blasi and Stefano Aliberti
Department of Pathophysiology and Transplantation, University of Milan, Cardio-Thoracic Unit and Cystic Fibrosis Adult Center, Fondazione IRCCS Cà Granda Ospedale Maggiore Policlinico, Via Francesco Sforza 35, 20122 Milan, Italy

Luigi Codecasa
Villa Marelli Institute, Niguarda Ca' Granda Hospital, 20122 Milan, Italy

James D. Chalmers
Scottish Centre for Respiratory Research, University of Dundee, Dundee DD1 9SY, UK

Michael R. Loebinger
Host Defence Unit, Royal Brompton and Harefield NHS Foundation Trust, London, UK Imperial College London, London SW3 6NP, UK

Stephanie Everaerts, Lieven J. Dupont and Wim Janssens
Department of Respiratory Diseases, University Hospitals Leuven, Herestraat 49, B-3000 Leuven, Belgium
Department of Chronic Diseases, Metabolism & Aging, Laboratory of Respiratory Diseases, KU Leuven, Herestraat 49, B-3000 Leuven, Belgium

Kristina Vermeersch and Bart M. Vanaudenaerde
Department of Chronic Diseases, Metabolism & Aging, Laboratory of Respiratory Diseases, KU Leuven, Herestraat 49, B-3000 Leuven, Belgium

Katrien Lagrou
Department of Laboratory Medicine, University Hospitals Leuven, Herestraat 49, B-3000 Leuven, Belgium
Department of Microbiology and Immunology, KU Leuven, Herestraat 49, B-3000 Leuven, Belgium

Marc Miravitlles
Pneumology Department, Hospital Universitari Vall d'Hebron, Ciber de Enfermedades Respiratorias (CIBERES), 08035 Barcelona, Spain

Antonio Anzueto
Department of Medicine, Division of Pulmonary Diseases/Critical Care Medicine, The University of Texas Health Science Center at San Antonio, San Antonio, TX 78229, USA
Pulmonary Section, The South Texas Veterans Health Care System, Audie L. Murphy Memorial Veterans Hospital Division, Pulmonary Diseases Section (111E), 7400 Merton Minter Boulevard, San Antonio, TX 78229, USA

Alessandra Bragonzi
Division of Immunology, Transplantation and Infectious Diseases, IRCCS San Raffaele Scientific Institute, Milano 20132, Italy
Infections & Cystic Fibrosis Unit, San Raffaele Scientific Institute, 20132 Milan, Italy

Moira Paroni
Infections and Cystic Fibrosis Unit, IRCCS San Raffaele Scientific Institute, 20132 Milan, Italy
Department of Biosciences, University of Milan, 20133 Milan, Italy

Luisa Pirone, Patrizia Paganin and Annamaria Bevivino
Territorial and Production Systems Sustainability Department, ENEA, Italian National Agency for New Technologies, Energy and Sustainable Economic Development, Casaccia Research Center, 00123 Rome, Italy

Ivan Coladarci and Fiorentina Ascenzioni
Biology and Biotechnology Department "Charles Darwin", Sapienza University of Rome, 00185 Rome, Italy

Nicola Ivan Lorè
Division of Immunology, Transplantation and Infectious Diseases, IRCCS San Raffaele Scientific Institute, Milano 20132, Italy
Vita-Salute San Raffaele University, Milano 20132, Italy

Noemi Veraldi, Elisa Calzi and Annamaria Naggi
Istituto di Ricerche Chimiche e Biochimiche "G. Ronzoni", Milano 20133, Italy

Camilla Riva, Barbara Sipione, Lorenza Spagnuolo, Ida De Fino, Medede Melessike and Cristina Cigana
Division of Immunology, Transplantation and Infectious Diseases, IRCCS San Raffaele Scientific Institute, Milano 20132, Italy

Diego J. Maselli, Holly Keyt and Marcos I. Restrepo
Division of Pulmonary Diseases & Critical Care Medicine, South Texas Veterans Health Care System, San Antonio, TX 78229, USA
University of Texas Health at San Antonio, San Antonio, TX 78240, USA

Beata Shiratori, Jingge Zhao, Haorile Chagan-Yasutan and Yugo Ashino
Division of Disaster-Related Infectious Diseases, International Research Institute of Disaster Science, Tohoku University, 2-1 Seiryo-machi, Aoba-ku, Sendai, Miyagi 980-8575, Japan

Masao Okumura and Takashi Yoshiyama
Department of Respiratory Medicine, Fukujuji Hospital, Japan Anti-Tuberculosis Association, 3-1-24 Matsuyama, Kiyose, Tokyo 204-8533, Japan

Hideki Yanai, Kazue Mizuno and Tadashi Idei
Department of Clinical Laboratory, Fukujuji Hospital, Japan Anti-Tuberculosis Association, 3-1-2 4 Matsuyama, Kiyose, Tokyo 204-8533, Japan

Chie Nakajima and Yasuhiko Suzuki
Division of Global Epidemiology, Research Center for Zoonosis Control, Hokkaido University, North 20, West 10, Kita-ku, Sapporo, Hokkaido 001-0020, Japan

Toshio Hattori
Department of Health Science and Social Welfare, Kibi International University, 8 Igamachi, Takahashi 716-8508, Japan

Giovanni Bacci and Alessio Mengoni
Department of Biology, University of Florence, Florence 50019, Italy

Ersilia Fiscarelli, Vanessa Tuccio and Vincenzina Lucidi
Cystic Fibrosis Microbiology and Cystic Fibrosis Center, "Bambino Gesù" Children's Hospital and Research Institute, Rome 00165, Italy

Nicola Segata
Centre for Integrative Biology, University of Trento, Trento 38123, Italy

Giovanni Taccetti and Daniela Dolce
Department of Pediatric Medicine, Cystic Fibrosis Center, Anna Meyer Children's University Hospital, Florence 50139, Italy

Patrizia Morelli and Alessandra De Alessandri
Cystic Fibrosis Center, IRCCS G. Gaslini Institute, Genoa 16146, Italy

Index

www.ingramcontent.com/pod-product-compliance
Lightning Source LLC
LaVergne TN
LVHW082154200926
848484LV00008B/2161
* 9 7 9 8 8 8 7 4 0 4 3 5 6 *